FIRST AID FOR THE®

Obstetrics & Gynecology Clerkship

Fifth Edition

SHIREEN MADANI SIMS, MD
Associate Professor and Clerkship Director
Vice Chair for Education
Department of Obstetrics and Gynecology
University of Florida College of Medicine
Gainesville, Florida

SARAH DOTTERS-KATZ, MD, MMHPE
Associate professor and clerkship director
Department of Obstetrics and Gynecology
Duke University School of Medicine
Durham, North Carolina

LATHA GANTI, MD, MS, MBA, FACEP
Professor of Emergency Medicine and Neurology
University of Central Florida College of Medicine
Vice Chair for Research and Academic Affairs
HCA UCF Emergency Medicine Residency of Greater Orlando
Orlando, Florida

MATTHEW KAUFMAN, MD
Associate Director
Department of Emergency Medicine
Richmond University Medical Center
Staten Island, New York

Mc
Graw
Hill

New York   Chicago   San Francisco   Athens   London   Madrid   Mexico City
New Delhi   Milan   Singapore   Sydney   Toronto

First Aid for the®: Obstetrics & Gynecology Clerkship, Fifth Edition

1 2 3 4 5 6 7 8 9   LWI   27 26 25 24 23 22

ISBN 978-1-264-26493-3
MHID 1-264-26493-3

NOTICE

Medicine is an ever-changing science. As new research and clinical experience broaden our knowledge, changes in treatment and drug therapy are required. The authors and the publisher of this work have checked with sources believed to be reliable in their efforts to provide information that is complete and generally in accord with the standards accepted at the time of publication. However, in view of the possibility of human error or changes in medical sciences, neither the authors nor the publisher nor any other party who has been involved in the preparation or publication of this work warrants that the information contained herein is in every respect accurate or complete, and they disclaim all responsibility for any errors or omissions or for the results obtained from use of the information contained in this work. Readers are encouraged to confirm the information contained herein with other sources. For example and in particular, readers are advised to check the product information sheet included in the package of each drug they plan to administer to be certain that the information contained in this work is accurate and that changes have not been made in the recommended dose or in the contraindications for administration. This recommendation is of particular importance in connection with new or infrequently used drugs.

This book was set in Electra LT Std by MPS Limited.
The editors were Bob Boehringer and Kim J. Davis.
The production supervisor was Catherine Saggese.
Project management was provided by Poonam Bisht, MPS Limited.

This book is printed on acid-free paper.

Library of Congress Cataloging-in-Publication Data

Names: Ganti, Latha, author. | Kaufman, Matthew, author. | Sims, Shireen
    Madani, author. | Dotters-Katz, Sarah K., author.
Title: First aid for the obstetrics & gynecology clerkship / Latha Ganti,
    Matthew Kaufman, Shireen Madani Sims, Sarah Dotters-Katz.
Other titles: First aid for the obstetrics and gynecology clerkship
Description: Fifth edition. | New York : McGraw Hill, [2022] | Includes
    index. | Summary: "Each of the chapters in this book contain the major
    topics central to the practice of obstetrics and gynecology and closely
    parallel the medical student learning objectives of the American
    Professors of Gynecology and Obstetrics and this book also targets the
    obstetrics and gynecology content on the USMLE Step 2 examination"—
    Provided by publisher.
Identifiers: LCCN 2021035943 (print) | LCCN 2021035944 (ebook) | ISBN
    9781264264933 (paperback ; alk. paper) | ISBN 9781264266500 (ebook)
Subjects: MESH: Obstetrics | Clinical Clerkship | Gynecology | Study Guide
Classification: LCC R839 (print) | LCC R839 (ebook) | NLM WQ 18.2 | DDC
    610.71/1—dc23
LC record available at https://lccn.loc.gov/2021035943
LC ebook record available at https://lccn.loc.gov/2021035944

McGraw Hill books are available at special quantity discounts to use as premiums and sales promotions or for use in corporate training programs. To contact a representative, please visit the Contact Us pages at www.mhprofessional.com.

Contents

Introduction

This clinical study aid was designed in the tradition of the *First Aid* series of books, formatted in the same way as the other titles in this series. Topics are listed by bold headings to the left, while the "meat" of the topic comprises the middle column. The outside margins contain mnemonics, diagrams, summary or warning statements, "pearls," and other memory aids. These are further classified as "exam tip" noted by the ♟ symbol, "ward tip" noted by the ♆ symbol, and "typical scenario" noted by the ♀ symbol, and "zebra alerts" noted by ▌ ▌ ▌.

The content of this book is based on the recommendations by the American Professors of Gynecology and Obstetrics (APGO) and the American College of Obstetricians and Gynecologists (ACOG) for the obstetrics and gynecology (OB/GYN) curriculum for third-year medical students. Each of the chapters contains the major topics central to the practice of OB/GYN and closely parallels APGO's medical student learning objectives. This book also targets the OB/GYN content on the USMLE Step 2 examination.

The OB/GYN clerkship can be an exciting hands-on experience. You will get to deliver babies, assist in surgeries, and see patients in the clinic setting. You will find that rather than simply preparing you for the success on the clerkship exam, this book will also guide you in the clinical diagnosis and treatment of the many interesting problems you will see during your OB/GYN rotation.

Acknowledgments

We would like to thank the following faculty for their help in the preparation of the fifth edition of this book:

Eugene C. Toy, MD
Assistant Dean for Educational Programs
Director, Doctoring Courses
Professor and Vice Chair of Medical Education
Department of Obstetrics and Gynecology
McGovern Medical School at University of Texas Health Science Center
UTHealth at Houston
Houston, Texas

Patti Jayne Ross, MD
Clerkship Director
Department of Obstetrics and Gynecology
The University of Texas–Houston Medical School
Houston, Texas

How to Contribute

To continue to produce a high-yield review source for the obstetrics and gynecology clerkship, you are invited to submit any suggestions or corrections. Please send us your suggestions for:

- New facts, mnemonics, diagrams, and illustrations
- Low-yield facts to remove

For each entry incorporated into the next edition, you will receive personal acknowledgment. Diagrams, tables, partial entries, updates, corrections, and study hints are also appreciated, and significant contributions will be compensated at the discretion of the authors. Also, let us know about material in this edition that you feel is low yield and should be deleted. You are also welcome to send general comments and feedback, although due to the volume of e-mails, we may not be able to respond to each of these.

The preferred way to submit entries, suggestions, or corrections is via electronic mail. Please include name, address, school affiliation, phone number, and e-mail address (if different from the address of origin). If there are multiple entries, please consolidate into a single e-mail or file attachment. Please send submissions to:

firstaidclerkships@gmail.com

Otherwise, please send entries, neatly written or typed (Microsoft Word) to:

Bob Boehringer
Executive Editor
McGraw Hill Education
1325 Avenue of the Americas, 7th Floor
New York, NY 10019

All entries become the property of the authors and are subject to editing and reviewing. Please verify all data and spellings carefully. In the event that similar or duplicate entries are received, only the first entry received will be used. Include a reference to a standard textbook to facilitate verification of the fact. Please follow the style, punctuation, and format of this edition if possible.

How to Succeed in the Obstetrics & Gynecology Clerkship

One of the best parts of obstetrics and gynecology (OB/GYN) is the opportunity to be with patients during some of the best moments of their lives but also the worst moments. Thus, be thoughtful about what you are walking into when you enter an exam room or a delivery. Realize that, though this might be the 15th patient you have seen today, this is the patient's first visit to talk about her new cancer diagnosis or her recent miscarriage after 10 years of trying to get pregnant. Remember that getting to be part of a patient's delivery is a privilege—though you may see many deliveries during your block, this might be the only one she ever has.

Being present with your patients during these moments is not always fun or easy. If you are feeling emotionally overwhelmed, reach out to your resident, your team, or your clerkship director—you are not the first or the last person. And, it is OK to cry with your patients, both in happiness and in sadness.

How to Behave on the Wards

BE ON TIME

Most OB/GYN teams begin rounding between 5 and 7 AM. If you are expected to "pre-round," you should give yourself at least 10 minutes per patient to see the patient, review the chart, and learn about the events that occurred overnight. Like all working professionals, you will face occasional obstacles to punctuality, but make sure this is infrequent. When you first start a rotation, try to show up at least 15 minutes early until you get the routine figured out.

DRESS IN A PROFESSIONAL MANNER

You must dress in a professional, conservative manner. Wear a white coat over your clothes unless discouraged (i.e., when you are on labor and delivery or in the operating room). Recommended attire (professional versus scrubs) can vary based on rotation and clinical site, so it is a question that should be addressed to the team on the first day of the rotation.

Men should wear long pants covering the ankle, dress shoes, a long-sleeved collared shirt, and a tie. No jeans, no sneakers, no short-sleeved shirts. Facial hair should be well groomed.

Women should wear long pants or knee-length skirt or dress, and a top with a modest neckline. No jeans, no sneakers, no bare midriffs, no open-toed shoes.

Both men and women may wear scrubs occasionally, during overnight call, in the operating room, or in the labor and delivery unit. You never know what to expect on labor and delivery; so, as a general guideline, always keep a spare pair of scrubs available on your hospital-issued scrub card. Operating room attire such as masks, hats, and shoe covers should only be worn in the operating or delivery room and should be discarded as soon as those areas are exited. Scrubs should not be worn outside the hospital (i.e., between home and the hospital). Because there are a lot of bodily fluids on labor and delivery—be sure to put on shoe covers before any vaginal or cesarean delivery.

ACT IN A PLEASANT MANNER

The rotation is often difficult, stressful, and tiring. You will have a smoother experience if you are nice to be around. Be friendly, introduce yourself to everyone—including unit secretaries, nurses, medical assistants, and scrub techs- ("Hi, My name is XXX and I am the medical student") and try to learn everyone's name.

Be aware of your demeanor and reactions. It is always good to approach each rotation with an open mind, but there will be times when you are bored or just not in the mood. Try to appear interested and engaged to attendings and residents. When someone is trying to teach you something, be respectful and look grateful, not tortured. If you seem uninterested, that attending or resident is unlikely to try to take the time to teach you again.

A crucial aspect of being a good doctor is to always treat patients professionally and with respect. It is a good idea to start exhibiting this behavior at the student level. Be thoughtful about the language you use to describe patients. Your relationship with patients is one factor that is used to assess your performance in all clerkships. Thus, having a good rapport with your patients is usually noted by attendings and residents, and this is likely to be reflected in your final evaluations. However, if a resident or attending spots you behaving in an impolite or unprofessional manner, it will damage your evaluation quicker than any incorrect answer on rounds ever could. Also, be nice to the nurses, medical assistants, unit secretaries, clerkship administrator, etc.—really nice! If they like you, they will make your life a lot easier and make you look good in front of the residents and attendings.

BE AWARE OF THE HIERARCHY

The way in which this will affect you will vary from hospital to hospital and team to team, but it is always present to some degree. In general, address your questions regarding ward functioning to interns or residents when the attending isn't present. Address your medical questions to residents or attendings; make an effort to be somewhat informed on your subject prior to asking. But don't ask a question just to show off what you know. It is annoying to everyone and is always very obvious. You are more likely to make a favorable impression by seeming interested and asking real questions when they come up.

Don't be afraid to ask questions, but be conscious of the time and number of questions asked during rounds, so that everyone can finish their work and go home at a reasonable time. Do not ask questions during high acuity situations; wait until things have settled down. Do not ever answer a question from an attending that was clearly directed at one of the residents or another student.

ADDRESS PATIENTS AND STAFF IN A RESPECTFUL WAY

Address patients as Sir or Ma'am, or Mr., Mrs., or Miss. Don't address patients as "honey," "sweetie," etc. Although you may feel that these names are friendly, patients may think you have forgotten their name, that you are being inappropriately familiar, or both. Address all physicians as "doctor," unless told otherwise. While your resident may tell you to call them by their first name, remember to call them "doctor" in front of patients.

BE HELPFUL TO YOUR RESIDENTS

Take responsibility for the patient you have been assigned. You should aim to know everything there is to know about her including her history, test results, details about her medical problems, prognosis, and general plan of care. Keep your interns or residents informed of new developments that they might not be aware of or had time to look up themselves (i.e., lab results, imaging reads, consultant recommendations). Communicate with the nurses prior to rounds to make sure you are aware of overnight or other new developments.

Work independently and try to anticipate the needs of your team and your patients. If during rounds, the attending or chief resident says, "lets get a CBC today"—that means it is your job to be sure that gets done. Add a "check box" to your list to ensure that it gets ordered and also that you note the results. Then, follow up with your resident once you see the result.

If you have the opportunity to make a resident look good, take it. If a new complication develops with a patient, make sure to tell the resident about it so they can be best prepared to take care of the patient and answer questions from the attending. Look up recent literature, if appropriate, and share it with your team (ideally before discussing with the attending). Don't hesitate to give credit to a resident for some great teaching in front of an attending. These things make the resident's life easier; he or she will be grateful, and the rewards will come your way.

After rounds, assess what needs to be done for your patients, and take ownership of their care. Pay attention to what was discussed on rounds so you can know what information to obtain or what follow-up phone calls to make. Volunteer to do things that will help out (call a consult, update a family member, update the list with "to dos," etc.). Observe and anticipate—if a resident asks you to so something one day, be sure you have it done without asking the next day. If a resident is always hunting around for some tape to perform a dressing change during rounds, get some tape ahead of time and be prepared to help.

RESPECT PATIENTS' RIGHTS

1. All patients have the right to have their personal medical information kept private. This means do not discuss the patient's information with their family members without that patient's consent, and do not discuss any patient in hallways, elevators, or cafeterias. Do not post any patient information on social media platforms under any circumstances.
2. All patients have the right to refuse treatment. This means they can refuse treatment by a specific individual (you, the medical student) or of a specific type (e.g., Pap test). Patients can even refuse lifesaving treatment. The only exceptions to this rule are a patient who is deemed to not have the capacity to make decisions or understand situations—in which case a healthcare proxy should be sought—or a patient who is suicidal or homicidal.
3. All patients should be informed of the right to seek advance directives on admission. This is often done by the admissions staff, in a booklet. If your patient is chronically ill or has a life-threatening illness, address the subject of advance directives with the assistance of your attending.

TAKE INITIATIVE

Be self-motivated. Volunteer to help with procedures or difficult tasks. Volunteer to look up the answer to a question that your team didn't know that answer to, and then share with your team. Volunteer to follow or care for additional patients if you feel able. Volunteer to stay late to push with a patient or help transport a patient to a study. Offer to help clean up a patient after a delivery and to help position and transfer patients in the OR. Give more of yourself unsolicited.

BE A TEAM PLAYER

Help other medical students with their tasks; share information you have learned. When the nights students come on—sign out your patients to them, and in the morning—get signout/handoff from them about the patients you are going to follow that day. Make your fellow medical students look good if you have the opportunity. Support your supervising intern or resident whenever possible. Never steal the spotlight, steal a procedure, or make a fellow medical student look bad. Don't complain—no matter how hard you have worked or how many hours you have been at the hospital.

BE HONEST

If you don't understand, don't know, or didn't do it, make sure you are honest about it. Never say or document information that is false (i.e., don't say "bowel sounds normal" when you did not listen).

KEEP PATIENT INFORMATION HANDY

Use a clipboard, notebook, index cards, or patient list to keep patient information, including a miniature history and physical, labs, and test results at hand. However, remember to place these notes/lists in the shredder bin at the end of your shift. Because they contain patient information—you cannot dispose of them in the normal trash.

PRESENT PATIENT INFORMATION IN AN ORGANIZED MANNER

Here is a template for the "bullet" presentation:

This is a [age]-year-old GXPXXX patient with a history of [**major history such as abdominal surgery, pertinent OB/GYN history**] who presented on [**date**] with [**major symptoms, such as pelvic pain, fever**] and was found to have [**working diagnosis**]. [**Tests done**] showed [**results**]. Yesterday the patient [**state important changes or important events in the last 24 hours, new plan, new tests, new medications**]. This morning the patient feels [**state the patient's words**], **vital signs significant for** [**add abnormal vitals**], the physical exam is significant for [**state major findings**]. **In sum, the patient is** [**restate your one liner**] [**then give assessment of how patient is doing**] Plan is [**state plan**].

The newly admitted patient generally deserves a longer presentation following the complete history and physical format. Other patients may just require an overnight update in the SOAP (Subjective, Objective, Assessment, Plan) format.

Some patients have extensive histories. The whole history can and probably should be present in the admission note, but in a ward presentation it is often too much to absorb. In these cases learn how to generate a good summary that maintains an accurate picture of the patient and includes the most pertinent information. This usually takes some thought, but it is worth it. Think about presenting like telling a story.

DOCUMENT INFORMATION IN AN ORGANIZED MANNER

A complete medical student initial history and physical is thorough and organized. Make sure you are not just checking boxes in a template in the electronic medical record. You should be thinking about every section of the history you take and documenting appropriately (see page 7). READ and review your note before you send it to your resident or preceptor. Often the electronic medical record auto-populates incomplete things as "not on file."

For example, it is very poor form to send a note to your preceptors that says, "PMH: not on file."

How to Organize Your Learning

One of the best things about the OB/GYN clerkship is that you get to see a lot of patients. The patient is the key to learning and is the source of most satisfaction and frustration on the wards. Starting OB/GYN can make you feel like you're in a foreign land. A lot of your studying from the preclinical years and your experiences on other clerkships do not necessarily help much. The learning curve is very steep. You have to start from scratch in some ways, and it will help enormously if you can skim through this book before you start. Get some of the terminology straight, get some of the major points down, and it won't seem so overwhelming. Also, remember, your residents and attendings know that it is new for you. Jot down questions or acronyms that you don't know and ask what they mean during some down time (or look them up yourself).

SELECT YOUR STUDY MATERIAL

We recommend:

- This review book, *First Aid for the® Obstetrics & Gynecology Clerkship*, 5th edition.
- A full-text online journal database, available through your institution's library.
- An online peer-reviewed resource, such as Up-To-Date®, which is now available in most hospitals and academic centers.

AS YOU SEE PATIENTS, NOTE THEIR MAJOR SYMPTOMS AND DIAGNOSIS FOR REVIEW

Your reading on the symptom-based topics above should be done with a specific patient in mind. For example, if a postmenopausal patient comes to the office with increasing abdominal girth and is thought to have ovarian cancer, read about ovarian cancer that night. It helps to have a real patient in mind to "hang" a diagnosis on for improved recall.

How to Prepare for the Clinical Clerkship and USMLE Step 2 Exam

If you have read about your core topics in OB/GYN, you will know a great deal about medicine. You should also be familiar with the clerkship educational objectives (see the course syllabus), and can always review the Association of Professors of Gynecology and Obstetrics (APGO) Medical Student Educational Objectives, 11th edition. This is available free to students at the APGO website under "Student Resources." To study for the clerkship exam, we recommend:

2–3 weeks before exam: Read this entire review book, taking notes.
10 days before exam: Read the notes you took during the rotation on your core content list and the corresponding review book sections. Begin doing

practice test questions through whatever resource you prefer (i.e., the U Wise test questions at the APGO website).

5 days before exam: Read this entire review book, concentrating on lists and mnemonics. Continue working through practice test questions.

2 days before exam: Exercise, eat well, skim the book, and go to bed early.

1 day before exam: Exercise, eat well, review your notes and the mnemonics, and go to bed on time. Do not have any caffeine after 2 PM.

Other helpful studying strategies are detailed below.

STUDY WITH FRIENDS

Group studying can be very helpful. Other people may point out areas that you have not studied enough and may help you focus on the goal. If you tend to get distracted by other people in the room, limit this to less than half of your study time.

STUDY IN A BRIGHT ROOM

Find the room in your house or in your library that has the best, brightest light. This will help prevent you from falling asleep. If you don't have a bright light, get a halogen desk lamp.

EAT LIGHT, BALANCED MEALS

Make sure your meals are balanced, with lean protein, fruits and vegetables, and fiber. A high-sugar, high-carbohydrate meal will give you an initial burst of energy for 1–2 hours, but then you'll drop.

TAKE PRACTICE EXAMS

The point of practice exams is not so much the content that is contained in the questions but the training of sitting still for 3 hours and trying to pick the best answer for each and every question. You can also use practice questions to assess where the gaps in your knowledge are in order to guide your future studying.

Terminology

A LITTLE HELPFUL TERMINOLOGY

Terminology—We talk a lot about Gs and Ps—Below is an explanation of that.

When you present, you will say, G#P#[1]#[2]#[3]#[4] (you may see this written as GFPAL):

G is for (gravidity) 3 = total number of pregnancies, including normal and abnormal intrauterine pregnancies, abortions, ectopic pregnancies, and hydatidiform moles. (*Remember, if patient was pregnant with twins,* **G = 1.**)

P is short is for parity and describes the outcome of those pregnancies—but you will see 4 numbers listed after the P. A good mnemonic to remember this is FPAL: "Florida Power And Light."

WARD TIP

A good way to elicit information about previous pregnancies is to ask—"How many times have your been pregnant?" then, "What happened in your first pregnancy?" What happened in your second pregnancy?," and so on.

#[1] or F→ for **fullterm** deliveries, all deliveries after 37 weeks, independent of if the fetus survived or had an intrauterine fetal demise (IUFD). (*Remember, if patient delivered twins, F = 1 because we are talking about deliveries not number of babies.*)

#[2] or P→ for **preterm** deliveries, all deliveries after 20 weeks but before 37 weeks, independent of if the fetus survived or had an IUFD. (*Remember, if patient delivered twins, P = 1 because we are talking about deliveries not number of babies.*)

#[3] or A→ for **abortions**; in this case abortions is number of pregnancies that were lost before the 20th gestational week—includes miscarriage, anembryonic gestation, elective terminations, and IUFD < 20 weeks.

#[4] or L→ for total **living** children and if equal to the number of successful pregnancy outcomes. (*Remember, if patient was pregnant with twins, L = 2.*)

High-Yield Facts in Obstetrics

Reproductive Anatomy

An adequate knowledge of the normal female anatomy is essential in obstetrics and gynecology. Each time a physician delivers a baby or performs a gynecologic surgery, he or she must be well versed in the anatomy of the region. This chapter will discuss the major structures of the pelvis. The major blood supply to the pelvis is from the **internal iliac artery (hypogastric artery)** and its branches. The lymphatics drain to the inguinal, pelvic, or para-aortic lymph nodes. The major parasympathetic innervation is via **S2, S3, and S4,** which forms the pudendal nerve. The major sympathetic innervation is via the aortic plexus, which gives rise to the **internal iliac plexus.**

Vulva

 A 30-year-old G1P1 patient presents to the emergency department with a lump in the vulva and acute onset of pain for 2 days. The pain has gradually ↑, and she is unable to sit. She reports no fever, chills, nausea, or vomiting. She has no medical problems and takes no medications. On exam, the right labium majorum is swollen. A 4 × 4-cm fluctuant tender mass is palpated at the 8 o'clock position; no drainage is noted. What is the most likely diagnosis? What is the best treatment?

Answer: Bartholin's gland abscess. The best treatment is incision and drainage followed packing, or placement of Word catheter. If it recurs, consider marupialization. Can consider broad-spectrum antibiotics. If the patient is postmenopausal with recurrent Bartholin's abscess or cysts, consider carcinoma and obtain a biopsy.

The vulva consists of all structures visible externally from the pubis to perineum. It includes the labia majora, labia minora, mons pubis, clitoris, vestibule of the vagina, vestibular bulb, and the greater vestibular glands (see Figure 1-1). The vestibule itself contains the urethral opening, vaginal opening, bilateral Bartholin gland ducts, and bilateral Skene's (paraurethral) glands. The blood supply, lymphatics, and nerve supply of the vulva are detailed in Table 1-1.

- **Clitoris:** Composed of a glans, a corpora, and two crura. Rarely exceeds 2 cm in length, and normal diameter is 1.5 cm. Homologuous to the male penis.
- **Bartholin glands:** Located at 4 o'clock and 8 o'clock of the vaginal orifice and are typically nonpalpable. They function in secreting mucous to provide vaginal lubrication and are homologous to the bulbourethral glands in males.
- **Skene's glands:** Ducts of these glands open on either side of the urethral orifice.

Vagina

The vagina is a tubular, muscular structure that extends from the vulva to the cervix. Exteriorly, the vaginal orifice is located anterior to the perineum and posterior the urethra. The blood supply, lymphatics, and nerve supply to the vagina are listed in Table 1-2.

Cervix

The cervix is actually a part of the uterus. It is the specialized narrow inferior portion of the uterus that is at the apex of the vagina.

EXAM TIP

Bartholin gland blockage causes a cyst or abscess.
  Most often:
  Cysts: Asymptomatic
  Abscesses: Painful

WARD TIP

A pudendal nerve block can provide pain relief at the time of a vaginal delivery.

EXAM TIP

Remember from embryology that the upper vagina comes from the paramesonephric ducts and merges with the lower vagina, which originates from urogenital sinus—because of this, they have different blood and lymphatic supply.

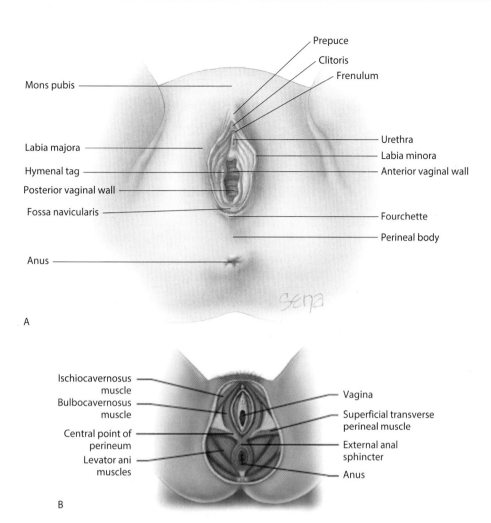

FIGURE 1-1. **(A) External female genitalia.** (Reproduced, with permission, from Cunningham FG, Leveno KJ, Bloom SL, et al. *Williams Obstetrics.* 23rd ed. New York: McGraw-Hill Education; 2010: Figure 2-2.) **(B) Perineal anatomy.** (Reproduced, with permission, from Ganti L. *Atlas of Emergency Medicine Procedures.* New York: Springer Nature; 2016.)

TABLE 1-1. **Vulvar Anatomy**

Blood supply	Branches of the external and internal pudendal arteries, which are subdivisions of the hypogastric artery (internal iliac)
Lymphatics	Medial group of superficial inguinal nodes
Nerve supply	Pudendal Nerve: it branches into:
	▪ **Anterior vulva:** Ilioinguinal nerves and the genital branch of the genitofemoral nerves.
	▪ **Posterior vulva:** Perineal nerves and posterior cutaneous nerves of the thigh.

COMPONENTS

The cervix can be further subdivided into:

- **Portio vaginalis:** Portion of the cervix projecting into the vagina
- **External os:** Lowermost opening of the cervix into the vagina
- **Ectocervix:** Portion of the cervix exterior to the external os
- **Endocervical canal:** Passageway between the external os and the uterine cavity
- **Internal os:** Uppermost opening of the cervix into the uterine cavity

TABLE 1-2.   Vaginal Anatomy

Blood supply	**Hypogastric artery (anastomotic network):**
	Vaginal branch of the uterine artery is the primary supply to the vagina.
	Middle rectal and inferior vaginal branches of the hypogastric artery (internal iliac artery) are secondary blood supplies.
	Anastomoses with cervical arteries.
Lymphatics	Upper 2/3rd: Obturator plexus, iliac nodes
	Lower 1/3rd: Superficial inguinal nodes
Nerve supply	**Hypogastric plexus:** Sympathetic innervation
	Pelvic nerve: Parasympathetic innervation

CERVICAL EPITHELIUM

 A 36-year-old G3P3 patient has an abnormal Pap test, showing a low-grade squamous intraepithelial lesion (LSIL). The colposcopic biopsy shows cervical intraepithelial neoplasia II. She undergoes a loop electroexcision procedure (LEEP). What portion of the cervix must be completely excised to ensure proper treatment?

Answer: The transformation zone should be completely excised because that is where the majority of cervical cancers arise.

Both **columnar** and **stratified nonkeratinized squamous** epithelia cover the cervix.

- The stratified nonkeratinized squamous epithelium covers the ectocervix.
- The columnar epithelium lines the endocervical canal.
- The **squamocolumnar junction** is where the two types of epithelium meet.
- The **transformation zone** is the area of metaplasia where columnar epithelium changes to squamous epithelium. It is the most important cytologic and colposcopic landmark, as this is where over 90% of cervical neoplasias arise.

BLOOD SUPPLY

Cervical and vaginal branch of the uterine artery, which arises from the internal iliac artery

NERVE SUPPLY

Hypogastric plexus

Uterus

The uterus is a muscular organ that lies posterior to the bladder and anterior to the rectum in the pelvis of a nonpregnant patient. In pregnancy, the uterus enlarges with the growth of the fetus and progressively becomes an abdominal as well as a pelvic organ. The blood supply, lymphatics, and nerve supply of the uterus are detailed in Table 1-3.

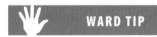
WARD TIP

Colposcopy: Magnified view of the cervix, vagina, and vulva

EXAM TIP

Total hysterectomy = Uterus and cervix are removed (ovarian status unknown). Supracervical hysterectomy = Uterus removed, cervix retained (ovarian status unknown).

Although you may hear patients refer to a "partial hysterectomy," this is not a term used to describe a hysterectomy. When patients say this, they usually mean that the ovaries were retained. To describe removal of the ovaries and Fallopian tubes, you would say, "bilateral salpingo-oophorectomy."

TABLE 1-3. Uterine Anatomy

Blood supply	**Uterine arteries:** Arise from hypogastric artery (internal iliac artery)
	Ovarian arteries: Arise from the aorta and anastamose with uterine vasculature
Lymphatics	Obturator plexus, iliac node
Nerve supply	**Superior hypogastric plexus**
	Inferior hypogastric plexus
	Common iliac nerves

COMPONENTS OF THE UTERUS

- **Fundus:** Uppermost region of uterus
- **Corpus:** Body of the uterus
- **Cornua:** Part of uterus that connects to the fallopian tubes bilaterally
- **Cervix:** Inferior part of the uterus that protrudes into the vagina

HISTOLOGY

- **Myometrium:** The smooth muscle layer of uterus. It is subdivided into three layers:
  1. Outer longitudinal.
  2. Middle oblique.
  3. Inner longitudinal.
- **Endometrium:** The mucosal layer of the uterus made up of columnar epithelium.

Fallopian (Uterine) Tubes

The fallopian tubes extend from the superior lateral aspects of the uterus through the superior fold of the broad ligament laterally to the ovaries. The blood supply for the fallopian tubes comes from the ovarian and uterine arteries. Pelvic plexus (autonomic) and ovarian plexus are the nervous supply to the fallopian tubes.

ANATOMIC SECTIONS, FROM LATERAL TO MEDIAL

- **Infundibulum:** The most distal part of the uterine tube. Gives rise to the fimbriae. Helps to sweep the egg that is released from the ovary into the tube.
- **Ampulla:** Widest section. This is where fertilization takes place.
- **Isthmus:** Narrowest part. This is where tubal sterilizations are performed.
- **Intramural part:** Pierces uterine wall and connects to the endometrial cavity.

Ovaries

The ovaries lie on the posterior aspect of the broad ligament and fallopian tubes. They are attached to the broad ligament by the mesovarium and are

WARD TIP

The ureter travels under the uterine artery. Think "water under the bridge."

WARD TIP

The tubes are occluded at the isthmus for permanent sterilization via laparoscopy, via mini infra-umbilical incision immediately postpartum, or at the time of cesarean delivery. Alternatively, they may be completely removed as part of a sterilization procedure (bilateral salpingectomy).

WARD TIP

Most common location for ectopic pregnancy = Ampulla of fallopian tube.

WARD TIP

No peritoneum around ovaries leads to fast dissemination of ovarian cancer in the abdomen.

Blood Supply of Ovaries

Aorta → Bilateral ovarian arteries

Left ovarian vein → Left renal vein

Right ovarian vein → Inferior vena cava

not covered by peritoneum. Each ovary functions in ova development and hormone production. The blood supply to both ovaries comes from the ovarian arteries which arise from the aorta at the level of L1. Ovarian veins drain into the inferior vena cava on the right side and the renal vein on the left. The ovaries are covered by tunica albuginea, a fibrous capsule. The tunica albuginea is covered by germinal epithelium.

Ligaments of the Pelvic Viscera

 A 22-year-old G2P1001 patient at 32 weeks' gestation reports sharp stabbing lower abdominal pain. The pain worsens with walking and improves with rest. She has no loss of fluid, vaginal bleeding, fever, trauma, sick contacts, or recent travel. Her last intercourse was 3 weeks ago. Fetal movement is present. Non-stress test (NST) is reassuring, and no contractions are noted. Her cervix is closed on exam. Urinalysis (UA) is negative. What is this patient's most likely diagnosis?

Answer: Round ligament pain. Round ligament pain is a diagnosis of exclusion. The round ligaments begin near the uterine cornua, pass through the inguinal canal, and terminate in the labia majora. The key finding is worsening pain with movement and improvement with rest. It can be treated with acetaminophen, belly belt, and rest.

Some ligaments of the pelvis act only as support structures, but others also carry the blood supply for essential organs.

- **Broad ligament:** Peritoneal fold extends from the lateral pelvic wall to the uterus and adnexa. Contains the fallopian (uterine) tube, round ligament, uterine and ovarian blood vessels, lymph, ureterovaginal nerves, and ureter (see Figure 1-2).
- **Infundibulopelvic (IP) ligament (aka suspensory ligament of the ovary):** Contains the ovarian artery and vein and connects the ovary to the pelvic wall.
- **Round ligament:** The remains of the gubernaculum; it extends from the corpus of the uterus down and laterally through the inguinal canal and terminates in the labia majora.
- **Cardinal ligament (Mackenrodt ligament):** Extends from the cervix (near the level of the internal cervical os) and lateral vagina to the pelvic

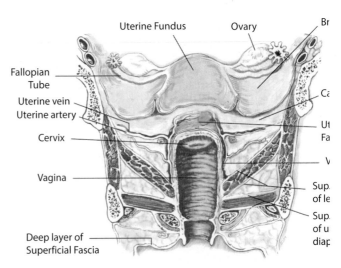

FIGURE 1-2. Supporting structures of the pelvic viscera. (Reproduced, with permission, from Lindarkis NM, Lott S. *Digging Up the Bones: Obstetrics and Gynecology*. New York: McGraw-Hill; 1998:2.)

side wall; the most **important support** structure of the uterus. It contains the uterine artery and vein.

- **Uterosacral ligaments:** Each ligament extends from an attachment posterolaterally to the supravaginal portion of the cervix and inserts into the fascia over the sacrum. Provides some support to the uterus.

Muscles

Various muscles of the pelvis make up the perineum. Most of the support is provided by the pelvic and urogenital diaphragms.

- **Pelvic diaphragm** forms a broad sling in the pelvis to support the internal organs. It is composed of the levator ani complex (iliococcygeus, puborectalis, pubococcygeus muscles) and the coccygeus muscles.
- **Urogenital diaphragm** is external to the pelvic diaphragm and is composed of the deep transverse perineal muscles, the constrictor of the urethra, and the internal and external fascial coverings. It helps maintain urinary continence.
- **Perineal body** is the central tendon of the perineum, which provides much of the support. The median raphe of the levator ani, between the anus and vagina. Bulbocavernosus, superficial transverse perineal, and external anal sphincter muscles converge at the central tendon.

BLOOD SUPPLY

Internal pudendal artery and its branches, inferior rectal artery, and posterior labial artery.

NERVE SUPPLY

Pudendal nerve, which originates from S2, S3, and S4 levels of the spinal cord.

Pelvis

The adult pelvis is composed of four bones: the sacrum, the coccyx, and two innominate bones. The innominate bones are formed from the fusion of the ilium, ischium, and pubis (see Figure 1-3).

- **Sacrum:** Consists of five vertebrae fused together to form a single wedge-shaped bone. It articulates laterally with two iliac bones to form the

 EXAM TIP
The artery of Sampson runs through the round ligament.

 WARD TIP
Most hysterectomies start by ligation and transection of the round ligament.

 EXAM TIP
Most common site for ureteral injury during hysterectomy = Level of cardinal ligament (ureter passes under the uterine artery).

 WARD TIP
Pelvic organ prolapse is caused by a defect in the pelvic diaphragm.

 WARD TIP
The perineal body is cut when episiotomy is performed.

WARD TIP
Pelvimetry assesses the shape and capacity of the pelvis in relation to the ability of a baby to pass through it.

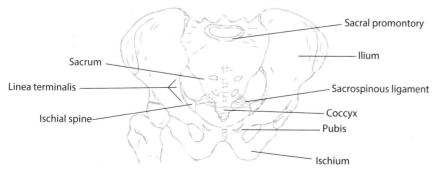
FIGURE 1-3. Bony pelvis.

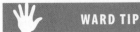

sacroiliac joints. The **sacral promontory** is the first sacral vertebrae, and it can be palpated during a vaginal exam. It is an important landmark for clinical pelvimetry.

- **Coccyx:** Composed of four vertebrae fused together to form a small triangular bone that articulates with the base of the sacrum.
- **Ischial spines:** Extend from the middle of the posterior margin of each ischium.

PELVIC SHAPES

There are four major shapes: **gynecoid, android, platypelloid,** and **anthropoid**. These shapes are differentiated based on the measurements of the pelvis. Gynecoid is the ideal shape for vaginal delivery, having a round to slightly oval pelvic inlet. (See Chapter 5, "Intrapartum," Table 5-5.)

Diagnosis of Pregnancy

It is essential to make an accurate diagnosis of pregnancy and establish the estimated date of delivery (EDD), because this determines the patient's future prenatal care. This chapter will discuss how to diagnose pregnancy, including symptoms of pregnancy, use of human chorionic gonadotropin (hCG), fetal heart rate (FHR), and ultrasound (US).

Naegele's Rule

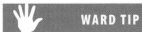 A 25-year-old G0P0 patient presents with a report of absent menses for 2 months. Prior to this, she had regular menses every 28 days, lasting for 4 days each month. She is sexually active and reports using condoms regularly. What is the best test to evaluate her condition?

Answer: Urine pregnancy test (UPT). Pregnancy must be considered in any patient of reproductive age with a report of amenorrhea or irregular menses, even if she is using contraception. Including or excluding pregnancy will significantly impact the differential diagnoses.

Naegele's rule is used to calculate the estimated date of confinement (EDC; i.e., due date or EDD) ±2 weeks.

- First day of patient's last menstrual period (LMP), minus 3 months, plus 7 days, plus 1 year.
- Example: If LMP = July 20, 2021, then EDC = April 27, 2022

Signs and Symptoms of Pregnancy

A patient's body goes through drastic physiologic changes from the day she conceives to weeks after the delivery of her baby. It is important to differentiate the normal physiologic changes of pregnancy from other pathological conditions. This section will discuss signs and symptoms that are indicative of pregnancy.

- **Cessation of menses:** Pregnancy is highly likely if 10 or more days have passed from the time of expected menses in a patient who previously had regular cycles.
- **Breast changes:**
  - ↑ breast tenderness.
  - ↑ in breast size.
  - Nipples become larger, more pigmented, and more erectile.
  - Areolae become broader and more pigmented.
  - Colostrum may be expressed from the nipples later in pregnancy.
- **Skin changes (more common later in gestation):**
  - Striae gravidarum (aka stretch marks): Reddish, slightly depressed streaks on the abdomen, breast, and thighs.
  - Linea nigra: Midline of the abdominal wall becomes darkly pigmented.
  - Chloasma or melasma gravidarum (aka mask of pregnancy): Irregular brown patches of varying size on the face and neck.
  - Angiomas: Red elevation at a central point with branching vasculature present on the face, neck, chest, and arms due to estrogens.
- **Uterine changes:**
  - The uterus ↑ in size throughout the pregnancy (its size correlates to gestational age). By week 12, it is about the size of a grapefruit, and the fundus of the uterus becomes palpable above the pubic symphysis (see Table 2-1).

WARD TIP

Naegele's rule assumes two things:
1. A normal gestation is 280 days.
2. All patients have a 28-day menstrual cycle.

These are BIG assumptions that are rarely true.

WARD TIP

When determining the EDC, use the first day of bleeding of the LMP.

WARD TIP

Use Naegele's rule to calculate the EDD from the LMP.

EDC = (LMP + 1 year + 7 days) − 3 months

WARD TIP

A nonpregnant cervix feels like the cartilage of the nose. A pregnant cervix feels like the lips of the mouth. Hegar's sign = Softening of the cervix.

WARD TIP

At 20 weeks, the uterus is at umbilicus, which is usually ~20 cm from the symphysis. The uterus grows 1 cm/week. Thus, the fundal height in centimeters should be equal to the gestational age in weeks.

TABLE 2-1. Fundal Height During Pregnancy

WEEKS PREGNANT	FUNDAL HEIGHT
12	Barely palpable above pubic symphysis
15	Midpoint between pubic symphysis and umbilicus
20	At the umbilicus
28	8 cm above the umbilicus
32	6 cm below the xyphoid process
36	2 cm below xyphoid process
40	4 cm below xiphoid process[a]

[a]Due to engagement and descent of the fetal head, the fundal height at 40 weeks is typically less than the fundal height at 36 weeks.

- **Cervical changes:** Cervix becomes softer much closer to onset of labor.
- **Vaginal mucosa discoloration:** With pregnancy and ↑ blood flow, the vagina appears dark bluish or purplish red.
- **Perception of fetal movement:** A primigravida may report fetal movement as early as 20 weeks' gestation, and a multipara at 18 weeks' gestation. More common to feel movement consistently at 22–24 weeks for a primigravida.
- **Nausea and/or vomiting** (aka morning sickness): Nausea and/or vomiting occurs in approximately 70–85% of pregnancies, most notably at 4–12 weeks' gestation. Morning sickness is a misnomer—though it frequently occurs in the morning, it really can occur throughout the day.
- **Hyperemesis gravidarum** is persistent and severe nausea and vomiting that occurs early in pregnancy. It results in weight loss, dehydration, acidosis (from starvation), alkalosis (from loss of HCl in vomitus), and hypokalemia. These patients often need hospitalization for IVF and IV antiemetics.
- **Hair growth changes:** Prolonged anagen (the growing hair phase).
- **Urologic changes:** ↑ pressure from the enlarging uterus results in ↑ urinary frequency, nocturia, and bladder irritability.

WARD TIP

Chadwick's sign: Bluish discoloration of the vaginal and cervical mucosa due to vascular congestion in pregnancy.

WARD TIP

Quickening: First fetal movements felt by the mother.

Human Chorionic Gonadotropin (hCG)

A 25-year-old patient presents with vaginal spotting and right lower quadrant pain. Her abdomen is slightly tender to palpation in the right lower quadrant. There is minimal dark blood in the vaginal vault, and her cervix is closed. Quantitative serum hCG is 4000 mIU/mL. A transvaginal ultrasound (TVUS) shows no evidence of pregnancy inside the uterus. What is the most likely diagnosis?

Answer: Ectopic pregnancy. A gestational sac should be seen inside the uterus on a TVUS with an hCG level of 1500 mIU/mL. If the pregnancy is not seen in the uterus, then an investigation must be carried out for an ectopic pregnancy.

Detection of hCG in the mother's serum and urine is used to diagnose pregnancy. This section discusses the various aspects of the hormone, as well as how it is used in the diagnosis of abnormal pregnancies.

OVERVIEW

- hCG can be detected in maternal serum and urine.
- It is a glycoprotein made by trophoblasts.
- Composed of two subunits—α and β:
    - α subunit is similar in luteinizing hormone (LH), follicle-stimulating hormone (FSH), and thyroid-stimulating hormone (TSH).
    - β subunits are unique: Urine and serum tests are based on antibody specificity to β subunit of hCG.
- **Function:** Helps sustain the corpus luteum during the **first 7 weeks**. After the first 7 weeks, the placenta takes over and makes its own hormones to sustain the pregnancy.
- Can be detected in the maternal serum or urine 6–12 days after fertilization (3–3.5 weeks after the LMP).
- ↑ by 66–100% every 48 hours prior to 10 weeks. In general, hCG should double every two days.
- Peaks at 10 weeks' gestation.
- Nadirs at 14–16 weeks.
- Keep in mind that pregnancy tests detect not only hCG produced by the syncytiotrophoblast cells in the placenta **but also:**
    - Hydatidiform mole.
    - Choriocarcinoma.
    - Germ cell tumors.
    - hCG produced by breast cancers and large cell carcinoma of the lung.
- A gestational sac can be visualized with TVUS when hCG levels are >1500. If hCG is >1500 and no evidence of intrauterine pregnancy, think *ectopic pregnancy*.

PREGNANCY TEST USING HCG

hCG can be detected in plasma and urine. Each test has specific uses, which are discussed below.

Urine hCG

- Preferred method to diagnose normal pregnancy.
- Total urine hCG closely parallels plasma concentration.
- First morning specimens are more accurate. hCG concentration is higher in the morning.
- Urine Assays detect 25 mIU/mL of hCG, and diagnose pregnancy with 95% sensitivity by 1 week after the first missed menstrual period.
- **False negatives** may occur if:
    - The test is performed too early (i.e., before the first missed period).
    - The urine is very dilute.
- **False positives** may occur with:
    - Proteinuria (confirm with plasma hCG).
    - Urinary tract infection (UTI).

Plasma hCG is used when quantitative information is needed. However, it is important to note that this is not useful in routine pregnancies because it does not provide additional information or change management. See Table 2-2.

 EXAM TIP
hCG is a glycoprotein hormone composed of α and β subunits.

 EXAM TIP
The hCG α subunit is identical to that in LH, FSH, and TSH.

 EXAM TIP
Plasma hCG levels should double every 48 hours prior to 10 weeks.

 EXAM TIP
If β-hCG does not rise as expected, consider some form of abnormal pregnancy, including: ectopic pregnancy, spontaneous abortion, or missed abortion.

 WARD TIP
Testing hCG before the time of a missed period usually should not be done due to a very low sensitivity.

 WARD TIP
hCG → supports corpus luteum → produces progesterone → supports early pregnancy.

 WARD TIP
Serial hCGs are used to follow and make prognosis of first-trimester bleeding.

WARD TIP
Normal fetal heart rate ranges from 110 to 160 bpm.

TABLE 2-2.   Plasma hCG Uses

ASSOCIATED WITH PREGNANCY	NOT RELATED TO ONGOING PREGNANCY
*Delineate between normal and abnormally growing pregnancy in first trimester prior to US evidence of pregnancy.	*Monitor trophoblastic tumors (see Chapter 30).
*Screen for aneuploidy in first or second trimester.	
*Assess/follow pregnancy status in setting of early first-trimester bleeding.	

Fetal Heart Rate (FHR)

Hearing or seeing the fetal heartbeat confirms the presence of a viable pregnancy. Electronic Doppler device can detect fetal heart tones as early as 10 weeks' gestation.

Ultrasound (US)

US is a noninvasive tool that serves multiple purposes in the setting of a pregnancy.
Figure 2-1

INDICATIONS FOR ULTRASOUND

- Confirm an intrauterine pregnancy (especially important if an ectopic is suspected).
- Document the viability of embryo. Fetal cardiac activity can be seen when the embryo measures ≥5 mm.

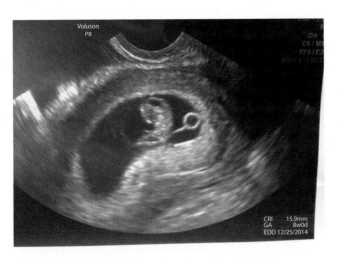

FIGURE 2-1.   Ultrasound of early first trimester fetus with yolk sac. Measurement of crown-rump length (CRL) used to estimate gestational age.

EXAM TIP

Up to 14 weeks, the crown-rump length is predictive of gestational age within 4 days.

WARD TIP

Verification of an intrauterine pregnancy does not ensure a normal pregnancy, just rules out ectopic pregnancy.

ZEBRA ALERT

Heterotopic pregnancy is when there is an intrauterine pregnancy AND an ectopic pregnancy at the same time.

WARD TIP

Early pregnancy US is more precise in establishing the EDC:
US done in T1 can vary by ±4 days.
US done in T2 can vary by ±14 days.
US done in T3 can vary by ±21 days.

- Diagnose multiple gestations.
- Estimate gestational age.
- Screen for fetal structural anomalies.

During a low risk normal pregnancy, a patient should have two USs. One in the first trimester to verify her dating/date the pregnancy if her periods are irregular or not 28 days or she isn't sure of her last menstrual period and one at 18–20 weeks to look at fetal anatomy.

It is also important to remember that an US is a radiologic study similar to a computed tomography (CT) scan or a cardiac magnetic resonance imaging (MRI). However, for many patients, they view the US very differently. This is the time when they get to see the baby for the first time or to find out gender—not a radiologic study looking for abnormalities.

LIMITATIONS

The US dating becomes progressively less accurate after 20 weeks' gestation. The US measures the size of the fetus, not the gestational age. There is more and more biologic variation in how a fetus grows as the pregnancy progresses which leads to decrease in accuracy of US dating. The US is also more challenging with increasing maternal body mass index.

Once pregnancy is diagnosed, by urine or serum pregnancy test, an US soon after is helpful to ensure pregnancy location, viability, and good dating. However, for patients with a live intrauterine pregnancy who are in the first trimester, the first visit with their obstetrics (OB) provider usually does not occur until 9–10 weeks' gestation.

Physiology of Pregnancy

Pregnancy causes changes in the female body from the time of conception. The body prepares not only for the development and growth of a fetus but also for delivery. These alterations can potentially lead to serious complications during pregnancy.

Conception

OVULATION

Ovulation is necessary for normal fertilization to occur:
- The ovum must leave the ovary and be carried into the fallopian tube.
- The unfertilized ovum is surrounded by its zona pellucida.
- This oocyte has completed its first meiotic division and carries its first polar body.

FERTILIZATION

Fertilization typically occurs within 24 hours after ovulation in the ampulla of the fallopian tube:
- The sperm penetrates the zona pellucida of the ovum. The male and female nuclear material combine to form a single cell called a zygote.
- Fertilization signals the ovum to complete meiosis II and to discharge an additional polar body.

PREIMPLANTATION

- The zygote starts to undergo cleavage (divide). At the 16 cells' stage, it is called a **morula**.
- The morula divides to form a multicellular **blastomere**.
- The blastomere passes from the fallopian tube into the uterine cavity.
- The embryo develops into a **blastocyst** as it freely floats in the endometrial cavity after conception (see Table 3-1).
- Each cell of the preimplantation embryo is totipotent; each cell can form all different types of cells in the embryo.

IMPLANTATION

- On day 5–6 after ovulation, the blastocyst adheres to the endometrium with the help of adhesion molecules on the secretory endometrial surface.
- After attachment, the endometrium proliferates around the blastocyst.

PLACENTATION

- During week 2 after ovulation, cells in the outer cell mass differentiate into **trophoblasts**.
- Trophoblastic shell forms the initial boundary between the embryo and the endometrium.
- The trophoblasts nearest to the myometrium form the placental disk; the other trophoblasts form the chorionic membranes.

WARD TIP

Fertilization occurs in the ampulla of the fallopian tube.

EXAM TIP

Human chorionic gonadotropin (hCG) is detectable in maternal serum after implantation has taken place, approximately 8–11 days after conception.

EXAM TIP

The decidua produces steroids and proteins that are related to the maintenance and protection of the pregnancy from immunologic rejection.

TABLE 3-1.   Embryology

Week	Preembryonic Period
1	Fertilization and start of implantation.
2	Formation of yolk sac and embryonic disk.
3	First missed menstrual period; formation of primitive streak and neural groove.

Embryonic Period

4	Primitive heartbeat; crown-rump length (CRL) approximately 4.0 mm.
5	Hand and foot plates develop.
6	Hand plates develop digital rays; upper lip, nose, and external ear formed.
7	Umbilical herniation (intestines begin growth outside abdominal cavity).
8	Human appearance; tail has disappeared; CRL approximately 30 mm.

Previable Fetal Period

9	Eyes closing or closed.
10	Intestines in abdomen; thyroid, pancreas, and gallbladder development.
11	Fetal kidneys begin excreting urine into amniotic fluid; fetal liver begins to function; baby teeth formed in sockets.
12	Sex distinguishable externally; fetal breathing movements begin; colonic rotation; fetus active; first trimester ends.
14	Head and neck take an erect, straight-line alignment.
16	↑ fetal activity; ultrasound can determine sex; myelination of nerves and ossification of bones begin.
18	Egg cells, ovaries, and uterus develop in females.
20	Head and body (lanugo) visible; testes begin descent in males.
22	Fetus can hear, will reflexively move in response to loud noise.

Viable Fetal Period

24	Fetal lungs develop alveoli and secrete surfactant, fetus generally capable of breathing air by week 27.
28	Third trimester begins; eyelids unfuse; muscle tone ↑.
30	Cerebral gyri and sulci, which began to form in week 26, are now prominent and begin accelerated formation.
32	Fetal immune system functioning and capable of responding to mild infections.
34	Vernix thickens.
36	Fetus capable of sucking; meconium present in fetal intestines.
40	Due date.

POSTIMPLANTATION

- The endometrium, or lining of the uterus, during pregnancy is termed *decidua*.
- Maternal RBCs may be seen in the trophoblastic lacunae in the second week postconception.

THE PLACENTA

The placenta continues to adapt over the second and third trimesters. It is the primary producer of steroid hormones after 7 weeks' gestation. The human placenta is **hemochorionic**; transfer of materials between mother and fetus is via maternal blood coming in contact with placental villi. There is no direct mixing of maternal and fetal blood.

Reproductive Tract

UTERUS

- The uterus is a thin-walled, muscular structure that is capable of expanding to hold the fetus, placenta, and amniotic fluid.
- Enlargement of the uterus is due to hypertrophy and hyperplasia of the myometrial smooth muscle.
- Early in pregnancy, this process is primarily stimulated by estrogen. As pregnancy progresses, ↑ in uterine size is due to mechanical distention.
- Throughout the pregnancy, the myometrial muscle cells will spontaneously contract.
  - These contractions, also known as Braxton Hicks contractions, are spontaneous and irregular with an intensity ranging from 5 to 25 mm Hg.
  - They may ↑ in frequency during the last month of pregnancy.
- Perfusion of the placenta depends on uterine blood flow, which comes from uterine and ovarian arteries.
- Blood flow ↑ as a result of vasodilation from the effects of estradiol and progesterone.
- Blood vessels lie between the various layers of uterine muscle. These muscle cells contract after delivery thereby constricting the blood vessels.

CERVIX

- The cervix is composed of smooth muscle and connective tissue. ↓ amount of collagen and accumulation of water cause the cervix to soften and become cyanotic.
- Other changes include ↑ in vascularity of the entire cervix and hypertrophy and hyperplasia of the glands.
- ↑ in gland activity leads to the formation of a mucous plug.
  - The mucous plug is composed of immunoglobulins and cytokines, which act as a barrier to bacteria.
  - Cervical effacement causes expulsion of the mucous plug as the cervical canal shortens in labor.

VAGINA

The vagina also undergoes changes during pregnancy in preparation for labor/delivery.

- The tissue becomes more vascular leading to a purplish tinge—Chadwick's sign.
- The vaginal walls prepare for distention by increasing the thickness of the mucosa, loosening of the connective tissue, and hypertrophy of smooth muscle cells.
- The vaginal secretions become thicker with a white color due to influence of progesterone. Additionally, the secretions are more acidic in nature as a result of ↑ *Lactobacillus acidophilus*. This inhibits growth of most pathogens and favors growth of yeasts.

SKIN

The skin undergoes changes in pigmentation and vascularity as a result of pregnancy.
- The ↑ in pigmentation is due to melanocyte-stimulating hormone, estrogen, and progesterone.
  - Linea nigra: Dark line/discoloration of the abdomen that runs from umbilicus to pubis.
  - Darkening of the nipple and areola.
  - Facial chloasma/melasma: Light to dark brown hyperpigmentation in exposed areas (face or neck).
- High levels of estrogen cause vascular spiders and palmar erythema.
- Certain dermatologic conditions are unique to pregnancy. See Table 3-2.

BREASTS

- Breasts may ↑ in size and become painful.
- After a few months of pregnancy, the breast may express a thick, yellow fluid called colostrum.

WATER METABOLISM

- Water retention is a normal part of pregnancy. Often, pitting edema of the ankles and legs is seen in pregnant women, especially at the end of the day. This is due to several factors, including:

WARD TIP

Patients with a normal pre-pregnancy weight are recommended to gain 25–35 lb during pregnancy.

WARD TIP

Though there are some increased caloric needs, pregnancy does not mean "eating for two."

EXAM TIP

If pre-pregnancy body mass index (BMI) is <19, weight gain should be 28–40 lb, while those with a BMI > 25 should gain 15–25 lb during the pregnancy. If the BMI is >30, the weight gain should be 11–20 lb.

TABLE 3-2.   Pruritic Dermatologic Disorders Unique to Pregnancy

DISEASE	ONSET	PRURITUS	LESIONS	DISTRIBUTION	INCIDENCE	↑ INCIDENCE FETAL MORBIDITY/MORTALITY	INTERVENTION
Pruritic urticarial papules and plaques of pregnancy (PUPPP) (polymorphic eruption of pregnancy)	T2–T3	Severe	Erythematous urticarial papules and plaques	Abdomen, thighs, buttocks, occasionally arms and legs	Common (1:160–1:300)	No	Topical steroids, antipruritic drugs (hydroxyzine, diphenhydramine, calamine lotion
Intrahepatic cholestasis of pregnancy (bile not properly excreted from the liver)	T3	Severe	Excoriations common	Generalized, palms, soles	Common (1–2%)	Stillbirth	Check serum bile acids, liver function tests, antipruritics, ursodeoxycholic acid, fetal testing

The placental hormone human placental lactogen (HPL) is thought to contribute to development of GDM because it causes insulin resistance.

The optimal time to screen for gestational diabetes (GDM) is at 26–28 weeks' gestation. This is when HPL levels peak. NOTE: Patients at high risk (h/o GDM, strong family history, BMI > 30) for GDM should also be screened at new obstetrics (OB) visit.

Normal pregnancy state is:
- Hyperlipemic
- Glycosuric
- Anabolic

Maternal blood volume ↑ more if having twins or higher order gestations, as compared to singleton.

If a mother has beta-thalassemia trait/disease or sickle cell trait/disease, test the father to determine the risk of inheritance for the fetus.

- ↑ venous pressure in the lower extremities due to compression of the vena cava and pelvic veins by the gravid uterus.
- ↓ in interstitial colloid osmotic pressure.
- ↑ hydration of connective tissue leading to laxity and swelling of connective tissue and joints that mainly occur in third trimester.

CARBOHYDRATE METABOLISM

- **First 20 weeks:**
  - Insulin sensitivity ↑ in first half of pregnancy.
  - Lower fasting glucose levels allow for glycogen synthesis and fat deposition.
- **After 20 weeks:**
  - Insulin resistance develops and plasma insulin levels rise.
  - Higher levels of both insulin and glucose stimulate utilization of glucose and lipids for energy.
  - As a result, pregnant women will have mild fasting hypoglycemia, postprandial hyperglycemia, and hyperinsulinemia.

Hematologic Changes

 A 29-year-old G3P2103 patient delivers a 7-lb 6-oz baby girl at 38³ᐟ⁷ weeks. The estimated blood loss for the delivery was 950 mL. Vitals remain within normal limits while her hemoglobin ↓ from 12 g/dL to 10 g/dL. What is the explanation for the patient's response to the large blood loss?

Answer: The patient remained hemodynamically stable despite a large blood loss due to the normal ↑ in blood volume that takes place in the second trimester. The ↑ in blood volume buffers the anticipated blood loss at the time of delivery.

BLOOD VOLUME

- Maternal blood volume ↑ during pregnancy by 50%. ↑ blood volume is needed to:
  - Meet the demands of the enlarged uterus.
  - Protect the mother and the fetus against impaired venous return.
  - Protect the mother from blood loss at the time of delivery.
- Expanded volume is composed of plasma and erythrocytes but proportionately more plasma. ↑ erythrocyte production is reflected by ↑ reticulocyte count.
- Both hemoglobin and hematocrit ↓ slightly.
  - Hemoglobin averages 12.5 g/dL.
  - Levels below 11.0 g/dL, especially late in pregnancy, should be considered abnormal.

IRON

- Iron requirements ↑ in pregnancy to about 1000 mg/day.
- Most of the iron is used for hematopoiesis, especially in the last half of pregnancy.
- The amount of iron from the diet is insufficient to meet the needs of the pregnancy, so many patients will need to take supplemental iron. The most common side effect of this supplementation is constipation.

TABLE 3-3 **Coagulation Cascade Changes in Pregnancy**

FACTORS THAT INCREASE	FACTORS THAT DECREASE
Fibrinogen	Protein S
Protein C resistance	Platelet count (decreases slightly)
Factors II, VII, VIII, X, XII, XIII	
von Willebrand factor	

IMMUNOLOGY

- During pregnancy, humoral and cell-mediated immunological functions are suppressed. During T3:
  - ↑ granulocytes, ↑ CD8 T lymphocytes.
  - ↓ in CD4 T lymphocytes, ↓ monocytes.
- The leukocyte count varies during normal pregnancy. Usually, it ranges from 5000/μL to 12,000/μL. During labor, counts can rise up to 25,000/μL; however, it averages 14,000–16,000/μL.
- Markers of inflammatory states such as leukocyte alkaline phosphatase, C-reactive protein, and erythrocyte sedimentation rate (ESR) also rise physiologically.

EXAM TIP

Physiologic anemia of pregnancy develops due to greater expansion of intravascular volume than red blood cell (RBC) increase.

COAGULATION

A 36-year-old G3P2002 patient at 32 weeks' gestation presents with a sudden onset of shortness of breath, dyspnea, and palpitations that has been ongoing for 1 hour and is now worsening. She reports no sick contacts, cough, fever, or leg swelling. She has no medical conditions and has a negative family history. On exam, she is afebrile, pulse is 120, respirations 25, and BP 120/80. She appears to be in distress. There are absent breath sounds on the right side. Her legs show 1+ pitting edema bilaterally. Fetal heart rate is reassuring. Pulse oximetry is 75% on room air. What is the most likely diagnosis?

Answer: Pulmonary embolus (PE). Estrogen causes an ↑ in clotting factors, resulting in a hypercoagulable state in pregnancy. Pregnant patients are at ↑ risk for PE and deep venous thrombosis (DVT) during the pregnancy and immediately after delivery.

Cardiovascular System

- Changes in cardiac function begin in the first 8 weeks of pregnancy (see Table 3-4).
- Cardiac output (CO) is ↑ as early as the fifth week of pregnancy due to:
  - ↓ systemic vascular resistance (SVR).
  - ↑ heart rate (HR).

EXAM TIP

↑ CO = ↓ SVR + ↑ HR.

WARD TIP

Patients with hypertensive heart disease may develop progressive or sudden deterioration in pregnancy.

Respiratory System

- As a result of the expanding uterus, diaphragm rises about 4 cm, the subcostal angle widens, and thoracic circumference ↑ about 6 cm.

TABLE 3-4. Cardiac Changes in Pregnancy

PHYSIOLOGY CHANGES	NORMAL EXAM CHANGES
Heart rate increases.	Heart is displaced to left and upward.
Stroke volume increases.	Systolic ejection murmur present.
Systemic venous resistance goes WAY down.	Blood pressure nadirs at 20–24 weeks, then increases until term.
Cardiac output goes up.	

TABLE 3-5. Respiratory Physiology in Pregnancy

PARAMETER	DEFINITION	PREGNANCY-RELATED CHANGE
Tidal volume	Normal **volume** of air displaced between normal inhalation and exhalation	Increases
Minute ventilation	The **volume** of gas inhaled (inhaled **minute volume**) or exhaled (exhaled **minute volume**) from a person's lungs per **minute**.	Increases
Functional residual capacity	Volume of air present in the **lungs** at the end of passive expiration	Decreases

Normal acid-base status in pregnancy = Compensated respiratory alkalosis (more CO_2 blown off).

- Respiratory rate unchanged (see Table 3-5).
- Normal acid-base status in pregnancy is **respiratory alkalosis** due to more CO_2 being blown off; pH = 7.45.

Urinary System

 A 31-year-old G1P0 patient at 24 weeks presents for a routine prenatal visit. She has no concerns. However, urinalysis showed large nitrites, large leukocytes, and small blood. What is the next step?

Answer: The patient should be empirically treated for asymptomatic bacteriuria. The antibiotics can be modified once the urine culture results are available. Due to the changes caused by progesterone, pregnant women are at ↑ risk for developing asymptomatic bacteriuria, and urinary tract infections (UTIs) can progress to pyelonephritis if left untreated. Pyelonephritis in pregnant women can lead to sepsis, respiratory failure, and fetal death; it is the most common non-obstetric cause for hospitalization in pregnancy, so prevention is key.

In pregnancy, the higher rate of renal clearance leads to reduced effective dose of antibiotics, anti-epiletic medications, and other medications that are renally cleared.

KIDNEYS

- ↑ glomerular filtration rate, creatinine clearance, and renal plasma flow.
- ↓ serum creatinine, blood urea nitrogen.
- Renal tubules lose some of their resorptive capacity: Amino acids, uric acid, and glucose are not completely absorbed. Sodium is retained in higher levels in the pregnant female.

URETERS

- Dilate due to compression from uterus at the pelvic brim and the effect of progesterone.
- Dilation R > L due to the dextroversion of the uterus.
- Dilated ureters cause ↑ glomerular size and ↑ fluid flow → enlarged kidneys.
- Decreased ureteral peristalsis and increased ureteral compression cause urinary stasis which can lead to asymptomatic bacteriuria and pyelonephritis.

BLADDER

- ↓ tone, ↑ capacity progressively during pregnancy.
- ↑ urinary frequency is due to bladder compression by an enlarged uterus.
- Stress incontinence develops as a result of relaxation of bladder supports.

Gastrointestinal Tract

- The stomach, appendix, and intestines are displaced upward by the enlarging uterus.
- Effects of progesterone:
    - ↓ lower esophageal sphincter tone → heartburn.
    - ↓ bowel peristalsis → constipation.
- **Hemorrhoids**, common in pregnancy, are caused by constipation and elevated pressure in veins below the level of the uterus.

LIVER

- **Alkaline phosphatase** activity in serum almost doubles during pregnancy. Serum aspartate transaminase, alanine transaminase, γ-glutamyl transferase, and bilirubin levels are slightly lower.
- Serum albumin ↓, but total albumin ↑ because of a greater volume of distribution.

GALLBLADDER

Contractility of the gallbladder is reduced, leading to an increased residual volume and cholestasis.
- Progesterone impairs gallbladder contraction by inhibiting cholecystokinin-mediated smooth muscle stimulation.
- Estrogen inhibits intraductal transport of bile acids, also contributing to cholestasis.

Endocrine System

PITUITARY GLAND

The pituitary gland ↑ in size and weight during pregnancy.

WARD TIP

Treat asymptomatic bacteriuria in pregnancy.

WARD TIP

Right hydronephrosis is a normal finding in pregnancy.

WARD TIP

Pain from appendicitis may occur much higher in the abdomen because the gravid uterus pushes the appendix up.

WARD TIP

Alkaline phosphatase is usually elevated in pregnancy because it is also made by the placenta.

EXAM TIP

Cholestasis with increased lipids and cholesterol leads to higher incidence of gallstones, cholecystitis, and biliary obstruction in pregnancy.

WARD TIP

Pitocin is a synthetic oxytocin. It is used to start or enhance labor.

Prolactin

- Main function is to ensure milk **production**.
- Levels ↑ throughout pregnancy due to estradiol.

Oxytocin

- Responsible for lactation, especially milk **letdown**.
- ↑ throughout the pregnancy.
- Released by nipple stimulation and infant crying.
- Causes uterine contractions.

THYROID GLAND

- Total thyroxine levels and thyroxine-binding globulin ↑ in response to high estrogen levels. However, *free* thyroxine remains normal and the mother remains euthyroid.
- Thyroid-stimulating hormone (TSH) is a sensitive marker for thyroid disease.
- The gland does not ↑ in size; therefore, all goiters need to be investigated.

PARATHYROID GLAND

- In the mother, parathyroid hormone ↓ in first trimester but then rises progressively during the remainder of the pregnancy. Estrogens block the action of parathyroid hormone on bone resorption, resulting in ↑ hormone levels, which allow the fetus to have adequate calcium supply.
- The fetus has ↑ calcitonin levels allowing for bone deposition.

CHAPTER 4

Antepartum

This chapter focuses on the care provided for the pregnant patient prior to delivery. The prenatal (or antepartum) course often influences the outcome of the pregnancy. During this time, patients are encouraged to maintain healthy practices and abstain from practices that are harmful for the pregnancy. Regular visits at specific intervals are used to screen patients and fetus for abnormal medical conditions that may develop.

Prenatal Care

The goal of prenatal care is as follows:
1. Determine the health status of mother and fetus.
2. Determine gestational age (GA).
3. Initiate plan for obstetrical care (routine versus high risk).
4. Lower the maternal/perinatal morbidity/mortality.
5. Enhance pregnancy, childbirth experience for patient/family.

DEFINITIONS

- **GA:** The time of pregnancy counting from the first day of the last menstrual period (LMP).
- **Developmental age:** The time of pregnancy counting from fertilization (rarely used term).
- **First trimester:** 0–12 weeks.
- **Second trimester:** 13–27 weeks.
- **Third trimester:** 28 weeks–birth.
- **Embryo:** Fertilization–8 weeks.
- **Fetus:** 9 weeks–birth.
- **Previable:** <22 weeks.
- **Periviable:** 22–24 weeks.
- **Preterm:** 20–36 weeks.
- **Term:** 37–42 weeks.

TERMINOLOGY OF REPRODUCTIVE HISTORY

The mother's pregnancy history is described in terms of gravidity (G) and parity (P).

- **Gravidity** is the total number of pregnancies, regardless of the outcome.
- **Parity** is the number of pregnancies that have reached a GA of ≥20 weeks. It can be further subdivided into term births, preterm births, abortions, and living children.
- A patient that is gravida 3, para 1201 (G3P1201) has been pregnant three times, has had one term birth, two preterm births, no abortions, and has one live child.

FREQUENCY OF OBSTETRIC VISITS

- <28 weeks: Every 4–6 weeks
- 28–36 weeks: Every 2–3 weeks
- 36–41 weeks: Once per week
- 41–42 weeks: Twice per week for fetal testing/plan for delivery
- See Table 4-1.

WARD TIP

Gravidity: The number of times a patient has been pregnant.
Parity: The number of times a patient has had a pregnancy that led to a birth after 20 weeks' gestation.

EXAM TIP

Parity: **FPAL** (Remember "Florida Power and Light")
Full term
Preterm
Abortuses (any loss before 20 weeks)
Living Children

TABLE 4-1. Prenatal Visits

First Visit	11–13 Weeks	16–20 Weeks	26–28 Weeks

1. History and physical (H&P)
2. Labs:
  ▪ Hct/Hgb
  ▪ Rh factor
  ▪ Blood type
  ▪ Antibody screen
  ▪ Pap smear
  ▪ *Gonorrhea* and *Chlamydia* cultures
  ▪ Urine analysis (protein, glucose, ketones)
  ▪ Urine culture
  ▪ Infection screen: Rubella, syphilis, hepatitis B, human immunodeficiency virus (HIV), tuberculosis (TB)
  ▪ Cystic fibrosis screen
  ▪ Hemoglobin electrophoresis (as needed)
3. Discuss plan for genetic testing.
	1. H&P
	2. Fetal exam:
	  ▪ Fetal heart tones
	3. Urine dip: Protein, glucose, leukocytes
	4. FTS or cfDNA
		1. H&P
		2. Fetal exam:
		  ▪ Fetal heart
		  ▪ Fundal height
		3. Urine dip: Protein, glucose, leukocytes
		4. Fetal ultrasound: Anatomy, dating
		5. Quad screen (if FTS or cfDNA not selected)
		6. Genetic amniocentesis (if indicated)
			1. H&P
			2. Fetal exam:
			  ▪ Fetal heart
			  ▪ Fundal height
			3. Labs:
			  ▪ Complete blood count
			  ▪ Ab screen (if Rh neg)
			  ▪ Diabetes screen
			  ▪ Urine dip: Protein, glucose, leukocytes
			4. Give anti D immunoglobulin if indicated (28 weeks)

Week 32	Week 36	Week 38	Week 39	Week 40

1. H&P
2. Fetal exam:
  ▪ Fetal heart
  ▪ Fundal height
3. Urine dip: protein, glucose, leukocytes
	1. H&P
	2. Fetal exam:
	  ▪ Fetal heart
	  ▪ Fundal height
	  ▪ Fetal presentation
	3. Urine dip: Protein, glucose, leukocytes
	4. Group B strep culture
	5. STD panel including HIV—required in some states
		1. H&P
		2. Fetal exam:
		  ▪ Fetal heart
		  ▪ Fundal height
		  ▪ Fetal presentation
		3. Urine dip: Protein, glucose, leukocytes
		4. Cervical exam (frequency is controversial)
			1. H&P
			2. Fetal exam:
			  ▪ Fetal heart
			  ▪ Fundal height
			  ▪ Fetal presentation
			3. Urine dip: Protein, glucose, leukocytes
				1. H&P
				2. Fetal exam:
				  ▪ Fetal heart
				  ▪ Fundal height
				  ▪ Fetal presentation
				3. Urine dip: Protein, glucose, leukocytes

FIRST VISIT

History

- Biographical: Age, ancestry, occupation, marital status.
- Obstetrical: Gravidity, parity, prior labor/deliveries (vaginal, cesareans), complications, infant status, birth weight.
- Menstrual: LMP, menstrual irregularities.
- Contraceptive use: What type and when was it last used?
- Medical: Asthma, diabetes, hypertension, thyroid disease, cardiac disease, seizures, rubella, previous surgeries, sexually transmitted infections, allergies, medications, smoking, alcohol, recreational drugs.
- Family history: Multiple gestations, diabetes, hypertension, bleeding disorders, congenital cardiac anomalies, developmental delay, genetic conditions, anesthetic problems.
- Helpful to get family and social history from the partner.

EXAM TIP

Remember that alcohol use has the highest correlation with congenital abnormalities.

Physical Exam

- Vitals: Blood pressure (BP), weight, height, temperature, heart rate.
- Head, neck, heart, lungs, back.
- Pelvic:
  - External genitalia: Bartholin's gland, condyloma, herpes, other lesions.
  - Vagina: Discharge, inflammation.
  - Cervix: Polyps, growths.
  - Uterus: Masses, irregularities, size compared to GA.
  - Adnexa: Masses.

SUBSEQUENT VISITS

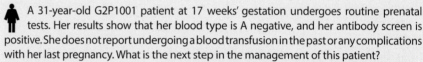

A 31-year-old G2P1001 patient at 17 weeks' gestation undergoes routine prenatal tests. Her results show that her blood type is A negative, and her antibody screen is positive. She does not report undergoing a blood transfusion in the past or any complications with her last pregnancy. What is the next step in the management of this patient?

Answer: The next step is to identify the antibody. There are many types of antibodies, and in a patient that is Rh negative, it should not be assumed that she has Rh antibodies.

History

As the patient progresses through pregnancy, some questions are asked at each visit (Table 4-2).

Physical Exam

After thorough initial exam, each subsequent exam must record four findings:
- BP
- Urine dip for protein, glucose, leukocytes
- Fundal height
- Fetal heart rate (FHR)

Routine Timed Tests

Certain prenatal tests should occur at specific times during pregnancy (see Table 4-1).

GENETIC SCREENING FOR ANEUPLOIDY

All patients should be offered aneuploidy screening. However, prior to ordering, they should be counseled on what the test is looking for / why it is being obtained. Also, all of the tests below are screening tests, and diagnosis should be confirmed with amniocentesis or chorionic villus sampling (CVS).

TABLE 4-2. Prenatal Visit Questions

Ask About at Each Visit:	Ask if Has preX or Risk Factors for preX	Ask if Not Established in Third Trimester
Fetal movement (>20 weeks)	Headache	Feeding plan (breast/bottle)
Vaginal bleeding	Vision changes	Contraception plan
Leakage of fluid	Nausea/vomiting	Desire for circumcision if male fetus
Contractions/cramping	RUQ pain	
New questions or concerns		Intrapartum anesthesia plan

- First-trimester options:
    - Cell-free DNA (cfDNA)—blood test
        - Screens for Down syndrome, trisomy 13, trisomy 18, and sex chromosome aneuploidy.
        - Sequencing of cell-free (actually placental) DNA in the maternal circulation.
        - In low risk patients, the positive predictive value of this test is about 50% for T13 and T18.
    - First-trimester screen (FTS)—blood test and ultrasound (US)
        - Screens for Down syndrome, trisomy 13, and trisomy 18.
        - Includes: Fetal nuchal translucency (NT) measured via US and maternal serum pregnancy-associated plasma protein A (PAPP-A) and free β-human chorionic gonadotropin (β-hCG).
        - In Down syndrome, the NT is ↑, PAPP-A ↓, free β-hCG ↑.
- Second-trimester screening options:
    - Quad screen (range 15–21 weeks).
        - Screens for Down syndrome, trisomy 13, and trisomy 18.
        - Includes: Unconjugated estriol (uE3), α-fetoprotein, β-hCG, inhibin A.
    - US for anatomy (18–20 weeks)
        - Screens for Down syndrome, trisomy 13, trisomy 18, and other congenital anomalies.
        - RECOMMENDED in all pregnancies.

FUNDAL HEIGHT

As the fetus grows, the leading edge of the uterus or the fundus grows superiorly in the abdomen, toward the maternal head. Fundal height (in centimeters) roughly corresponds to GA (in weeks). It is measured from the pubic symphysis to the top of the fundus:

- Uterus at level of pubic symphysis: 12 weeks
- Uterus between pubic symphysis and umbilicus: 16 weeks
- Uterus at the level of umbilicus: 20 weeks
- Uterine height correlates to weeks' gestation: 20–36 weeks

Fundal height (cm) should correlate to GA (weeks) ±2. If not, consider inaccurate dating (most common), fibroids, maternal habitus, multiple gestations, or possible growth aberrations. Beyond approximately 36 weeks' gestation, the fundal height may not correspond to the GA due to the fetal descent into the pelvis.

Fetal Surveillance

When a patient is diagnosed with a medical condition that increases the risk of intrauterine fetal demise (IUFD), or when the fetus is diagnosed with a condition that increases the risk of IUFD, several tests can be used to monitor the status of the fetus. They include non-stress test (NST), biophysical profile (BPP), the modified BPP (mBPP), and Doppler ultrasonography. In general, these are started in T3, but may be done earlier. These tests assess for chronic uteroplacental insufficiency and cannot predict acute events. The choice and frequency of testing depend on indication, GA, medical condition, and experience of the practitioner. The higher the risk of stillbirth, the more frequent the testing should occur.

FETAL MOVEMENT COUNTS

Fetal movement counts, or kick counts, may be performed at home by the patient in order to monitor the fetal status. The patient should select a time at which the

WARD TIP

When "size not equal to dates" is identified, order an US to better assess fetal growth.

WARD TIP

Intrauterine fetal demise (IUFD) is a medical term, stillbirth is a "lay term."

WARD TIP

Intrauterine growth restriction (IUGR) can be used synonymously with fetal growth restriction (FGR).

fetus usually is active, usually after a meal or at night before bed. The level of activity differs for each baby, and most have sleep cycles of 20–40 minutes.

There are several ways to assess fetal movements:
- Ask the patient to record daily how long it takes the fetus to make 10 movements. For most, this is usually achieved in about 2 hour.
- Alternatively, ask the patient to record the number of fetal movements in 1 hour three times per week.
- While doing kick counts, the patient should be in a quiet place and focused on the fetus (not multi-tasking).
- For both of these strategies, a physician should be contacted if there is a change from the normal pattern or number of movements recorded.

NON-STRESS TEST (NST)

- The NST evaluates four components of the FHR tracing:
- Baseline: Normal is 110–160 beats/min.
- Variability: Beat-to-beat variation of the FHR. Presence of variability reflects an intact and mature brain stem and heart (see Table 4-3).
- Decelerations:
  - Early deceleration: Vagally mediated, caused by head compression usually at cervical dilation of 4–7 cm.
  - Variable deceleration: Caused by cord compression.
  - Late deceleration: Reflects uteroplacental insufficiency.

TABLE 4-3. Variability

	ABSENT	MINIMAL	MODERATE	MARKED
Beat-to-beat variation	0 (like an EKG flatline)	≤5 bpm	>5 bmp to <25 bmp	>25 bmp
Causes	Fetal metabolic acidosis, congenital anomalies,	Fetal metabolic acidosis, central nervous system (CNS) depressants, fetal sleep cycles, congenital anomalies, prematurity, preexisting neurologic abnormality	ABSENCE of acidaemia	Normal variant, exaggerated autonomic response to poor oxygenation
Example				

bpm, beats per minute

- Acceleration: At least two accelerations of at least 15 beats/min above baseline for 15 seconds in a 20-minute period. Presence of accelerations = fetal well-being. Reactive NST = two or more accelerations over 20 minutes.
    - Uterine contractions are also recorded to help interpret the NST.
- Preterm fetuses are frequently nonreactive:
    - 24–28 weeks: Up to 50% nonreactive.
    - 28–32 weeks: 15% nonreactive.
- An NST usually takes 20 minutes to complete. If the NST is nonreactive, the baby may be asleep. If this is suspected, ask the patient to eat or drink to make the baby active; if not reactive within 1–2 hours, then additional testing may need to be performed.

CONTRACTION STRESS TEST (CST)

The CST assesses how the fetus reacts to uterine contractions by looking for changes in the FHT related to contractions. The CST is usually an inpatient procedure because CST requires uterine stimulation, usually with pitocin or nipple stimulation. They are potentially risky since contractions are induced and may lead to fetal distress. Clinically, because a cesarean section after labor is associated with increased morbidity, a CST maybe used when there is concern for placental insufficiency (i.e., the fetus will not tolerate labor). Some examples might be a very growth restricted fetus or a term patient who had late decelerations on an NST done for a chronic condition.

During a CST, the FHR and the contractions are recorded simultaneously. During a contraction, the blood flow to the placenta briefly ↓. A well-oxygenated fetus can compensate, and there are no decelerations in the FHR. If the fetus is already compromised with low levels of oxygen, the contraction may cause a late deceleration in FHR, which reflects uteroplacental insufficiency and thus, hypoxemia in the fetus.

- Patient is placed in lateral recumbent position and contractions are stimulated.
    - Administration of oxytocin (pitocin).
    - Nipple stimulation (2-minute self-stimulation through clothes every 5 minutes).
- Adequate contractions:
    - Occur three times in 10 minutes.
    - Last at least 40 seconds.
- Interpreted as the presence or absence of late decelerations:
    - **Negative:** No late or significant variable decelerations.
    - **Positive:** Late decelerations following 50% or more of contractions.
    - **Equivocal:** Intermittent late decelerations or significant variable decelerations.
    - **Unsatisfactory:** Fewer than three contractions in 10 minutes.
- Contraindications:
    - History of extensive uterine surgery or previous cesarean delivery.
    - Known placenta previa.

EXAM TIP

A reactive NST has two or more accelerations over 20 minutes.

ULTRASOUND (US)

Routinely, in a low-risk pregnancy, a patient should have two USs. One early in the pregnancy (first trimester) to estimate GA and confirm viability, and a second US at 18–20 weeks to assess fetal anatomy. Figures 4-1 to 4-4 show common images obtained in an anatomy US.

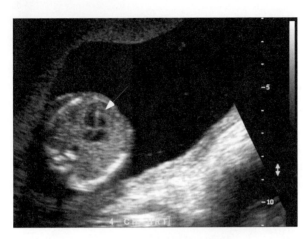

FIGURE 4-1.   Normal four-chamber heart.

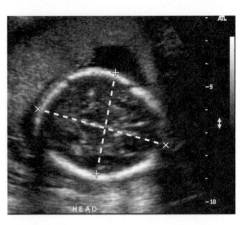

FIGURE 4-2.   Measurement of biparietal diameter.

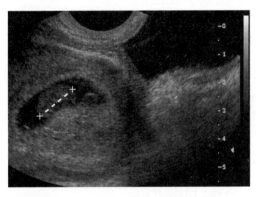

FIGURE 4-3.   Measurement of crown-rump length.

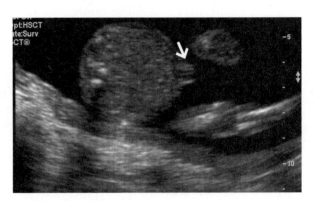

FIGURE 4-4.   Umbilical cord insertion.

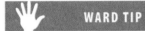

WARD TIP

When can a baby's heartbeat be detected with Doppler?
- 10–12 weeks of gestation.
- Fetal heart starts beating at 22–24 days.

In high risk or complicated pregnancies, more USs can be performed to monitor fetal growth in the late second and third trimesters, measure the maternal cervical length (16–22 weeks), assess amniotic fluid volume, check placenta location, and assess fetal presentation. US can also be used to measure blood flow in the umbilical artery for fetuses that are growth restricted or to assess for fetal anemia. In rare cases, US is used to guide diagnostic procedures during pregnancy such as CVS, amniocentesis, or intrauterine transfusion (Figures 4-5 to 4-7).

BIOPHYSICAL PROFILE (BPP)

- A BPP is the combination of the NST and an US exam, for a total of five components:
  1. NST: Appropriate variation of FHR with a reactive NST.
  2. Breathing: ≥1 episode of rhythmic breathing movements of 30 seconds or more within 30 minutes.
  3. Movement: ≥3 discrete body or limb movements within 30 minutes.
  4. Muscle tone: ≥1 episode of extension with return to flexion or opening/closing of a hand.
  5. Determination of amniotic fluid volume: Single vertical pocket of amniotic fluid measuring ≥2 cm is considered adequate* [or an amniotic fluid index (AFI) >5 cm].

*In the presence of oligohydramnios (largest pocket of amniotic fluid ≤2 cm), further investigation is required.

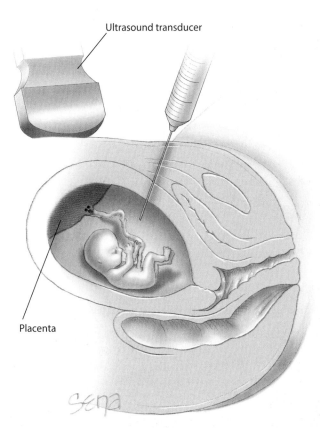

FIGURE 4-5. Amniocentesis. (Reproduced, with permission, from Cunningham FG, Leveno KJ, Bloom SL, et al. *Williams Obstetrics.* 23rd ed. New York: McGraw-Hill; 2010:299.)

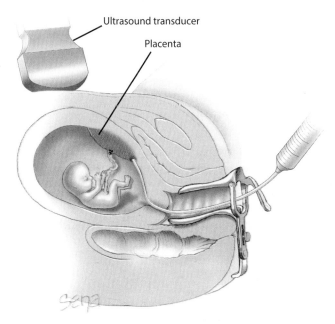

FIGURE 4-6. Transcervical CVS. (Reproduced, with permission, from Cunningham FG, Leveno KJ, Bloom SL, et al. *Williams Obstetrics.* 23rd ed. New York: McGraw-Hill; 2010:300.)

- Each category is given a score of 0 or 2 points:
    - 0: Abnormal, absent, or insufficient.
    - 2: Normal and present as previously defined.
    - Total possible score is 10 points.
    - Normal score: 8–10.
    - Equivocal: 6.
    - Abnormal: ≤4.

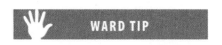

WARD TIP

mBPP = NST + AFI

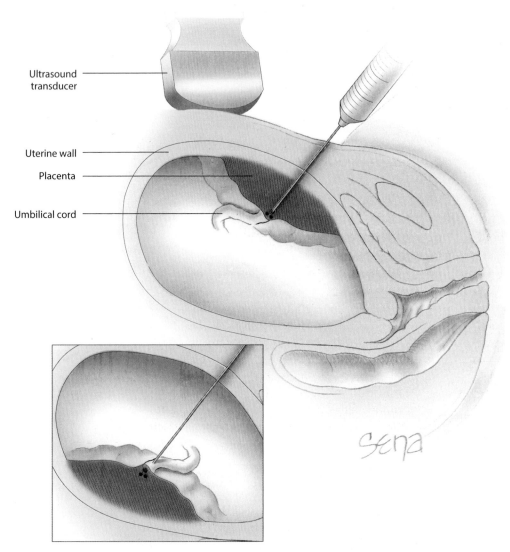

Ultrasound transducer

Uterine wall

Placenta

Umbilical cord

FIGURE 4-7. **Cordocentesis also known percutaneous umbilical blood sampling.** (Reproduced, with permission, from Cunningham FG, Leveno KJ, Bloom SL, et al. *Williams Obstetrics.* 23rd ed. New York: McGraw-Hill; 2010:301.)

MODIFIED BIOPHYSICAL PROFILE (mBPP)

- An mBPP includes two components: an NST and an AFI.
- Normal amniotic fluid volume varies and ↑ with GA. The peak volume is 800–1000 mL at 36–37 weeks' gestation. In the late T2 or T3, amniotic fluid volume represents fetal urine output. If there is uteroplacental insufficiency and ↓ oxygenation to the fetus, the fetus preferentially shunts blood to the brain and heart, leaving the fetal kidneys underperfused. This results in ↓ fetal urine output and, as a result, ↓ amniotic fluid. Therefore, the AFI is used as a measure of chronic uteroplacental function.
- The AFI is the sum of amniotic fluid measured in four quadrants of the uterus via the US (upper right, upper left, lower right and lower left).
  - AFI 6–24 cm: Normal. Median AFI is 8–18 between weeks 20 and 35, after which values ↓.
  - AFI ≤5 cm: Abnormal (oligohydramnios).
  - AFI ≥25 cm: Abnormal (polyhydramnios).
- **Oligohydramnios:**
  - Most common cause: ruptured membranes.

- May be associated with uteroplacental insufficiency and can see concurrent intrauterine growth restriction (IUGR) 60% of the time.
- Evaluate for genitourinary malformations or other fetal anomalies.
- **Polyhydramnios:**
  - Many causes, including:
    - Fetal malformation (anencephaly, esophageal or intestinal atresia).
    - Genetic disorders.
    - Maternal diabetes.
    - Multiple gestation.
    - Fetal anemia.
    - Viruses.
  - Associated with uterine overdistention, resulting in:
    - Preterm labor.
    - PROM.
    - Fetal malposition.
    - Uterine atony.

WARD TIP

Most common cause of oligohydramnios = rupture of membranes.

Screening for Congenital Anomalies

Screening for fetal abnormalities can include testing during the first and second trimesters, and the tests can be noninvasive. Commonly used techniques are maternal serum screens and US. Diagnostic testing is invasive and includes amniocentesis(amnio) or/and CVS. It is important to understand and to ensure that patients understand that a screening test is NOT diagnostic—it provides a risk estimate, but not a yes/no answer. Screening for aneuploidy should be offered to all patients.

Cell-Free DNA (cfDNA)

- cfDNA is a serum screen performed after 10 weeks. It is a screening test and requires further invasive diagnostic tests if the results are abnormal.
- cfDNA screens for trisomy 21 (Down syndrome), trisomy 18, trisomy 13, and sex chromosome aneuploidies by using next-generation sequencing of cfDNA in the maternal circulation.
- The sensitivity is 98–99% for detection of T21 in a high-risk patient.

EXAM TIP

Down (trisomy 21)
β-hCG ↑
PAPP-A ↓
NT ↑

FIRST-TRIMESTER SCREEN (FTS)

- The FTS is performed between weeks 11 and 13. It is a screening test and may require further diagnostic tests if the results are abnormal.
- The FTS combines a maternal blood screening test with a fetal US evaluation to identify risk for Down syndrome (trisomy 21). It can also detect Edwards syndrome (trisomy 18).
- The results of maternal hormone levels and fetal US, along with the mother's age, are combined to determine risk factors. The following is assessed in the FTS:
  - Maternal serum: Free or total β-hCG, PAPP-A.
  - US at 11–13 weeks' gestation: NT—measurement of fluid under the baby's skin at the level of the neck (see Figure 4-8).
  - In the case of Down syndrome, β-hCG will be ↑ and PAPP-A will be ↓, and the NT will be thick (>0.3 mm).
- The FTS has a sensitivity of 85% for Down syndrome.

EXAM TIP

Fifty percent of fetuses with T21 have a normal US.

EXAM TIP

A targeted US evaluates the fetus for congenital structural abnormalities that may or may not correlate with abnormal serum screening findings.

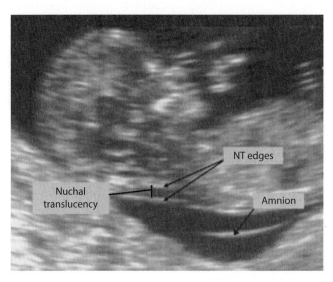

FIGURE 4-8. Nuchal translucency measurement. (Reproduced, with permission, from Cunningham FG, Leveno KJ, Bloom SL, et al. *Williams Obstetrics.* 23rd ed. New York: McGraw-Hill, 2010:351.)

QUAD SCREEN

 A 19-year-old G1P0 patient at 16 weeks' gestation based on an unsure LMP has an ↑ risk for Down syndrome on her second-trimester quad screen. Her blood pressure is within normal limits, urine protein is negative, and fetal heart tones are 148 bpm. The fundus is palpated 2 cm above the umbilicus. What is the most likely cause of the abnormal quad screen? What diagnostic tests can confirm the screening test?

Answer: The most common cause for the abnormal quad screen is incorrect estimation of GA. This patient's fundal height indicates that her pregnancy is further than what her LMP indicates. The next step is to perform an US to confirm the GA of the fetus and recalculate the quad screen. If the quad screen is abnormal with correct dating, the patient should undergo genetic counseling and be offered genetic testing.

The quad screen is a test of maternal serum that evaluates the risk a patient has for delivering a baby with Down syndrome (trisomy 21), Edwards syndrome (trisomy 18), or neural tube defects (NTDs). If the quad screen shows an ↑ risk for any of the screened conditions, further diagnostic tests may be performed to confirm the findings. See Table 4-4 for a summary of quad screen results.

- Ideally performed at 16–18 weeks' gestation (range is 15–21 weeks).
- Sensitivity: 81%.
- Evaluates four maternal serum analytes:
    - Maternal serum α-fetoprotein (MSAFP).
    - Unconjugated estriol (uE3).
    - hCG.
    - Inhibin A.
- Abnormal quad screen → confirm dates (US) and recalculate in needed → if still abnormal → genetic counseling + targeted US if there are abnormal findings on US or if desired by the patient → diagnostic procedure (amniocentesis) → karyotype analysis.
- Most common cause of abnormal quad screen: Incorrect dates, can also be due to twins.

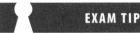

EXAM TIP

Most neural tube defects are thought to be polygenic or multifactorial.

EXAM TIP

If there is high α-fetoprotein at 16 weeks, a neural tube defect is a likely diagnosis. Low α-fetoprotein is associated with certain chromosomal defects (e.g., trisomy 21 or trisomy 18).

TABLE 4-4. Quad Screen Summary

	DOWN (TRISOMY 21)	EDWARDS (TRISOMY 18)	NTD
uE3	↓	↓	Normal
AFP	↓	↓	↑
β-hCG	↑	↓	Normal
Inhibin A	↑	↓	Normal

AFP, α-fetoprotein; β-hCG, β-human chorionic gonadotropin; NTD, neural tube defect; ue3, unconjugated estriol.

TABLE 4-5. AFP-Related Findings

HIGH AFP	LOW AFP
NTD	Chromosomal trisomies: Down syndrome (trisomy 21), Edwards syndrome (trisomy 18)
Abdominal wall defects (gastroschisis and omphalocele)	Molar pregnancy
Underestimation of GA	Overestimation of GA
Placental abruption	High maternal weight
Multiple gestation	Fetal death
Fetal death	

MATERNAL SERUM A-FETOPROTEIN (MSAFP)

- MSAFP is first produced in the yolk sac and then by the fetal gastrointestinal tract and liver.
- Normally, it passes by diffusion through the chorion and amnion. It begins to rise at 13 weeks and peaks at 32 weeks.
- In general, MSAFP levels >2.0–2.5 multiples of the median (MOM) warrant further investigation, as they are suspicious of NTDs. Causes of abnormal MSAFP are in Table 4-5.
- MSAFP screening is most accurate between 16 and 18 weeks. MSAFP can be drawn in isolation for patients who had a cfDNA or FTS or can be part of the quad screen.

GENETIC TESTING

Genetic testing is not required for every pregnancy, but current guidelines recommend offering all pregnant patients genetic testing, regardless of risk status. There are specific circumstances where the risk of a genetic abnormality is particularly high, and where genetic testing should be more strongly recommended.

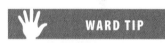

WARD TIP

What can US determine?
- Diagnosis of early pregnancy.
- Determination if fetus is still viable in the setting of vaginal bleeding in early pregnancy.
- Determination of GA and assessment of fetal size.
- Diagnosis of fetal malformation (cleft lip, polydactyly, club foot, fetal sex, NTDs, abdominal wall defects, abdominal renal anomalies).
- Placental localization.
- Polyhydramnios and oligohydramnios.

AMNIOCENTESIS

- Amniocentesis is the most frequently employed technique used to obtain fetal cells. A needle is placed through the maternal abdominal wall and uterus with US guidance (see Figure 4-6). Amniotic fluid is obtained for various purposes. Usually done at 15–20 weeks, but can be done until delivery, even in the setting of IUFD. Usually amniocentesis is done for genetic assessment, but the fluid can also be sent for Gram stain, culture, polymerase chain reaction (PCR) to assess for infection if clinically indicated.
- **Karyotype:** Fetal cells obtained via amniocentesis are cultured and an evaluation of the chromosomes is performed in the following circumstances: Fetal anomaly suspected on US. Abnormal serum genetic screen or family history of congenital abnormalities. Most commonly, if the amnio is normal, the cells will be sent for **microarray** to look for smaller genetic abnormalities. Because live cells are needed to grow out the cells for a karyotype, a microarray can also be helpful in cases of IUFD where living cells are not present.
- **Risks to amniocentesis:**
  - Pain/cramping.
  - Vaginal spotting (resolves spontaneously).
  - Amniotic fluid leakage in <1% of cases.
  - Symptomatic amnionitis in <1 in 1000 patients.
  - **Rate of fetal loss is 1/1000.**

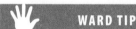

EXAM TIP

Microarray looks for microdeletions.

CHORIONIC VILLUS SAMPLING (CVS)

- CVS is a diagnostic technique in which a small sample of chorionic villi is taken transcervically or transabdominally and analyzed (see Figure 4-7).
- Typically done between 9 and 12 weeks' gestation.
- Information on fetal genetics (karyotype and microarray).
- Biochemical assays or DNA tests can be done earlier than amniocentesis.
- **Complications:** Fetal loss 1/500
  - Preterm delivery.
  - PROM.
  - Fetal injury, especially limb abnormalities if performed before 9 weeks' gestation.

WARD TIP

Advanced maternal age (>35 years at delivery) is the most common indication for prenatal genetic testing.

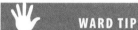

WARD TIP

Chromosomal abnormalities occur in 0.6% of all live births, account for 5% of stillbirths and 50–60% of spontaneous abortions.

Differences Between CVS and Amniocentesis

- **CVS:**
  - Transvaginal or transabdominal aspiration of placental cells in the intrauterine cavity.
  - Done at 9–12 weeks.
  - Evaluates chromosomal abnormalities and genetic disorders.
  - Higher risks (fetal loss has 1/500, limb defects if done <9 weeks), diagnosis accuracy is comparable to amniocentesis.
- **Amniocentesis:**
  - Transabdominal aspiration of amniotic fluid using US-guided needle.
  - Evaluates chromosomal abnormalities and genetic disorders.
  - Done at 15–20 weeks.

WARD TIP

Body Mass Index (BMI)
   BMI ≥30: Obese
   25.0–29.9: Overweight
   18.5–24.9: Normal
   <18.5: Underweight

Nutritional Needs of the Pregnant Patient

Proper nutritional habits are important for every patient; this is especially true for those who are pregnant. ↑ energy needs and specific vitamins are required by the mother to supply the appropriate nutrients essential to the normal development of the fetus. Without proper dietary control, certain common deficiencies and complications in both mother and baby may occur.

DIET

- The average patient must consume an additional **300 kcal/day** beyond baseline needs and an additional **500 kcal/day when breast-feeding**.
- High protein (70–75 g/day), low simple carbohydrates and fats, high fiber.

FOLIC ACID

 A 32-year-old G3P2002 patient at 16 weeks' gestation presents for initial obstetric visit. She reports that her last child born 3 years ago has spina bifida. What dose of folic acid she should take to reduce her risk of having another child with NTD?

Answer: Patients with a previous child with an NTD should take 4 mg/day of folic acid starting at least 6 weeks before conception and continuing through 12 weeks of pregnancy.

- ↑ dietary folate is required to prevent NTDs.
- For low-risk patients, **400 μg/day** is recommended. Ideal if started at least 6 weeks before pregnancy. This amount is contained in every prenatal vitamin.
- If previous child with NTD, need folic acid 4 mg/day, starting 6 weeks prior to conception and through T1.

MINERALS

- In total, **30 mg of elemental iron per day is recommended in T2 and T3**. Total of 1-g iron is needed for pregnancy (500 mg for ↑ RBC mass, 300 mg for fetus, 200 mg for GI losses). Many prenatal vitamins have extra iron in them for this reason. Iron is very constipating. Thus, for patients who need extra iron, also offer stool softeners.
- The recommended dietary allowance (RDA) for calcium is ↑ in pregnancy to 1200 mg/day and may be met adequately with diet alone.
- The RDA for zinc is ↑ from 15 to 20 mg/day.

VEGETARIANS

- **Lacto-ovovegetarians** in general have no nutritional deficiencies, except possibly iron and zinc.
- **Vegans** must consume sufficient quantities of vegetable proteins to provide all essential amino acids normally found in animal protein. Supplementation of zinc, vitamin B_{12}, and iron is necessary.

PICA

Occasionally seen in pregnancy, pica is the compulsive ingestion of nonfood substances with little or no nutritional value, such as ice, clay (geophagia), or starch (amylophagia).

Common Questions

Pregnancy is a complicated time for most patients. Their bodies undergo a transformation which entails many physiologic adaptations. These changes

EXAM TIP

How is IUGR monitored? Serial US for fetal growth, antenatal testing, and Doppler studies of the umbilical artery.

WARD TIP

What should be taken to prevent NTDs? Folic acid 400 μg/day or 0.4 mg/day. Patients with a history of an affected fetus/neonate need 4 mg.

WARD TIP

Prenatal vitamins are often large pills that cause many women nausea in the first trimester, thus many women switch to gummy prenatal vitamins, which contain the same ingredients except do not have the extra iron.

WARD TIP

The neural tube is nearly formed by the time of the first missed period. Starting folic acid supplementation when pregnancy is diagnosed is too late to prevent NTDs.

WARD TIP

Pregnant patients develop iron deficiency anemia due to the ↑ hematopoietic demands of both mother and baby.

WARD TIP

Pica may occur during pregnancy, but all normal dietary and nutritional needs must be met and the substances consumed should be nontoxic (ice). Advise patients against the consumption of nonedible and possibly toxic items, such as dirt or laundry detergent.

may be alarming to some patients, and a provider must be able to discern between normal pregnant physiology and pathophysiologic changes, which may require further investigation or immediate attention in a hospital setting.

CAFFEINE IN PREGNANCY

- Contained in coffee, tea, chocolate, cola beverages.
- Ingestion of caffeine (>300 mg/day or >3–4 servings per day) may ↑ risk of early spontaneous abortion among nonsmoking patients carrying fetuses of normal karyotype. This risk ↑ according to amount of caffeine ingested.

EXERCISE

- No data exist to indicate that a pregnant patient must ↓ the intensity of her exercise or lower her target heart rate.
- Patients who exercised regularly before pregnancy may and can continue. Exercise may relieve stress, ↓ anxiety, ↑ self-esteem, modulate weight gain, and shorten labor.
- The form of exercise should be one with low risk of trauma, particularly abdominal (water exercises are ideal). Avoid contact sports or activities where patient could hit the abdomen or fall. New and intense exercise regimens should not be started in pregnancy.
- Exercise that requires prolonged time in the supine position should be approached with caution in T2 and T3.
- Exercise should be stopped if patient experiences oxygen deprivation (manifested by extreme fatigue, dizziness, or shortness of breath).
- Relative contraindications to exercise include:
  - Active heavy vaginal bleeding.
  - Cervical insufficiency.
  - Rupture of membranes.
  - Pregnancy-induced hypertension/preeclampsia/eclampsia.

NAUSEA AND VOMITING (N&V)

- Recurrent N&V in T1 occurs in 50% of pregnancies.
- If severe, can result in dehydration, electrolyte imbalance, and malnutrition.

HEARTBURN

- Occurs in 30% of pregnancies.
- **Etiology:**
  - Normal relaxation of lower esophageal sphincter (due to progesterone).
  - Mechanical forces.
- **Treatment:**
  - Elimination of spicy/acidic foods.
  - Small, frequent meals.
  - Decreasing amount of liquid consumed with each meal.
  - Limiting food and liquid intake a few hours prior to bedtime.
  - Sleeping with head elevated on pillows.
  - Antacids and H_2-receptor inhibitors.

CONSTIPATION

- Common in pregnancy (due to progesterone)
- **Management:**
  - Increase intake of high-fiber foods
  - Increase PO hydration

WARD TIP

Hyperemesis gravidarum: Excessive vomiting during pregnancy + dehydration + electrolyte imbalances. A **hypochloremic alkalosis** may occur. What is the treatment? IVF, antiemetics.

WARD TIP

"Morning sickness" can occur day or night.

WARD TIP

Pregnancy is a hypercoagulable state, and there is an ↑ in clotting factor levels.

- ▪ Use of psyllium-containing products (e.g., Metamucil) and stool softeners
- ▪ Use enemas, strong cathartics, and laxatives with caution and hydration

VARICOSITIES

- ▪ Common in pregnancy, particularly in lower extremities and vulva.
- ▪ Can cause chronic pain and superficial thrombophlebitis.
- ▪ **Management:**
  - ▪ Avoidance of garments that constrict at the knee and upper leg.
  - ▪ Use of support stockings.
  - ▪ ↑ periods of rest with elevation of the lower extremities.

> **WARD TIP**
>
> Hypercoagulable state and mechanical compression of venous blood flow from the lower extremities cause increased risk of thrombosis.

HEMORRHOIDS

- ▪ Varicosities of the rectal veins are common in pregnancy.
- ▪ **Management:**
  - ▪ Cool sitz baths.
  - ▪ Stool softeners.
  - ▪ ↑ fluid and fiber intake to prevent constipation.
  - ▪ Hemorrhoidal ointment to ↓ swelling, itching, and discomfort.
  - ▪ Topical anesthetic spray or steroid cream for the severe pain of thrombosed hemorrhoids.

> **WARD TIP**
>
> Most hemorrhoids improve after delivery.

> **WARD TIP**
>
> Hemorrhoidectomy can be performed safely during pregnancy if necessary.

LEG CRAMPS

- ▪ Occur in 50% of pregnant patients, typically at night and in T3.
- ▪ Most commonly occur in the calves.
- ▪ Massage and stretching of the affected muscle groups is recommended.

BACKACHE

- ▪ Typically progressive in pregnancy (30–50%)
- ▪ **Management:**
  - ▪ Minimizing time standing
  - ▪ Wearing a support belt over the lower abdomen
  - ▪ Acetaminophen for pain as needed
  - ▪ Exercises to ↑ back strength
  - ▪ Supportive shoes and avoidance of high heels
  - ▪ Gentle back massage
  - ▪ Heating pad to back

ROUND LIGAMENT PAIN

- ▪ Sharp, bilateral or unilateral groin pain: "Stabbing"
- ▪ Frequently occurs in T2
- ▪ May ↑ with sudden movement/change in position

SEXUAL INTERCOURSE

- ▪ There are no restrictions during the normal pregnancy.
- ▪ Nipple stimulation, vaginal penetration, and orgasm may cause release of oxytocin and prostaglandins, resulting in uterine contractions.
- ▪ Contraindications:
  - ▪ Ruptured membranes.
  - ▪ Placenta previa.

TABLE 4-6. **Clinical Scenarios where Genetic Testing Should Be Offered**

BASED ON A PATIENT'S HISTORY	BASED ON SOMETHING IN CURRENT PREGNANCY
Previous child with abnormal karyotype	Fetal structural abnormality on sonogram
Known parental chromosome or genetic abnormality (balanced translocation or point mutation)	Second trimester unexplained fetal growth restriction (FGR)
	Abnormal genetic screening test

TABLE 4-7. **Risk Factors for IUGR**

MATERNAL	OBSTETRIC/FETAL
Tobacco use	Preeclampsia
Cocaine use	Multiple gestation
Alcohol use	Genetic abnormalities
Maternal vascular diseases	Placental infarction
History of IUGR in prior pregnancy	In utero infection
Maternal morbid obesity	

EMPLOYMENT

- Work activities that ↑ risk of falls/trauma should be avoided.
- Exposure to toxins/chemicals should be avoided.

TRAVEL

- The best time to travel is in T2. Patient is past possible complications of miscarriage in T1 and not yet encountered risk of preterm labor of T3.
- If prolonged sitting is involved, the patient should attempt to stretch her lower extremities and walk for 10 minutes every 2 hours. This is to avoid deep venous thrombosis (DVT).
- The patient should bring a copy of her medical record.
- Airplane travel in pressurized cabin presents no additional risk to the pregnant patient (if uncomplicated pregnancy). Air travel is not recommended after 36 weeks. All transportation security administration (TSA) screening techniques are safe in pregnancy.
- In underdeveloped areas or when traveling abroad, the usual precautions regarding ingestion of unpurified water and raw foods should be taken. Appropriate vaccines should be given.

IMMUNIZATIONS (TABLE 4-9)

- Influenza vaccine should be strongly recommended to every pregnant patient, regardless of GA.
- The TDaP (tetanus, diphtheria and pertussis) vaccine should be given in each pregnancy at 26–28 weeks, such that there is time for antibodies

TABLE 4-8. Management of N/V in First Trimester

MILD CASES	SEVERE CASES
Eating small frequent meals/snacks	All recommended interventions for mild cases
Ginger teas or candies	IVF with dextrose
Pyridoxine (vitamin B$_6$) ± doxylamine (antihistamine)	Promethazine
	Metoclopramide
Acupressure and acupuncture	Ondansetron >10 weeks

TABLE 4-9. Vaccine Safety in Pregnancy

SAFE	NOT WELL STUDIED IN PREGNANT WOMEN, SO DEFER UNTIL FURTHER RECOMMENDATIONS ISSUED	ADMINISTER ONLY IF RISK OUTWEIGHS BENEFIT	UNSAFE (LIVE)
Inactivated polio (IPV)	Human papillomavirus (HPV)	Yellow fever	Oral polio
Inactivated typhoid	Meningococcus (MPV4)	Anthra	Oral typhoid
Inactivated influenza	Pneumococcus (PPV)	Pertussis	Intranasal influenza
Diphtheria	Hepatitis A		Measles, mumps, rubella (MMR)
Tetanus			Varicella
Rabies			Bacillus Calmette-Guérin (BCG)
Meningococcus (MPSV4)			Shingles
Hepatitis B			

to cross the placenta and protect the neonate until it is old enough to be vaccinated.

- Live vaccines are not given in pregnancy.
- Live vaccines may be safely given to the children of pregnant patients.
- Immune globulins are safe in pregnancy and are recommended for patients exposed to measles, hepatitis A and B, tetanus, varicella (chickenpox), and rabies.

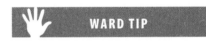

WARD TIP

Ideally, patients should avoid getting pregnant for 4 weeks after receiving live vaccines, such as measles, mumps, rubella (MMR), or varicella.

Notify the Physician

While many physiologic changes in pregnancy are uncomfortable, most are non-emergent. There are, however, some situations when a pregnant patient should contact her obstetrician immediately:

- Vaginal bleeding
- Leakage of fluid from the vagina
- Rhythmic abdominal cramping or back pain, >6/hr that does not improve with hydration and lying supine
- Progressive and prolonged abdominal pain
- Fever and chills

- Dysuria or abnormally cloudy urine (indicative of a urinary tract infection)
- Prolonged vomiting with inability to hold down liquids or solids for >24 hour
- Progressive, severe headache; visual changes; or generalized edema (pre-eclamptic symptoms)
- Seizure (eclampsia)
- Pronounced ↓ in frequency or intensity of fetal movements

Intrapartum

Duration of labor is typically shorter in the multiparous patient than in nulliparous patients.

There are three stages of labor and two phases of stage 1.

Labor is defined as contractions resulting in cervical change.

Three Stages of Labor

A 25-year-old G1P0 patient at 38 weeks' gestation presents to triage reporting contractions that have been increasing in strength and frequency over a 12-hour period. She does not have vaginal bleeding, leakage of fluid, or preeclampsia symptoms. She reports good fetal movement. Fetal heart rate (FHR) is reassuring. She is contracting every 2 minutes on the monitor. The cervical exam is 6 cm dilated, 50% effaced, 0 station, cephalic. What stage of labor is she in? If her labor progresses as expected, what should her cervical dilation be at the next vaginal exam (VE) in 2 hours?

Answer: She is in the active phase of the first stage of labor. Since she is a primigravida, her cervix should dilate at a minimum of 1.2 cm/hr. So, in 2 hours, she should be 8.4 cm (or 8–9 cm) dilated.

Labor is defined as regular contractions that result in cervical change. A patient can have contractions that do not cause cervical change as well as cervical change without contractions—neither of these are "labor." The progression of labor is illustrated in Figure 5-1.

FIRST STAGE

- The first stage of labor begins with onset of uterine contractions of sufficient frequency, intensity, and duration to result in effacement and dilation of the cervix, and ends when the cervix is completely dilated to 10 cm.
- The first stage of labor consists of **two phases:**
  1. **Latent phase:** Begins with the onset of labor and ends at approximately 4–6 cm cervical dilation.
     - Nulliparous: Prolonged if >20 hours.
     - Multiparous: Prolonged if >14 hours.
  2. **Active phase:** Rapid dilation. Begins at 4–6 cm dilation and ends at 10 cm.
     - Fetal descent begins at 7–8 cm of dilation in nulliparas and becomes most rapid after 8 cm.

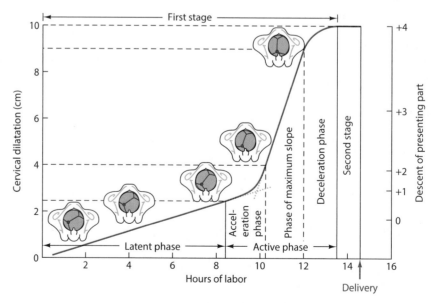

FIGURE 5-1. **Progression of labor.** (Reproduced, with permission, from DeCherney AH, Pernoll ML. *Current Obstetrics & Gynecologic Diagnosis & Treatment*. Norwalk, CT: Appleton & Lange; 1994:211.)

- Average duration of cervical dilation from 4 to 10 cm (minimal normal rate):
  - Nulliparous: <1.2 cm/hr.
  - Multiparous: <1.5 cm/hr.

SECOND STAGE

The second stage of labor is the stage of **fetal expulsion**. It begins when the cervix is fully dilated and ends with the delivery of the fetus.

Average Pattern of Fetal Descent

- Nulliparous: <2 hours (3 hours with epidural)
- Multiparous: <1 hours (2 hours with epidural)

THIRD STAGE

The main event of the third stage is **placental separation**. It begins immediately after the delivery of the fetus and ends with the delivery of the fetal and placental membranes.

- **Duration:** Usually <10 minutes; considered prolonged if >30 minutes.
- The three signs of placental separation are:
  1. Gush of blood from vagina
  2. Umbilical cord lengthening
  3. Fundus of the uterus rises up and becomes firm
  Know these! They are commonly asked at delivery.

True Labor versus False Labor

FALSE LABOR	TRUE LABOR
Occur at irregular intervals	Occur at regular intervals that shorten
Intensity remains the same	↑ in intensity
Discomfort in lower abdomen	Discomfort in lower abdomen
No cervical change	Cervix dilates
Relieved by medications	**Not** relieved by medications

Assessment of Patient in Labor

HISTORY

- Patients without prenatal care require a complete history and physical (H&P), and those with prenatal care require an update and focused physical. Prenatal record should be obtained when possible.

WARD TIP

Remember the three "Ps" that affect the duration of the active phase of labor:
- **Power** (strength and frequency of contractions)
- **Passenger** (size of the baby)
- **Pelvis** (size and shape of mother's pelvis)

WARD TIP

If progress during the active phase is slower than these figures, evaluation for adequacy of uterine contractions, fetal malposition, or cephalopelvic disproportion (CPD) should be done.

WARD TIP

Abnormalities of the second stage may be either protraction or arrest of descent (the fetal head descends <1 cm/hr in a nullipara and <2 cm/hr in a multipara).

WARD TIP

If 30 minutes have passed without placental expulsion, manual removal of the placenta may be required.

WARD TIP

What are the three signs of placental separation?
1. Gush of blood
2. Umbilical cord lengthening
3. Fundus of uterus rises and firms

WARD TIP

Bloody show is small amount of blood mixed with cervical mucus that is present with cervical dilation and effacement.

Blood supply to the uterus from uterine and ovarian arteries.

Normal blood loss for deliveries:

- Vaginal: ~500 cc
- Cesarean: ~1000 cc

What can cause a false-positive nitrazine test?

- Vaginal infections with *Trichomonas vaginalis* or *bacterial vaginosis*
- Blood
- Semen

- The following information should always be obtained from a laboring patient:
  - Time of onset and frequency of contractions.
  - Status of fetal membranes. Typical history for ruptured membranes: gush of fluid with continuous leakage. Color may be clear or yellow/green (meconium).
  - Presence/absence of vaginal bleeding. Bloody show is small amount of blood mixed with cervical mucus that is present with cervical dilation and effacement. It should be distinguished from vaginal bleeding.
  - Notation of fetal activity.
  - Symptoms of preeclampsia (headache, visual disturbances, right upper quadrant pain).
  - How long ago patient consumed food or liquids and how much [mostly in case the patient needs to undergo a cesarean delivery (CD)].

VAGINAL EXAM (VE)

- Perform a sterile **speculum** exam (SSE) first if:
  - Rupture of membranes (ROM) is suspected.
  - The patient is thought to be in preterm labor.
  - Placenta previa is present or suspected.
- Then, **sterile digital** vaginal exam (SVE) may be performed.

RUPTURE OF MEMBRANES (ROM)

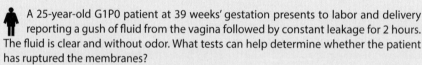

A 25-year-old G1P0 patient at 39 weeks' gestation presents to labor and delivery reporting a gush of fluid from the vagina followed by constant leakage for 2 hours. The fluid is clear and without odor. What tests can help determine whether the patient has ruptured the membranes?

Answer: Sterile speculum exam, testing for pooling, ferning, and nitrazine. If these are positive, the membranes are likely ruptured and the fluid noted on the exam is likely amniotic fluid.

Diagnosis of ROM

The patient's history alone is correct in 90% of patients. Urinary leakage or excess vaginal discharge can be mistaken for ROM.

Spontaneous rupture of membranes (SROM) most often occurs during the course of active labor.

- Perform a sterile speculum exam (how to rule in or rule out ROM):
  1. **Pooling:** The presence of fluid collection in the posterior fornix or in the posterior blade of the speculum (positive pooling).
  2. **Valsalva:** If pooling is not present, ask the patient to bear down and perform a Valsalva maneuver. Note if fluid is seen to come through the cervical os = Positive valsalva. Coughing can work here too.
  3. **Ferning:** Place a thin layer of the vaginal secretions or pooled fluid on a slide. View the dried amniotic fluid under a microscope for a characteristic ferning pattern made by the crystallized sodium chloride in the amniotic fluid (positive ferning). Confirms ROM in 85–98% of cases (see Figure 5-2A and B, B is a false fern and results when cervical mucous dries in the absence of amniotic fluid).
  4. **Nitrazine:** Place the vaginal fluid on nitrazine paper to assess the pH. If nitrazine paper turns blue, this indicates basic pH (positive nitrazine). Amniotic fluid has basic pH as compared to vaginal secretions that have acidic pH. Confirms ROM in 90–98% of cases. (See Table 5-1.)
- The presence of pooling, valsalva, ferning, and nitrazine indicates that the membranes are likely ruptured and the fluid noted on the exam is amniotic fluid.
- Fluid should also be examined for meconium.

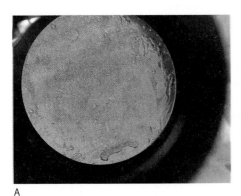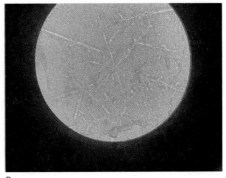

A   B

FIGURE 5-2. Ferning pattern. (A) depicts a "true" ferning pattern due to rupture of membranes. (B) depicts a "false fern" seen with cervical mucous, and not due to ROM.

TABLE 5-1. Types of ROM

ACRONYM	WORDS	DEFINITION
AROM	Artificial rupture of membranes	ROM performed by medical provider to augment or induce labor
SROM	Spontaneous rupture of membranes	ROM that occurs on its own during labor (or during induction)
PROM	Prelabor rupture of membranes	ROM that occurs prior to labor but after 37 weeks and 0 days
PPROM	Preterm prelabor rupture of membranes	ROM that occurs prior to labor and before 37 weeks

- Meconium staining is more common in term and postterm pregnancies than in preterm pregnancies.
- **Meconium aspiration syndrome (MAS):** Fetal stress, like hypoxia, leads to meconium in the amniotic fluid. With further fetal gasping, the meconium is inhaled into the fetal lungs, causing lung damage. At birth, the infant will present with respiratory distress and can develop pulmonary hypertension. Intubation does not provide adequate oxygenation due to the lung injury and pulmonary hypertension. Infants with MAS may require extracorporeal membranous oxygenation (ECMO) which bypasses the lungs in order to provide oxygen to the baby.

 WARD TIP

Vernix: The fatty substance consisting of desquamated epithelial cells and sebaceous matter that normally covers the skin of the term fetus. More common in early term infants.

 EXAM TIP

Meconium: A dark green fecal material that collects in the fetal intestines and is discharged at or near the time of birth.

CERVICAL EXAM

There are five parameters of the cervix that are examined: dilation, effacement, station, consistency, and position.

Dilation

Describes the size of the **opening** of the cervix at the internal os.

- **Ranges:** From zero to 10 cm dilated (closed to completely dilated). The presenting part of a term-sized infant can usually pass through a cervix that is fully dilated.
- **Determination of dilation:** The index and/or the middle fingers are inserted in the cervical opening and are separated as far as the cervix will allow. The distance (cervical dilation) between the two fingers is estimated.

 WARD TIP

Know this cervical exam stuff cold for the wards!

Effacement

Describes the **length of the cervix**. With labor, the cervix thins out and softens, and the length is reduced. The normal length is 3–4 cm outside of labor.

- **Terminology:** When the cervix shortens by 50% (to around 2 cm), it is said to be 50% effaced. When the cervix becomes as thin as the adjacent lower uterine segment, it is 100% effaced (think paper-thin).
- **Determination of effacement:** Palpate with finger and estimate the length from the internal to external os.

Station

Describes the degree of **descent** of the presenting part in relation to ischial spines, which are designated at 0 station.

- **Terminology** (two systems):
  1. The ischial spine is zero station, and the areas above and below are divided into thirds. Above the ischial spines are stations –3, –2, and –1, with –3 being the furthest above the ischial spines and –1 being closest. Positive stations describe fetal descent below the ischial spines. +3 station is at the level of the introitus, and +1 is just past the ischial spines.
  2. Very similar except that the areas above and below the ischial spines are divided by centimeters, up to 5 cm above and 5 cm below. Above are five stations or centimeters: –5, –4, –3, –2, and –1, with –5 being the 5 cm above the ischial spines and –1 being 1 cm above. Positive stations describe fetal descent below the ischial spines. +5 station is at the level of the introitus, and +1 is 1 cm past the ischial spines.
- If the fetus is vertex, the station should be determined by the location of the biparietal diameter (BPD), not the tip-top of the head, which may simply be caput and not the head at all. So, when the BPD is at the level of the ischial spines, the station is 0.

Consistency

Breakdown of collagen bonds in the cervix changes the consistency of the cervix progressively from firm to medium to soft, in preparation for dilation and labor. For some context: Firm consistency is described like the forehead would feel if pushed on, medium like the tip of the nose, and soft like the check.

Position

Describes the location of cervix with respect to the fetal presenting part. It is classified as one of the following:

- **Posterior:** Difficult to palpate because it is behind the presenting part, and usually high in the pelvis.
- **Midposition.**
- **Anterior:** Easy to palpate, low in pelvis, pointing forward.

During labor, the cervical position progresses from posterior to anterior.

BISHOP SCORE

WARD TIP

- **Vaginal prostaglandins** are inserted for ripening (softening) of cervix.
- **IV pitocin** is used to ↑ strength and frequency of contractions.

A 26-year-old G2P1001 patient at 41 weeks' gestation presents to the hospital for an induction of labor. Her dates are verified, and the infant is noted to be cephalic. Her cervical exam is 3 cm dilation, 70% effaced, –2 station, anterior position, and soft. What is her Bishop score? What is the likelihood of a successful vaginal delivery?

Answer: The Bishop score is 9 showing that she has a favorable cervix for induction of labor. Her chance of vaginal delivery is similar to those who present in spontaneous labor.

TABLE 5-2. Bishop Scoring System

FACTOR	0 POINTS	1 POINTS	2 POINTS	3 POINTS
Dilation (cm)	Closed	1–2	3–4	≥5
Effacement (%)	0–30	40–50	60–70	≥80
Station[a]	–3	–2	–1 to 0	+1 to +3
Consistency	Firm	Medium	Soft	—
Position	Posterior	Midposition	Anterior	—

[a]Station reflects −3 to +3 scale.

This is a scoring system that helps to determine the status of the cervix—favorable or unfavorable—for successful vaginal delivery.

- If induction of labor is indicated, the status of the cervix must be evaluated to help determine the method of labor induction that will be utilized. See Table 5-2 and section on Labor in this chapter.
- A score of ≥6 indicates that the probability of vaginal delivery with induction of labor is similar to that of spontaneous labor.

Assessment of the Fetus

LEOPOLD MANEUVERS

- Leopold maneuvers begin in late pregnancy to determine which way the baby is presenting in the uterus (Figure 5-3). Consist of four parts:

Lie

Lie describes the relation of the long axis of the fetus to that of the mother. A **longitudinal** (99% of term or near-term births) lie can be vertex (head first) or breech (buttocks first). The lie may be **transverse** or **oblique**.

Presentation/Presenting Part

Describes the portion of the fetus that is foremost within the birth canal. It is normally determined by palpating through the cervix on SVE.

- If the lie is longitudinal, the presentation is either the head (cephalic), buttocks (breech), brow, or face. The most common type of presentation is the **vertex presentation** in which the posterior fontanel is the presenting part.
- If the lie is transverse, the shoulder, back, or abdomen may be the presenting part.

Position

Refers to the relation of the presenting part to the right (R) or left (L) side of the birth canal and its direction anteriorly (A), transversely (T), or posteriorly (P)—described based on digital exam.

- The top of the **fetal skull** is composed of five bones: two frontal, two parietal, and one occipital. The anterior fontanel lies where the two frontal

WARD TIP

Anterior fontanel: Larger diamond shape

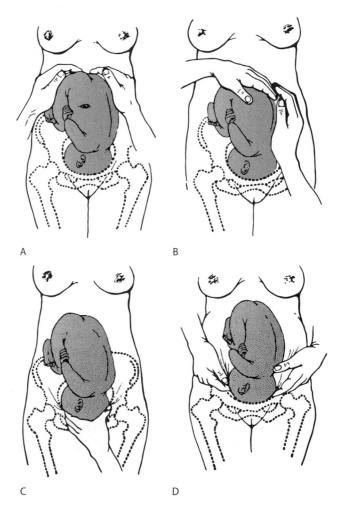

A   B

C   D

FIGURE 5-3.   Leopold maneuvers. (Reproduced, with permission, from Pernoll ML. *Benson & Pernoll's Handbook of Obstetrics and Gynecology.* 10th ed. New York: McGraw-Hill; 2001:159.)

Interpreting Fetal Positions
Fetal position is oriented based on the patient being supine (her symphysis anterior and coccyx posterior), and described based on the fetuses' head position in relation to the patient's own position. Figure 5-4 represents the mother's birth canal with the fetal head in various positions.

EXAM TIP

Ninety percent of babies presenting in the occiput posterior position spontaneously rotate to occiput anterior position.

and two parietal meet, and the posterior fontanel lies where the two parietal meet the occipital bone.
- For a cephalic presentation, the **occiput** is used as the reference point to determine the position.
- The **chin** is used as the reference point for face presentation. The **sacrum** is used as the reference point for breech presentation.

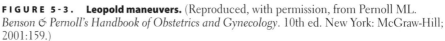
NORMAL PRESENTATION

Vertex Presentation (Occiput Presentation)

Vertex presentation is **most common** (96% of term or near-term presentations). The head is flexed so that the chin is in contact with the chest. The **posterior fontanel** is the presenting part. This creates the shortest diameter of the fetal skull that has to pass through the pelvis.

MALPRESENTATIONS

Face Presentation

In face presentation (0.3% of presentations at or near term), the fetal neck is sharply extended so the occiput is in contact with the fetal back. The face is the presenting part. Diagnosis is made by palpation of the fetal face on SVE.

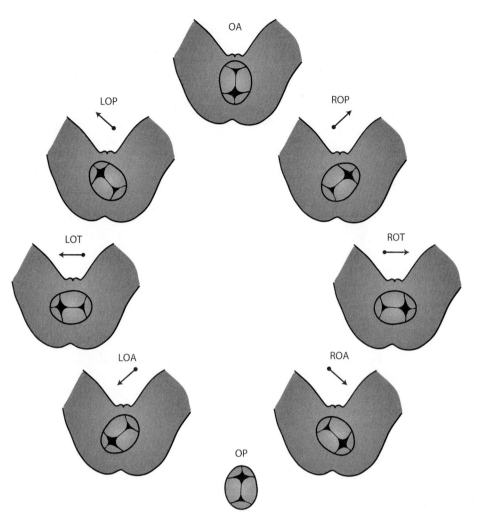

FIGURE 5-4.   Vertex positions.

Brow Presentation

The fetal head assumes a position such that the eyebrows present first. This forces a large diameter through the pelvis; usually, vaginal delivery is possible only if the presentation is converted to a face or vertex presentation.

Breech Presentations

In breech presentations, the presenting fetal part is the **buttocks**. Incidence: 3.5% at or near term but much greater in early pregnancy (14%). Those found in early pregnancy will often spontaneously convert to vertex as term approaches. Risk factors for breech presentation include congenital anomalies such as hydrocephalus or anencephaly, uterine anomalies, multiple gestation, placenta previa, oligohydramnios, polyhydramnios, and grand multiparity. Breech presentation can be diagnosed with Leopold Maneuvers, ultrasound, or digital exam. The safest way for a singleton breech fetus to delivery is by cesarean.

TYPES OF BREECH (SEE FIGURE 5-5)

- **Frank breech (65%):** The thighs are flexed (bent forward), and knees are extended (straight) over the anterior surfaces of the body (feet are in front of the head or face).
- **Complete breech (25%):** The thighs are flexed (bent) on the abdomen, and the knees are flexed (folded) as well.

WARD TIP

Vaginal delivery is possible only if the fetus is mentum anterior; mentum posterior cannot deliver vaginally—must be delivered by cesarean.

EXAM TIP

A pregnant patient presents at 31 weeks' gestation with a breech presentation. What is the next step? Recheck fetal presentation at 36 weeks and then offer external cephalic version if persistently breech. *Note:* If <34 weeks, malpresentation not uncommon and not significant.

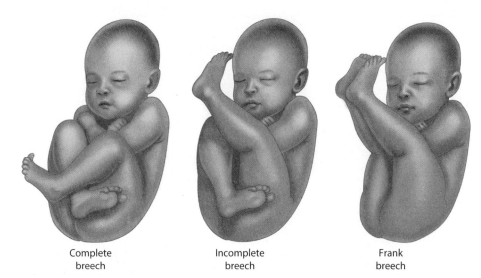

Complete   Incomplete   Frank
breech   breech   breech

FIGURE 5-5.   Types of breech presentations. (Reproduced, with permission, from Ganti L. *Atlas of Emergency Medicine Procedures*. New York: Springer Nature; 2016.)

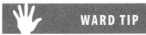

WARD TIP

A patient presents in labor at 6 cm with breech presentation, what is the safest mode of delivery? Cesarean.

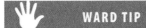

WARD TIP

Complete and incomplete breeches are not delivered vaginally due to risk of umbilical cord prolapse.

- **Incomplete (footling) breech (10%):** One or both of the hips are not flexed so that a foot lies below the buttocks.
- **External cephalic version:** Procedure that maneuvers the infant to a cephalic position by applying pressure through the maternal abdomen. Can be done if breech is diagnosed before onset of labor. Ideally performed at 37 weeks. The success rate is 50%, and the risks are placental abruption, FHR abnormalities, and reversion.

Cardinal Movements of Labor

The cardinal movements of labor are movements of the fetal head that allow it to pass through the birth canal. The movements are as follows: engagement, descent, flexion, internal rotation, extension, and external rotation (restitution). Delivery of the shoulders follows (see Figure 5-6).

ENGAGEMENT

The descent of the BPD (the largest transverse diameter of the fetal head, 9.5 cm) through the plane of the pelvic inlet. Can occur in late pregnancy or in labor. Clinically if the presenting part is at 0 station, the head is thought to be engaged in the pelvis.

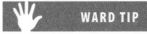

WARD TIP

Engagement is determined by palpation of the presenting part of the occiput.

DESCENT

Occurs when the fetal head passes down into the pelvis. It occurs in a discontinuous fashion. The greatest rate of descent is in the deceleration phase of the first stage of labor and during the second stage of labor.

WARD TIP

The fundal height ↓ at term due to engagement of the fetus.

FLEXION

Occurs when the chin is brought close to the fetal thorax. This passive motion facilitates the presentation of the smallest possible diameter of the fetal head to the birth canal.

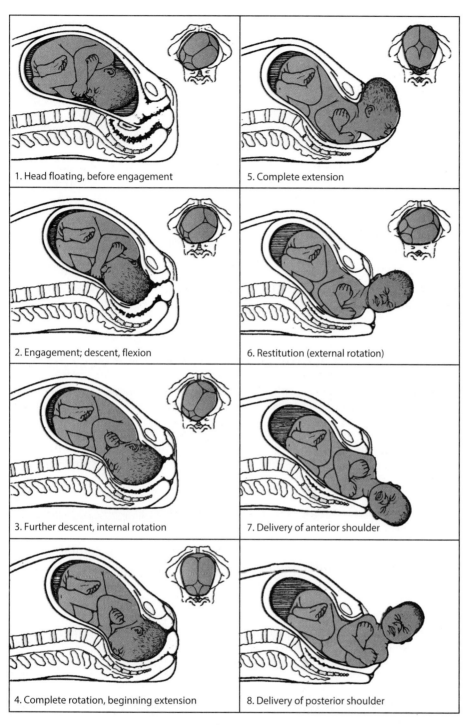

1. Head floating, before engagement

5. Complete extension

2. Engagement; descent, flexion

6. Restitution (external rotation)

3. Further descent, internal rotation

7. Delivery of anterior shoulder

4. Complete rotation, beginning extension

8. Delivery of posterior shoulder

FIGURE 5-6. Cardinal movements of labor. (Reproduced, with permission, from Cunningham FG, Leveno KJ, Bloom SL, et al. *Williams Obstetrics.* 22nd ed. New York: McGraw-Hill; 2005:418.)

INTERNAL ROTATION

Refers to turning of the head that moves the occiput gradually toward the symphysis pubis or less commonly toward the hollow of the sacrum.

EXTENSION

Extension moves the occiput toward the fetal back:

- Occurs after the fetus has descended to the level of the maternal vulva.
- This action brings the base of the occiput into contact with the inferior margin of the symphysis pubis, where the birth canal curves upward.
- The delivery of the fetal head occurs when it changes from the flexed to the extended position, curving under and past the pubic symphysis.

EXTERNAL ROTATION (RESTITUTION)

Occurs after delivery of the head, when the fetus resumes its normal "face-forward" position with the occiput and spine lying in the same plane. One shoulder is anterior behind the pubic symphysis, and the other is posterior.

EXPULSION

After external rotation, further descent brings the anterior shoulder to the level of the pubic symphysis. The shoulder is delivered under the pubic symphysis, and then the rest of the body is quickly delivered.

Normal Spontaneous Vertex Vaginal Delivery

DELIVERY OF THE HEAD

- Place your hands such that your pinkies abut the perineum. One hand above the fetal head and one below to control the delivery of the head.
- With maternal effort, the infant's head will deliver and restitute either to the left or to the right.

CHECKING FOR NUCHAL CORD

- Nuchal cord occurs when loops of umbilical cord wrap around the fetal neck. To check for this condition, following delivery of the head, a finger should be passed along the fetal neck to ascertain the presence of the cord.
- If nuchal cord is present, a finger should be slipped under the cord, and, if loose enough, the cord should be slipped over the infant's head.
- If the cord is wrapped tightly around the infant's neck, the remainder of the infant can be deliver, with attention to keeping the head as close to the perineum as possible as the body delivers.

DELIVERY OF SHOULDERS

- Most frequently, the shoulders appear at the vulva just after external rotation and are delivered spontaneously.
- Occasionally, the shoulders must be extracted:
    - The sides of the head are grasped with both hands and *gentle* downward traction is applied until the anterior shoulder descends from under the pubic arch.
    - Next, *gentle* upward traction is applied to deliver the posterior shoulder.

DELIVERY OF THE INFANT

- The rest of the infant is delivered with maternal pushing.
- Support the infant's head with one hand by grasping the neck, taking care not to grasp the throat.

- Support the infant's buttocks as they are delivered with the other hand.
- Transfer the infant's buttocks in the crook of the elbow of the hand that is holding the head. This frees the other hand to suction the baby and clamp and cut the cord. As long as the infant looks ok, delay clamping and cutting the cord for 30–60 seconds.
- Hand the baby to the nurse or pediatrician.

DELIVERY OF THE PLACENTA

- Obtain arterial pH if indicated, and venous blood for fetal blood typing.
- Monitor for signs of placental separation:
  - There is often a sudden gush of blood.
  - Uterus becomes globular and firmer.
  - The uterus rises in the abdomen after the bulk of the separated placenta passes into the vagina.
  - The umbilical cord lengthens, indicating descent of the placenta.
- Apply pressure with one hand in the suprapubic region and apply gentle traction on the umbilical cord to guide placenta out.
- Once placenta is past the introitus, grasp with hands and gently remove membranes. Inspect the placenta for intact cotyledons and three-vessel cord.
- Perform fundal massage to help the uterus contract down and ↓ the bleeding.

VAGINAL INSPECTION

Inspect patient for any lacerations or extensions of episiotomy that may need to be repaired. Look at:

- Vaginal walls
- Labia
- Perineum
- Circumferential cervix (if there is persistent bleeding without clear etiology)

PERINEAL LACERATIONS

The perineum and anus become stretched and thin, which results in ↑ risk of spontaneous lacerations to the vagina, labia, perineum, and rectum.

- **First degree:** Involve the fourchette, perineal skin, and vaginal mucosa, but not the underlying fascia and muscle.
- **Second degree:** First degree plus the fascia and muscle of the perineal body but *not* the anal sphincter.
- **Third degree:** Second degree plus involvement of the anal sphincter.
- **Fourth degree:** Extend through the rectal mucosa to expose the lumen of the rectum.

EPISIOTOMY

The incision of the perineum to aid delivery by creating more room. Not performed routinely, but can be performed in special cases such as shoulder dystocia or operative vaginal deliveries. The classification of episiotomy is the same as perineal lacerations. The incision can be either midline or mediolateral (Figure 5-7).

1. **Midline:** The incision is made in the midline from the posterior fourchette. Most common. ↑ the risk of a fourth-degree laceration.
2. **Mediolateral:** The incision is oblique starting from 5 o'clock or 7 o'clock position of the vagina. Causes more bleeding and pain.

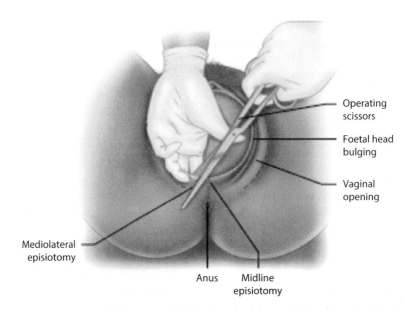

Operating scissors

Foetal head bulging

Vaginal opening

Mediolateral episiotomy

Anus   Midline episiotomy

FIGURE 5-7. Episiotomy technique. (Reproduced, with permission, from Ganti L. *Atlas of Emergency Medicine Procedures.* New York, NY: Springer Nature; 2016.)

POSTDELIVERY HEMOSTASIS

After the uterus has been emptied and the placenta delivered, hemostasis must be achieved:

- The primary mechanism is myometrial contraction leading to vasoconstriction.
- Fundal massage stimulates uterine contraction.
- Oxytocin (pitocin) is administered in the third stage of labor. It causes myometrial contractions and reduces maternal blood loss.
- Postpartum hemorrhage: Often defined as >1000 mL of blood loss either vaginal delivery or CD.

Management of Patients in Labor

STERILE VAGINAL EXAMS (SVEs)

SVEs should be kept to the minimum number required for the evaluation of a normal labor pattern, for example, every 4 hours in latent phase and every 2 hours in active phase. Sterile gloves and lubricant should be used.

MATERNAL VITAL SIGNS

Maternal blood pressure and pulse should be evaluated and recorded regularly, along with the exact frequency varies on labor stage and maternal condition.

OTHER CONSIDERATIONS

Usually, oral intake in active phase and second stage is limited to small sips of water, ice chips, popsicles, or hard candies (clear liquids).

Monitoring during Labor

During labor, uterine contractions and FHR are monitored closely.

UTERINE CONTRACTIONS

Uterine activity is monitored by external or internal uterine monitors.

- **External monitors:**
  - Accurately display the frequency of the contraction. Does not provide information about strength.
  - More commonly used.
- **Intrauterine pressure catheters (IUPC):**
  - Internal monitor that is threaded through the cervix and into the uterus after ROM.
  - Records frequency, duration, and strength of the contraction.
- Strength of contraction measured in **Montevideo units**.
  - Calculated by ↑ in uterine pressure above baseline multiplied by contraction frequency over 10 minutes.
  - If you have time, do not multiply—add every contraction.

FETAL HEART RATE (FHR)

The **FHR** can be assessed in two ways:

1. **Intermittent** auscultation with a fetal stethoscope or Doppler ultrasonic device.
2. **Continuous** electronic monitoring of the FHR and uterine contractions is most commonly used in United States. The standard fetal monitor tracing records the FHR on the top portion and the contractions on the bottom.
- **External (indirect) electronic FHR monitoring:** FHR is detected using a Doppler device placed on the maternal abdomen.
- **Internal electronic FHR monitoring (aka Fetal scalp electrope, FSE):** A bipolar spiral electrode is attached to the fetal scalp, which detects the peak R-wave voltage of the fetal electrocardiogram. This is more invasive and is used if closer fetal monitoring is required or if unable to trace FHR well externally. Can only place after ROM.

FHR Patterns

- The normal baseline for the FHR is 110–160 beats per minute (bpm). Baseline is described in multiples of 5 (e.g., baseline of 130 or 135, but not 132).
- Baseline rate refers to the most common heart rate over the last ≥10 minutes.
- Periodic changes above and below termed **accelerations** (↑ in HR) and **decelerations** (↓ in HR).
- A **reassuring NST** has two accelerations of at least 15 bpm above the baseline, lasting for at least 15 seconds, in 20 minutes. It indicates a well-oxygenated fetus with an intact neurological and cardiovascular system.

DEFINITIONS

- **Hypoxemia:** ↓ oxygen content in blood.
- **Hypoxia:** ↓ level of oxygen in tissue.

TABLE 5-3. Types of Decelerations

	EARLY DECELERATION	LATE DECELERATION	VARIABLE DECELERATION
Significance	Benign	Abnormal	Variable
Shape	U shaped	U shaped	Variable (often V or W shaped)
Onset	Gradual	Gradual	Abrupt
Depth	Shallow	Shallow	Variable
When	Nadir of decel = Peak of ctx	Start and end after the uterine ctx Nadir of decel after peak of ctx	Variable
Why	Head compression	Uteroplacental insufficiency	Cord compression
Initial treatment	None required	O₂, lateral decubitus position, Pitocin off, close monitoring	Amnioinfusion

Ctx, contraction; decel, deceleration; **gradual**, baseline to nadir >30 seconds; **abrupt**, baseline to nadir <30 seconds.

- **Acidemia:** ↑ concentration of hydrogen ions in the blood.
- **Acidosis:** ↑ concentration of hydrogen ions in tissue.
- **Asphyxia:** Hypoxia with metabolic acidosis. Goal of fetal monitoring during labor is to avoid metabolic acidosis and asphyxia, which can cause permanent neurological injury.

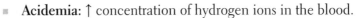

DECELERATIONS

A 32-year-old G2P1001 patient at 40 weeks' gestation presents to labor and delivery with contractions. She is noted to be 5 cm dilated, 50% effaced, −1 station, and cephalic. The monitor shows contractions every 2 minutes, and the FHR pattern shows a baseline of 150 bpm, minimal variability, and decelerations that nadir after the peak of the contractions. No accelerations are noted. What is the most likely cause of the findings on the FHR? What is the next step in management?

Answer: Uteroplacental insufficiency is the most likely cause for this patient's late decelerations. The patient should be turned on her left side to maximize oxygenation to the fetus. IV fluid bolus can be given. If her membranes are ruptured, a fetal scalp electrode and an IUPC (internal monitors) will help with the FHR monitoring.

Decelerations during labor have different interpretations depending on when they occur in relation to contractions. (See Table 5-3 and Figure 5-8.)

Early Decelerations

- Early decelerations are *normal* and are due to **head compression** during contractions or during maternal expulsive efforts.
- The nadir of the gradual deceleration corresponds to the peak of the contraction.

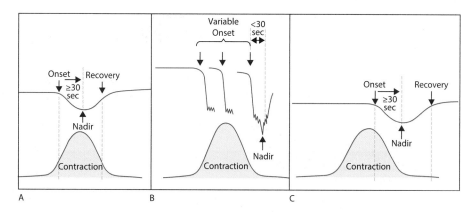

FIGURE 5-8. **Features of early (A), variable (B), and late (C) decelerations on fetal heart monitoring.** (Reproduced, with permission, from Cunningham FG, Leveno KJ, Bloom SL, et al. *Williams Obstetrics.* 22nd ed. New York: McGraw-Hill; 2005:452–454.)

▣ The effect is regulated by vagal nerve activation.
▣ No intervention is necessary. They are clinically benign.

Late Decelerations

▣ Late decelerations are *abnormal* and are due to **uteroplacental insufficiency** (blood without enough oxygen) during contractions.
▣ They are a gradual decrease below the baseline with onset, nadir, and recovery occurring after uterine contraction onset, peak, and recovery, respectively.

MANAGEMENT

▣ Change maternal position to the left lateral recumbent position.
▣ Give oxygen by facemask.
▣ Stop oxytocin (pitocin) infusion.
▣ Provide an IV fluid bolus.
▣ Consider tocolysis.
▣ Monitor maternal blood pressure. Treat hypotension with medications.
▣ SVE to assess for change in fetal station or position.
▣ If repetitive (>50% of the contractions have late decelerations) and no other reassuring finding present, consider delivery.

Variable Decelerations

▣ Variable decelerations are *abnormal* and reflect the fetal autonomic reflex response to umbilical cord compression.
▣ They can be seen with oligohydramnios or a nuchal cord.
▣ Abrupt deceleration that looks like a "V".
▣ They can occur at any time.

MANAGEMENT OF VARIABLE DECELERATIONS

▣ **Amnioinfusion:** Infuse normal saline into the uterus through the IUPC to alleviate cord compression.
▣ Change maternal position to side/Trendelenburg position.
▣ Plan delivery of fetus soon if worsening or nonreassuring.

Prolonged Decelerations

Isolated decelerations with fall in baseline by ≥15 bpm that last 2–10 minutes. Causes include:

▣ Uterine hyperactivity
▣ Maternal hypotension leading to transient fetal hypoxia
▣ Umbilical cord compression

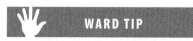

The left lateral recumbent position is best for maximizing cardiac output and uterine blood flow. (In the supine position, the vena cava and aortoiliac vessels may be compressed by the gravid uterus.)

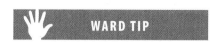

STOP when you see decelerations:
SVE.
Turn the patient to her left side.
Give the patient **O**xygen.
Pitocin off.

MANAGEMENT

- Stop oxytocin and prostaglandins.
- Change maternal position.
- Administer IV fluids.
- Correct hypotension with vasopressors.
- Administer maternal O_2.
- SVE to exclude cord prolapse, sudden cervical dilation, or fetal descent.

FETAL TACHYCARDIA

- Baseline HR >160 bpm for >10 minutes.
- Causes:
  - Fetal hypoxia
  - Intrauterine infection
  - Maternal fever
  - Drugs

FETAL BRADYCARDIA

- HR < 110 bmp.
- Causes:
  - Maternal beta-blocker therapy
  - Hypothermia
  - Hypoglycemia
  - Fetal heart block

SINUSOIDAL PATTERN

- Fluctuations in FHR baseline with regular amplitude and frequency.
- Associated with severe fetal anemia.

BEAT-TO-BEAT VARIABILITY (BTBV)

- **The single most important characteristic of the baseline FHR.**
- Variation of successive beats in the FHR BTBV is controlled primarily by the autonomic nervous system. ↑ in FHR is due to activation of the sympathetic nervous system. The ↓ in the FHR is due to the activation of the parasympathetic nervous system. The constant push and pull of the sympathetic and parasympathetic systems creates the BTBV, which indicates intact fetal CNS.
- At <28 weeks' gestational age, the fetus is neurologically immature; thus, ↓ variability is expected.
- Measured in a 10-minute window, with amplitude measured peak to trough in bpm.
  - Absent = Amplitude undetectable.
  - Minimal = Amplitude 0–5 bpm.
  - Moderate = Amplitude 6–25 bpm.
  - Marked = Amplitude >25 bpm.

Decreases in variability

The variability ↓ with:

- Fetal acidemia
- Fetal asphyxia
- Maternal acidemia

ZEBRA ALERT

Sinusoidal pattern is considered Cat III and requires immediate delivery, but is VERY rare.

- - - - - - - - - - - - - - -

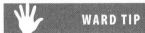 **WARD TIP**

If an FHR of 160 bpm lasts for ≥10 minutes, then tachycardia is present.

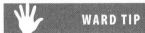 **WARD TIP**

Scalp stimulation is done between decelerations to elicit a reactive acceleration and rule out metabolic acidosis.

TABLE 5-4.   Classification of FHR Patterns

Cat I	ALL criteria must be present:
	▪ Baseline rate: 110–160 bpm
	▪ Moderate variability
	▪ No late or variable decelerations
	▪ ±early decelerations
	▪ ±accelerations
Cat III	Either (1) or (2):
	1. Absent variability PLUS any of following:
	▪ Recurrent late decelerations
	▪ Recurrent variable decelerations
	▪ Bradycardia
	2. Sinusoidal pattern
Cat II	Does not meet criteria for Cat I or Cat III.
	Significance is indeterminate.

- Drugs [narcotics, magnesium sulfate (MgSO$_4$), barbiturates, etc.]
- Acquired or congenital neurologic abnormality

Increases in variability

The variability can ↑ with mild fetal hypoxemia but may also be a normal variant.

Internal FHR monitoring is the best way to determine BTBV.

WARD TIP

Absent variability = **Fetal acidosis**, and delivery should be expedited.

Classification and Interpretation of FHR Patterns

- Three-tier FHR classification system:
  - Category I—normal FHR, minimal chance of fetal acidosis.
  - Category II—all patterns that are not Cat I or Cat III. Risk of acidosis varies widely.
  - Category III—abnormal, associated with increased chance of fetal acidosis and/or hypoxia (Table 5-4).

Abnormal Labor Patterns

ARREST OF DILATION

A 32-year-old G3P2002 patient at 38 weeks' gestation is admitted for active labor. Two hours ago her cervical exam was 5 cm/80% effaced/–2 station. Her exam now is 6 cm/80% effaced/–2 station. What is her labor pattern? What is the next step in management?

Answer: She has a protracted active phase. Since she is a multipara, she should dilate 1.5 cm/hr at a minimum and should have been 8 cm over a span of 2 hours. The next step in management is to determine if there are adequate contractions, if the fetal size and position are amenable for a vaginal delivery, and whether the pelvis is adequate for a normal vaginal delivery.

TABLE 5-5.   Abnormal Labor Patterns

LABOR PATTERN	NULLIPARAS	MULTIPARAS
Prolongation disorder (prolonged latent phase)	>20 hours	>14 hours
Protraction disorder		
1. Protracted active phase dilatation	<1.2 cm/hr	<1.5 cm/hr
2. Protracted descent	<1 cm/hr	<2 cm/hr
Arrest disorders		
1. Dilatation	>2 hours	>2 hours
2. Descent	>1 hour	>1 hour
3. Failure of descent (no descent in deceleration phase or second stage of labor)	>1 hour	>1 hour

Dystocia literally means difficult labor and is characterized by abnormally slow or no progress of labor.

- **Prolonged latent phase** (see Table 5-5).
- **Active phase abnormalities:** May be due to cephalopelvic disproportion (CPD), excessive sedation, conduction analgesia, and fetal malposition (i.e., persistent OP).
- **Protraction disorders:** A slow rate of cervical dilation or descent.
- **Arrest disorders:** Complete cessation of dilation or descent (see Table 5-5).
- With the diagnosis of protraction or arrest disorder of labor, assess the following:
  - Contraction strength: Use IUPC, then Start or ↑ pitocin to obtain stronger contractions.
  - Fetal size and position: Baby too big to pass through pelvis? Position abnormal?
  - Pelvis: Does pelvimetry indicate adequate pelvis?

WARD TIP

With the diagnosis of abnormal labor pattern, assess the three Ps:
- Power (contractions)
- Passenger (fetus)
- Pelvis

Pelvic Shapes

See Table 5-6.

Induction of Labor

INDICATIONS

Medically indicated induction of labor is performed when the benefits of delivery to either the maternal or fetal status outweigh the risks of continuing the pregnancy. See Table 5-7.

CONTRAINDICATIONS

Contraindications to induction include factors that are contraindications to vaginal delivery.

- **Maternal:**
  - Placenta or vasa previa
  - Classical CD

WARD TIP

In some cases, a preterm fetus may be delivered due to maternal illness.

TABLE 5-6. Pelvic Shapes

	GYNECOID	ANDROID	ANTHROPOID	PLATYPELLOID
	(circle)	(heart)	(vertical oval)	(horizontal oval)
Frequency	In 50% of all females	One-third of white women; one-sixth of nonwhite women	One-fourth of white women; one-half of nonwhite women	Rarest, <3% of women
Inlet shape	Round	Heart shaped	Vertically oriented oval	Horizontally oriented oval
Sidewalls	Straight	Convergent	Convergent	Divergent, then convergent
Ischial spines	Not prominent (diameter ≥ 10 cm)	Prominent (diameter < 10 cm)	Prominent (diameter < 10 cm)	Not prominent (diameter > 10 cm)
Sacrum	Inclined neither anteriorly nor posteriorly	Forward and straight with little curvature	Straight = Pelvis deeper than other three types	Well curved and rotated backward; short = Shallow pelvis
Significance	Good prognosis for vaginal delivery	Limited posterior space for fetal head → poor prognosis for vaginal delivery	Good prognosis for vaginal delivery; commonly seen with OP position	Poor prognosis for vaginal delivery

TABLE 5-7. Common Indications for Induction

MATERNAL[a]	FETAL	OBSTETRIC
Preeclampsia	IUGR	GA > 41 weeks (post term)
cHTN	IUFD	PPROM/PROM
Diabetes	Abnormal fetal testing/non-reassuring fetal status	Intra-amniotic infection
BMI > 40	Major fetal anomaly	Oligohydramnios/polyhydramnios
Elective		

[a]There are many more indications, these are just some of the most common reasons for IOL.

cHTN, chronic hypertension; IUFD, intrauterine fetal demise; IUGR, intrauterine growth restriction; PPROM, preterm prelabor rupture of membranes; PROM, prelabor rupture of membranes.

- Active genital herpes infection
- Previous myomectomy
- **Fetal:**
  - Fetal malpresentation
  - Cord prolapse

INDUCTION METHODS

Most patients who come in for induction have a low Bishop score and thus need cervical ripening. Cervical ripening is a process that makes the cervix softer, so it opens easier with contractions. Prostaglandins are a commonly used method for cervical ripening. Most common, is misoprostol, a synthetic PGE_1 analog. This medication can be given intravaginally or orally.

Another prostaglandin is a PGE_2 gel and vaginal insert. Both contain dinoprostone and are used for cervical ripening in patients at or near term. Prostaglandins are contraindication in patients with a prior CD. Cervical ripening can also be done mechanically. Most commonly, this occurs with a Foley balloon that is passed through the internal cervical os into the extra-amniotic space, inflated and rested with traction on the internal os to cause dilation. It is safe to use both pharmacologic and mechanical ripening at the same time.

Once the cervix is ripe, oxytocin, a synthetic polypeptide hormone, can be used to stimulate uterine contraction. It Acts promptly when given intravenously and has half-life about 5 minutes. This medication is a potent antidiuretic effects of oxytocin in high doses can cause water intoxication (i.e., hyponatremia), which can lead to convulsions, coma, and death. Oxytocin is related structurally and functionally to vasopressin or antidiuretic hormone. However, when used it is titrated slowly and closely in order to avoid uterine tachysystole (>5 contraction in 10 minutes).

EXAM TIP

Prostaglandins are contraindicated in patients with prior CD due to increased risk of uterine rupture.

Cesarean Delivery (CD)

The birth of a fetus through incisions in the abdominal wall (laparotomy) and the uterine wall (hysterotomy).

TYPES (SEE FIGURE 5-9)

1. Low-transverse cesarean section (LTCS):
   - Horizontal incision made in lower uterine segment.
   - Most common type performed.
2. Classical:
   - Vertical incision made in the contractile portion of uterine corpus.
   - Performed when:
     - Lower uterine segment is not developed (i.e., extreme prematurity).
     - Fetus is transverse lie with back down.

EXAM TIP

The CPD can lead to failure to progress and cesarean delivery (CD).

INDICATIONS

- Prior cesarean (elective repeat, previous classical)
- Arrest of dilation or arrest of descent
- Fetal malpresentation

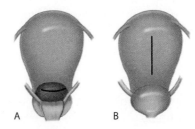

A   B

FIGURE 5-9.   Types of uterine incisions. (A) Low transverse. (B) Classical. (Reproduced, with permission, from Gabbe S, Niebyl J, Simpson J. *Obstetrics: Normal and Problem Pregnancies.* 5th ed. Philadelphia: Churchill Livingstone; 2007: Figure 19-3. Copyright © Elsevier.)

- Concern for fetal well-being (i.e., nonreassuring fetal heart tones)
- Uterine scars / prior myomectomy

Trial of Labor after Cesarean (TOLAC)

TOLAC is associated with a small **risk of uterine rupture** with poor outcome for mother and infant:

- Classical uterine incision: 3–10% risk.
- Low-transverse incision: 0.5–0.9% risk after 1 CD and 1–2% after 2 CD.
- Maternal and infant complications are ↑ with a failed trial of labor followed by CD.

CANDIDATES FOR TOLAC

- One or two prior LTCS.
- No other uterine scars or previous rupture.
- Physician immediately available throughout active labor capable of monitoring labor and performing an emergency CD.
- Availability of anesthesia and personnel for emergency CD.

CONTRAINDICATIONS TO TOLAC

- Prior classical or T-shaped incision or other transmyometrial uterine surgery
- Medical/obstetric complication that precludes vaginal delivery
- Inability to perform emergency CD because of unavailable surgeon, anesthesia, sufficient staff, or facility

Operative Vaginal Delivery

FORCEPS DELIVERY

Forceps are an important tool to allow for a vaginal delivery. The cervix must be fully dilated.

INDICATIONS

- Arrest of descent.
- Fetal distress.
- Maternal factors: exhaustion, heart disease, pulmonary edema, aneurysm, etc.
- After coming head for a breech delivery.

CONTRAINDICATIONS

- Presenting part is not engaged.
- Position of head is not precisely known.
- Membranes are not ruptured.
- Cervix is not fully dilated.
- Presence of CPD.

VACUUM DELIVERY

- Same indications and contraindications as forceps.
- A safe, effective alternative to forceps delivery.
- A vertex fetus is required.

WARD TIP

The most common reason for CD = Previous CD.

WARD TIP

The skin incision on the maternal abdomen does not tell you the type of uterine incision the patient received. For example, a patient may have a midline skin incision but a low-transverse uterine incision.

EXAM TIP

Remember, if a young patient has an 18- or 20-week-size uterus but a negative pregnancy test, the most likely diagnosis is a fibroid uterus.

ADVANTAGES

- Simpler to apply with fewer mistakes in application.
- Less anesthesia is necessary (local anesthetic may suffice).
- No increase in diameter of presenting head.
- Less maternal soft-tissue injury.

DISADVANTAGES

- Traction is applied only during contractions.
- Proper traction is necessary to avoid losing vacuum.
- Possible longer delivery than with forceps.
- Higher risk of neonatal cephalohematomas.

Pain Control during Labor and Delivery

Three essentials of obstetric pain relief are simplicity, safety, and preservation of fetal homeostasis.

LOWER GENITAL TRACT INNERVATION

During the second stage of labor, much of the pain arises from the lower genital tract:

- Painful stimuli from the lower genital tract are primarily transmitted by the **pudendal nerve**, which passes beneath the posterior surface of the sacrospinous ligament (just as the ligament attaches to the ischial spine).
- The sensory nerve fibers of the pudendal nerve are derived from the ventral branches of the second, third, and fourth sacral nerves.

NONPHARMACOLOGICAL METHODS OF PAIN CONTROL

Patients who are free from fear and who have confidence in their obstetrical staff require smaller amounts of pain medication:

- An understanding of pregnancy and the birth process
- Appropriate antepartum training in breathing
- Appropriate psychological support (e.g., by a friend or family member)
- Considerate obstetric care providers who instill confidence

INTRAVENOUS ANALGESIA AND SEDATION

Pain relief with an opiate or opioid plus an antiemetic is typically sufficient, with no significant risk to the mother or infant:

- Discomfort is still felt during uterine contractions but is more tolerable.
- Slight ↑ in uterine activity.
- Does *not* prolong labor.

LOCAL ANESTHESIA

Administered before an episiotomy or after a delivery to repair a laceration.

REGIONAL ANESTHESIA

Nerve blocks that provide pain relief for patients in labor and delivery without loss of consciousness.

Pudendal Block

- Local infiltration of the pudendal nerve with a local anesthetic agent (e.g., lidocaine) by obstetrician.
- Allows pinching of the lower vagina and posterior vulva bilaterally without pain.
- Effective, safe, and reliable method of providing analgesia for spontaneous delivery.
- Can be used along with epidural analgesia.
- **Complications:** Inadvertent intravascular injection will cause systemic toxicity, hematoma, infection.

Spinal (Subarachnoid) Block

- Introduction of local anesthetic into the subarachnoid space.
- Used for uncomplicated CD and vaginal delivery.
- Provides excellent relief of pain from uterine contractions.
- Preceded by infusion of 1 L of crystalloid solution to prevent hypotension.
- Complications:
  - Maternal hypotension (common).
  - Total spinal blockade.
  - Spinal (postpuncture) headache—worse with sitting or standing.
  - Bladder dysfunction.
- Contraindications:
  - Coagulation/hemostasis disorders.
  - Neurologic disorders.
  - Infection at the puncture site.
  - Surgical emergency.

Epidural Analgesia

- Injection of local anesthetic into the epidural or peridural space:
  - **Lumbar epidural analgesia:** Injection into a lumbar intervertebral space.
  - **Caudal epidural analgesia:** Injection through the sacral hiatus and sacral canal.
- Relieves pain of uterine contractions, abdominal delivery (block begins at the eighth thoracic level and extends to first sacral dermatome), or vaginal delivery (block begins from the tenth thoracic to the fifth sacral dermatome).
- Complications:
  - Inadvertent spinal blockade (puncture of dura with subarachnoid injection).
  - Ineffective analgesia.
  - Hypotension.
  - Seizures.
- Effects on labor:
  - Longer second stage of labor (no significant impact on first stage of labor).
- Contraindications:
  - Same as spinal contraindications above.

WARD TIP

Always pull back on the syringe prior to injection of anesthetic to look for blood flow into the syringe; if present, you are in a vessel and must reposition your needle.

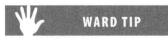

WARD TIP

When vaginal delivery is anticipated in 10–15 minutes, a rapidly acting agent is given through the epidural catheter to effect perineal analgesia.

WARD TIP

Prophylactic measures to avoid aspiration:
- Fasting for 6–8 hours
- Administer antacids
- Cricoid pressure before induction of anesthesia

GENERAL ANESTHESIA

General anesthesia should be only used as a last resort in setting of an emergency. This is because all anesthetic agents that depress the maternal CNS cross the placenta and depress the fetal CNS, and also because induction of general anesthesia can cause aspiration of gastric contents, resulting in airway obstruction, pneumonitis, pulmonary edema, and/or death. Thus, when clinically indicated, it should not be induced until all steps preparatory to actual delivery have been completed, so as to minimize transfer of the agent to the fetus, thereby avoiding newborn respiratory depression.

CHAPTER 6

Postpartum

The Puerperium of the Normal Labor and Delivery

The **puerperium** is the period between birth and 6 weeks after delivery. During this time, the reproductive tract returns anatomically to a normal non-pregnant state. It is also known as the fourth trimester.

UTERUS

Involution of the Uterine Corpus

Immediately after delivery, the fundus of the contracted uterus is slightly below the umbilicus. After the first 2 days postpartum, the uterus begins to shrink in size. Within 2 weeks, the uterus has descended into the cavity of the true pelvis. The contraction of the uterus immediately after delivery is critical for the achievement of hemostasis. "Afterpains" due to uterine contraction are common and respond very well to nonsteroidal anti-inflammatory drugs (NSAIDs). They typically ↓ in intensity by the third postpartum day.

Endometrial Changes

 A 27-year-old patient undergoes a spontaneous vaginal delivery and spontaneous placental delivery without lacerations. An hour later she has persistent vaginal bleeding. What is the likely diagnosis? What is the next step?
Answer: Most likely cause is uterine atony. Massage the fundus, which may feel boggy, and consider administration of uterotonics. Empty the bladder.

Within 2–3 days postpartum, the remaining decidua becomes differentiated into two layers:

1. Superficial layer becomes necrotic, sloughs off as vaginal discharge = *Lochia*.
2. Basal layer (adjacent to the myometrium) becomes new endometrium.

Lochia (lóke-ah) is a decidual tissue that contains erythrocytes, epithelial cells, and bacteria. See Table 6-1.

Placental Site Involution

Within hours after delivery, the placental site consists of many thrombosed vessels. Immediately postpartum, the placental site is the size of the palm of the hand and rapidly ↓ in size.

Changes in Uterine Vessels

Large blood vessels are obliterated by hyaline changes and replaced by new, smaller vessels.

TABLE 6-1. Lochia

Type	Description	When Observed
Lochia rubra	Red due to blood in the lochia	Days 1–3
Lochia serosa	More pale in color	Days 4–10
Lochia alba	White to yellow-white due to leukocytes and reduced fluid content	Day 11 →

CERVIX

- The external os of the cervix contracts slowly and has narrowed by the end of the first week. The multiparous cervix takes on a characteristic fish mouth appearance.
- As a result of childbirth, the cervical epithelium undergoes much remodeling. Some patients with cervical dysplasia will show regression after a vaginal delivery due to the remodeling of the cervix.

VAGINA

Gradually diminishes in size, but rarely returns to nulliparous dimensions:
- Rugae reappear by the third week.

PERITONEUM AND ABDOMINAL WALL

- The broad ligaments and round ligaments slowly return to the nonpregnant state.
- The abdominal wall is soft and flabby due to the prolonged distention and rupture of the skin's elastic fibers; it resumes pre-pregnancy appearance in several weeks.

URINARY TRACT

- The puerperal bladder has an ↑ capacity and is relatively insensitive to intravesical fluid pressure. Hence, overdistention, incomplete bladder emptying, and excessive residual urine are common and can result in a urinary tract infection (UTI).
- Between days 2 and 5 postpartum, "puerperal diuresis" typically occurs to reverse the ↑ in extracellular water associated with normal pregnancy.
- Dilated ureters and renal pelves return to their pre-pregnant state 6–8 weeks postpartum.

HEMATOLOGY/CIRCULATION

- **Leukocytosis** occurs during and after labor (up to 30,000/μL).
- During the first few postpartum days, the **hemoglobin** and **hematocrit** fluctuate moderately from levels just prior to labor.
- **Plasma fibrinogen** and the **erythrocyte sedimentation rate** may remain elevated for ≥1 week postpartum.
- The **cardiac output** is higher than during pregnancy for ≥48 hours postpartum due to ↓ blood flow to the uterus (much smaller) and ↑ systemic intravascular volume.
- By 1-week postpartum, the **blood volume** has returned to the patient's nonpregnant range.

BODY WEIGHT

Most patients approach their pre-pregnancy weight 6 months after delivery, but still retain approximately 1.4 kg of excess weight. About 5–6 kg is lost at the time of delivery due to uterine evacuation and normal blood loss. About 2–3 kg more is lost due to diuresis in the first week postpartum.

WARD TIP

The thinned-out lower uterine segment (that contained most of the fetal head) contracts and retracts over a few weeks and forms the uterine isthmus. The uterine isthmus is located between the uterine corpus above and the internal cervical os below.

WARD TIP

At the completion of involution, the cervix does not resume its pregravid appearance:
- Before childbirth, the os is a small, regular, pinpoint opening.
- After childbirth, the os is a horizontal slit.

WARD TIP

Instrument-assisted delivery and regional and general anesthesia are risk factors for postpartum urinary retention.

WARD TIP

All postpartum patients who cannot void should be assessed for urinary retention and may need catheterization to relieve the retention.

EXAM TIP

Risk of venous thromboembolism is highest in the postpartum period (compared to during pregnancy or at delivery).

EXAM TIP

The likelihood of cardiac overload is highest in the immediate postpartum period, due to the autotransfusion of blood.

Routine Postpartum Care

IMMEDIATELY AFTER LABOR

First Hour

- Take blood pressure (BP) and heart rate (HR) at least every 15 minutes.
- Monitor the amount of vaginal bleeding.
- Palpate the fundus to ensure adequate contraction. If the uterus is relaxed, it should be massaged through the abdominal wall until it remains contracted. Massaging the uterus leads to ↑ release of oxytocin, which helps promote uterine contraction.

FIRST SEVERAL HOURS

Early Ambulation

Patients are out of bed (OOB) within a few hours after delivery. Advantages include:
- **Reduced** frequency of puerperal venous thrombosis and pulmonary embolism (PE)
- ↓ bladder complications
- Less frequent constipation

If Episiotomy/Laceration Repair

- An ice pack should be applied for the first several hours to reduce edema and pain.
- At 24 hours postpartum, moist heat (e.g., via warm sitz baths) can ↓ local discomfort.
- The episiotomy/laceration is typically well healed and asymptomatic by week 3 of the puerperium. Sutures dissolve on their own and do not need to be removed.

Bladder Function

Ensure that the postpartum patient has voided within 4–6 hours of delivery. If not:
- This indicates further voiding trouble to follow.
- An indwelling catheter may be necessary.
- Bladder sensation and capability to empty may be diminished due to anesthesia.
- Consider a hematoma of the genital tract as a possible etiology.

THE FIRST FEW DAYS

Bowel Function

Encourage early ambulation and feeding to ↓ the possibility of constipation. Ask the patient about flatus. It is normal to not have a bowel movement (BM) prior to leaving the hospital, especially if they had a cesarean delivery.

If Third- or Fourth-Degree Laceration

Fecal incontinence may result, even with correct surgical repair, due to injury to the innervation of the pelvic floor musculature. Keep the patient on a stool softener and a low residue diet to avoid straining and ↓ risk of fistula formation. Avoid enemas or suppositories which can disrupt the repair.

Discomfort/Pain Management

During the first few days of the puerperium, pain may result from:

- Afterpains: Contractions of the uterus as it involutes. May increase with breast-feeding due to oxytocin release. Treat with NSAIDs.
- Episiotomy/laceration pain: NSAIDs or acetaminophen can help.
- Breast engorgement: Well-fitted with brassiere. NSAIDs. Pumping/nursing frequently can help as well.
- Postspinal puncture headache: Positional headache that is worse when upright, improved when lying down. Caffeine and hydration may help. Occasionally, patient may need a blood patch (performed by anesthesiologist).
- Constipation: Treat with stool softeners over 2–3 weeks. May discontinue iron supplementation if it worsens constipation.

Return to Normal Activity

Exercise may be initiated any time after vaginal delivery and after 2–4 weeks after cesarean delivery. Walking can start any time after either kind of delivery. Patients can drive once they are no longer taking narcotics and can slam on the break without abdominal pain. Patients who have had a cesarean should not lift more than 15 pounds for 2 weeks. Stairs can be climbed at any time postpartum.

Diet

- There are *no* dietary restrictions/requirements for patients in the postpartum period. Two hours postpartum, the mother should be permitted to eat and drink.
- Continue iron supplementation for a minimum of 3 months postpartum if tolerated.

Immunizations

- The non-isoimmunized D-negative mother whose baby is D-positive is given 300 μg of anti-D immune globulin within 72 hours of delivery.
- Mothers not previously immunized against/immune to rubella or varicella should be vaccinated prior to discharge. Rubella vaccine and varicella vaccine are not given during the pregnancy because they are live vaccines.
- If the patient did not receive during pregnancy, she may be offered vaccinations against influenza and pertussis (tetanus-diphtheria toxoid or Tdap) if these are out of date.

Postpartum Infection

A 30-year-old G1P1001 patient is postpartum day 1 from a vaginal delivery over an intact perineum. On rounds, she reports lower abdominal pain. She reports no cough, back pain, leg pain, dysuria, or breast pain. She had a temperature of 100.1°F (37.8°C) 4 hour ago, and now has a temperature of 101.0°F (38.3°C). Her lungs are clear, and her breasts are soft. There is no costovertebral angle tenderness (CVAT), suprapubic tenderness, or calf tenderness. She has fundal tenderness and foul-smelling lochia. She was admitted with ruptured membranes at 2-cm dilation and delivered after 30 hour in labor. Fetal heart tones were concerning for late decelerations, so she had internal monitors. She pushed for 3 hours before the infant was delivered. What is the most likely diagnosis? What risk factors did this patient have?

Answer: Endometritis. Fever, fundal tenderness, and foul-smelling lochia in the absence of other findings are consistent with endometritis. This patient's risk factors include prolonged rupture of membranes and internal monitors, and she likely had multiple vaginal exams during her long labor course.

WARD TIP

Kleihauer–Betke test detects fetal-maternal hemorrhage in Rh-negative mothers; 300 μg of anti-D immune globulin neutralizes 30 mL of fetal whole blood or 15 mL of Rh-positive RBCs.

WARD TIP

Cesarean delivery is an important risk factor for endometritis.

WARD TIP

Following delivery, the bladder and lower urinary tract remain somewhat hypotonic, resulting in residual urine and reflux, which predisposes to UTI.

ZEBRA ALERT

Group A strep causes a high fever and endometritis in the immediate postpartum and can be deadly.

EXAM TIP

Postpartum endometritis is usually polymicrobial.

WARD TIP

Postdelivery causes of fever:
The 6 Ws + B

- Wind: Atelectasis, 1–2 days postop
- Water: UTIs, 2–3 days postpartum
- Womb: Endometritis 1–7 days postpartum
- Wound: Surgical site infection (SSI)—cellulitis, purulence, fluctuance, tenderness; 5–7 days postpartum
- Cesarean: Abdominal incision
- Vaginal: Episiotomy/laceration
- Walking: Deep vein thrombosis (DVT) and subsequent PE (PE), 4–10 days postpartum
- Wonder drugs: Drug fever, 7–10 days postpartum
- Breast: Engorgement, mastitis, abscess, 3 days–4 weeks postpartum

EXAM TIP

Wound infection occurs in 4–12% of patients following cesarean delivery.

TYPES OF POSTPARTUM INFECTIONS

Endometritis (Metritis, Endomyometritis)

- A postpartum uterine infection involving the decidua, which may involve the myometrium and parametrial tissue.
- More common after cesarean delivery than vaginal delivery. Hypoxic tissue and foreign body (suture) with cesarean delivery increase risk for infection.
- Typically develops postpartum day 2–3.
- Treat with IV antibiotics until patient is afebrile for 24–48 hours.

CAUSES OF ENDOMETRITIS

- **Gram-positive cocci:** Group A, B, and D Streptococci
- **Gram-positive bacilli:** *Clostridium* species, *Listeria monocytogenes*
- **Aerobic gram-negative bacilli:** *Escherichia coli*, *Klebsiella*, *Proteus* species
- **Anaerobic gram-negative bacilli:** *Bacteroides bivius*, *B. fragilis*, *B. disiens*
- **Others:** *Mycoplasma hominis*, *Chlamydia trachomatis*

RISK FACTORS

- Prolonged rupture of membranes >18 hour
- Prolonged labor
- Cesarean delivery
- Colonization of the lower genital tract with certain microorganisms (i.e., Group B Streptococci [GBS], *C. trachomatis*, *M. hominis*, and *Gardnerella vaginalis*)
- Preterm labor and birth
- Multiple cervical exams
- Manual extraction of placenta
- Diabetes
- Chorioamnionitis
- Internal monitors

DIAGNOSIS

- Fever >100.4°F (38°C).
- Fundal tenderness with or without purulent drainage.
- Rule out other sources of fever/infection (i.e., pyelonephritis, mastitis).

MANAGEMENT

Broad-spectrum antibiotics

Urinary Tract Infection (UTI)

- Caused by catheterization, urinary stasis, birth trauma, conduction anesthesia, and frequent pelvic examinations.
- Presents with dysuria, frequency, urgency, and low-grade fever.
- Rule out pyelonephritis (CVAT, pyuria, and hematuria).
- Obtain a urinalysis and urinary culture (*E. coli* is isolated in 75% of postpartum patients).
- Treat with appropriate antibiotics.

Cesarean Delivery: SSI

> A 30-year-old G2P2002 patient is 2 weeks postoperative from a repeat cesarean delivery. She reports swelling around the incision site and ↑ tenderness. Her pain medications do not help. She reports a small amount of purulent malodorous drainage from the incision. She is tolerating her diet well and voiding spontaneously. On physical exam, she is afebrile. Her surgical site is indurated 2 cm around the incision and erythematous 3 cm around the incision. Purulent drainage is noted from a 1-cm opening at the right margin. What is the next step in management?
>
> **Answer:** Next step is to differentiate whether this is a superficial or deep SSI. The wound should be opened further and should be probed to evaluate whether the fascia is intact. Cultures should be obtained and the patient should receive antibiotics (usually IV).

EXAM TIP

Antibiotic prophylaxis with IV cefazolin should be given before every cesarean delivery.

WARD TIP

The more extensive the laceration/incision, the greater the chance of infection and wound breakdown.

SSI DIAGNOSIS

- Wound erythema and persistent tenderness, purulent drainage (may or may not have a fever).
- Management: Consider cultures from wound. Wound should be opened, drained, irrigated, and debrided. Antibiotics should be given along with wet-to-dry packing if infection is superficial. If a deeper infection is present or there is necrotic tissue, the wound May need debridement. In severe cases, this may require surgery/operating room. In mild cases, this can be done at the bedside.

Laceration or Episiotomy Infection

- RARE.
- Look for pain at the episiotomy site, disruption of the wound, and a necrotic membrane over the wound.
- Rule out the presence of a rectovaginal fistula with a careful rectovaginal exam.
- Open, clean, and debride the wound to promote granulation tissue formation.
- Sitz baths are recommended.
- Reassess for possible closure after granulation tissue has appeared.

Discharge from Hospital

VAGINAL DELIVERY

About 1–2 days postdelivery, if no complications. Return to the office at 4–6 weeks for postpartum exam.

CESAREAN DELIVERY (CD)

About 2–3 days postdelivery, if no complications. Return to the office in 4–6 weeks for postpartum exam.

*For patients with hypertensive disorders or mental health concerns can consider a 1-week check-in.

The patient should call the doctor or go to hospital if she develops:

- Fever >100.4°F (38°C).
- Excessive vaginal bleeding—soaking a >1 pad an hour for >1 hour: Suspicious for retained placenta.
- Lower extremity pain and/or swelling: Suspicious for DVT.
- Shortness of breath: Suspicious for PE.

Postpartum Intercourse

- After 6 weeks, intercourse may be resumed based on the patient's desire and comfort. A vaginal lubricant may improve comfort.
- Dangers of premature intercourse:
  - Pain due to continued uterine involution and healing of lacerations/episiotomy scars.
  - ↑ likelihood of hemorrhage and infection.

CONTRACEPTION

A 25-year-old G1P1001 patient is postpartum day 2 from a vaginal delivery. She is overall healthy and is breast-feeding. She wants contraception that is easy to use. She reports that she had used a combination oral contraceptive pill prior to conceiving this baby and had no bad side effects. She is afraid of needles. What is the best contraceptive option for this patient?

Answer: Long-acting reversible contraception (LARC), either intrauterine device (IUD) or contraceptive implant.

- Do not wait until first menses to begin contraception; ovulation may come before first menses.
- Typically start progesterone-only pills immediately postpartum and combined oral contraceptive pills can be started 6 weeks postpartum.
- See chapter "Contraception and Sterilization."

Lactational Amenorrhea: Method of Contraception

Lactational amenorrhea involves exclusive breast-feeding to prevent ovulation. It can be used as a contraceptive method. It is 98% effective for up to 6 months if:

- The mother is not menstruating.
- The mother is nursing >2–3 times per night, and more than every 4 hour during the day without other supplementation. Does not work with pumping—must be nursing.
- The baby is <6 months old.

Oral Contraceptive Pills in Postpartum

- **Combined oral contraceptive pills** may reduce the amount of breast milk, and very small quantities of the hormones are excreted in the milk. Start at 6 weeks to decrease venous thromboembolism (VTE) risk.
- **Progestin-only oral contraceptive pills** are 95% effective with typical use without substantially reducing the amount of breast milk. Need to take it the same time every day.

Depo-medroxyprogesterone

A progesterone-containing injection, given every 3 months, should not reduce breast milk production; 99% effective. Can increase risk of postpartum depression (PPD) in patients with known moderate to severe mental health concerns.

Intrauterine Device (IUD)

May be inserted immediately postpartum (higher risk of expulsion) after vaginal delivery or cesarean delivery or interval insertion 6 weeks postpartum. Lasts 3–10 years, depending on the device. Can be with or without hormones.

Progesterone Implants

A progestin-releasing implant is placed in the arm; lasts for 3 years. Can also be placed immediately postpartum.

Infant Care

Prior to discharge:
- Follow-up care arrangements should be made.
- All laboratory results should be reassuring, including:
  - Coombs' test.
  - Bilirubin.
  - Hemoglobin and hematocrit.
  - Blood glucose.
- Initial HBV vaccine should be administered.
- All screening tests required by law should be performed (e.g., testing for phenylketonuria [PKU] and hypothyroidism).
- Patient education regarding infant immunizations and well-baby care.

Breasts

LACTOGENESIS

Progesterone, estrogen, placental lactogen, prolactin, cortisol, and insulin act together to stimulate the growth and development of the milk-secreting machinery of the mammary gland:

- Midpregnancy: Lobules of alveoli form lobes separated by stromal tissue, with secretion in some alveolar cells.
- T3: Alveolar lobules are almost fully developed, with cells full of proteinaceous secretory material.
- Postpartum: Rapid ↑ in cell size and in the number of secretory organelles. Alveoli distend with milk.

MILK DEVELOPMENT

- At delivery, the abrupt, large ↓ in progesterone and estrogen levels allow for milk production. All vitamins, except vitamin K, are found in human

EXAM TIP

Nursing mothers rarely ovulate within the first 10 weeks after delivery. Non-nursing mothers typically ovulate 6–8 weeks after delivery.

WARD TIP

Colostrum is a yellow-colored liquid secreted by the breasts that contains minerals, protein, fat, antibodies, complement, macrophages, lymphocytes, lysozymes, lactoferrin, and lactoperoxidase.

milk, necessitating neonatal administration of vitamin K to prevent hemorrhagic disease of the newborn.

■ **Colostrum** can be expressed from the nipple almost immediately postpartum and is secreted by the breasts for 5 days postpartum. It has more minerals and protein than breast milk. It has less sugar and fat when compared to breast milk. Antibodies in colostrum protect the infant against enteric organisms.

MATURE MILK AND LACTATION

■ Colostrum is composed of protein, fat, carbohydrates (lactose), secretory IgA, and minerals.
■ Milk comes in within the first week postpartum and is composed of protein, fat, carbohydrates (lactose), and water.
  ■ Protein: Colostrum > milk.
  ■ Fat: Milk > colostrum.
  ■ Carbs: Milk > colostrum.
■ Colostrum is gradually converted to mature milk by 4 weeks postpartum. Subsequent lactation is primarily controlled by the repetitive stimulus of nursing and the presence of prolactin.
■ Breast engorgement with milk is common on days 2–4 postpartum:
  ■ May be painful.
  ■ Often accompanied by transient temperature elevation. See Table 6-2.
  ■ Also occurs in non-breast-feeding patients.
■ Suckling stimulates the neurohypophysis to secrete oxytocin in a pulsatile fashion, causing contraction of myoepithelial cells and small milk ducts, which leads to milk expression.

LACTATION SUPPRESSION

A 26-year-old patient who is 4-weeks postpartum presents with a 1-day history of fever of 100.9°F (38.3°C) and breast tenderness. She has been breast-feeding without problems and reports no other symptoms. Her left breast has a 4-cm area of induration and erythema at the 3 o'clock position that is tender to palpation. Milk expressed from that breast is white. What is the most likely diagnosis? What is the treatment?

Answer: Mastitis. Focal area of breast infection and fever approximately 1 month postpartum is consistent with mastitis. The patient should be started on dicloxacillin.

Patients who do not want to breast-feed or who have an intrauterine fetal demise (IUFD) should wear a supportive bra, breast binder, or "sports bra." Pharmacologic therapy with bromocriptine is not recommended due to its associations with strokes, myocardial infarction, seizures, and psychiatric disturbances. Cold compresses can help as well. Patients should avoid warm/hot showers, as this will increase engorgement. Cold green cabbage leaves in the bra also help with milk suppression.

BREAST FEVER

TABLE 6-2.   Breast-Associated Fevers

	ENGORGEMENT	MASTITIS	ABSCESS
Time frame	2–4 days postpartum	Anytime while lactating (usually >3–4 weeks postpartum)	Anytime while lactating
Presentation	Bilaterally painful, swollen, and firm breasts	Focal erythema and induration, streaking on the breast	Fluctuant tender mass on the breast
Causative agents	Milk collecting in breast	Staph aureas, MRSA, coag negative staph	Staph aureas, MRSA, coag negative staph
Management	supportive bra, 24-hour demand feedings, ice packs	Treat with dicloxacillin for 7–10 days	Treat with broad-spectrum antibiotics and incision and drainage or ultrasound-guided needle aspiration
Continue breast-feeding?	Yes	Yes	Yes

MRSA, Methicillin resistant *Staphylococcus aureus*

BREAST-FEEDING

Human milk is the ideal food for neonates for the first 6 months of life. Breast-fed infants are less prone to enteric infections than are bottle-fed babies.

Recommended Dietary Allowances

Lactating patients need an extra 500 nutritious calories per day. Food choices should be guided by the Food Guide Pyramid, as recommended by the U.S. Department of Health and Human Services/U.S. Department of Agriculture.

Benefits

- Uterine involution: Nursing accelerates uterine involution (increases oxytocin).
- Immunity:
  - Colostrum and breast milk contain secretory IgA antibodies against *E. coli* and other potential infections.

WARD TIP

CMV, HBV, and HIV are excreted in breast milk.

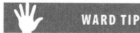
- Milk contains memory T-cells, which allow the fetus to benefit from maternal immunologic experience.
- Colostrum contains interleukin-6, which stimulates an ↑ in breast milk mononuclear cells.
- Nutrients: All proteins and essential and nonessential amino acids available are absorbed by babies .
- Gastrointestinal (GI) maturation: Milk contains epidermal growth factor, which may promote growth and maturation of the intestinal mucosa.

Contraindications to Breast-Feeding

Mothers with the following infections:
- HIV infection.
- Active herpes simplex virus lesions on the breast.
- Tuberculosis (active, untreated).
- Breast-feeding not contraindicated:
  - Cytomegalovirus (CMV): Both the virus and antibodies are present in breast milk.
  - Hepatitis B virus (HBV): If the infant receives hepatitis B immune globulin.
  - Hepatitis C: No documented evidence that breast-feeding spreads hepatitis C.
  - **Medications:** Mothers ingesting the following contraindicated medications (not an exhaustive list):
  - Bromocriptine can suppress lactation.
  - Antineoplastic drugs such as cyclophosphamide (alkylating agent) or doxorubicin (anthracycline).
  - In most situations, the pros and cons of any medication must be weighed against the potential benefit to the mother.
- **Radiotherapy:** Mothers undergoing radiotherapy should not breast-feed. However, if the agent is being used as a diagnostic agent (i.e., CT with contrast), breast-feeding does not need to be interrupted.

Postpartum Psychiatric Disorders

MATERNITY/POSTPARTUM BLUES

 A 25-year-old G1P1001 patient presents 1-week postpartum with tearfulness, inability to sleep, fatigue, and decreased appetite. She has good support at home and is still very involved in taking care of her infant. What is the most likely diagnosis? What therapy should be offered?
Answer: Postpartum blues. She should be given supportive therapy with monitoring for more severe signs of depression.

A self-limited, mild mood disturbance due to biochemical factors and psychological stress:
- Affects 50% of patients.
- Begins within 3–6 days after delivery.
- Usually resolves within 2 weeks.
- May be related to progesterone withdrawal.
- Can also manifest with anxiety.

TREATMENT

- Supportive—acknowledgment of the mother's feelings and reassurance.
- Monitor for the development of more severe symptoms (i.e., PPD or psychosis).

POSTPARTUM DEPRESSION (PPD)

Similar to minor and major depression that can occur at any time:
- Classified as "PPD" if it begins within 3–6 months after childbirth.
- Eight to fifteen percent of postpartum patients develop PPD within 2–3 months.
- Up to 70% recurrence.

PPD is diagnosed using a validated screening tool such as the Edinburgh postnatal depression score (EPDS). This is scored out of 30 points, and a score of >12 is considered diagnostic for PPD. However, even the patient who has a lower score who endorses symptoms of PPD should be treated for the disease (Figure 6-1).

SYMPTOMS

Symptoms are the same as major depression.

NATURAL COURSE

- Gradual improvement over the 6-month postpartum period.
- The mother may remain symptomatic for months to years.

TREATMENT

- Pharmacologic intervention is typically required:
  - Antidepressants [selective serotonin reuptake inhibitors (SSRI) most commonly].
  - Electroconvulsive therapy in very severe cases.
- Mother should be co-managed with a psychiatrist or counselor (i.e., for psychotherapy to focus on any maternal fears or concerns).

POSTPARTUM PSYCHOSIS

- Mothers cannot discern real versus unreal (can have periods of lucidity). Hearing voices, seeing things.
- Occurs in 1–4 in 1000 births.
- Peak onset: 10–14 days postpartum, but may occur months later.

RISK FACTORS

- History of psychiatric illness
- Family history of psychiatric disorders
- Younger age
- Primiparity

COURSE

Variable and depends on the type of underlying illness; often 6 months.

TREATMENT

- Psychiatric care
- Pharmacologic therapy
- Hospitalization (in most cases)

Postpartum Thyroid Dysfunction

Postpartum thyroiditis is a transient lymphocytic thyroiditis in 5–10% of patients during the first year after childbirth. The **two clinical phases** of postpartum thyroiditis are **thyrotoxicosis** and **hypothyroidism** (see Table 6-3).

WARD TIP

Criteria for Major Depression/PPD
Two-week period of depressed mood or anhedonia nearly every day plus four of the following. Symptoms must cause distress and not attributable to substance use or other medical condition.
1. Significant weight loss or weight gain without effort (or ↑ or ↓ in appetite)
2. Insomnia or hypersomnia
3. Psychomotor agitation/retardation
4. Fatigue or loss of energy
5. Feelings of worthlessness/excessive or inappropriate guilt
6. ↓ ability to concentrate/think
7. Recurrent thoughts of suicide/death

Edinburgh Postnatal Depression Scale[1] (EPDS)

Name: _____   Address: _____

Your Date of Birth: _____   _____

Baby's Date of Birth: _____   Phone: _____

As you are pregnant or have recently had a baby, we would like to know how you are feeling. Please check the answer that comes closest to how you have felt **IN THE PAST 7 DAYS**, not just how you feel today.

Here is an example, already completed.

I have felt happy:
- ☐ Yes, all the time
- ☒ Yes, most of the time   This would mean: "I have felt happy most of the time" during the past week.
- ☐ No, not very often   Please complete the other questions in the same way.
- ☐ No, not at all

In the past 7 days:

1. I have been able to laugh and see the funny side of things
   - ☐ As much as I always could
   - ☐ Not quite so much now
   - ☐ Definitely not so much now
   - ☐ Not at all

2. I have looked forward with enjoyment to things
   - ☐ As much as I ever did
   - ☐ Rather less than I used to
   - ☐ Definitely less than I used to
   - ☐ Hardly at all

*3. I have blamed myself unnecessarily when things went wrong
   - ☐ Yes, most of the time
   - ☐ Yes, some of the time
   - ☐ Not very often
   - ☐ No, never

4. I have been anxious or worried for no good reason
   - ☐ No, not at all
   - ☐ Hardly ever
   - ☐ Yes, sometimes
   - ☐ Yes, very often

*5 I have felt scared or panicky for no very good reason
   - ☐ Yes, quite a lot
   - ☐ Yes, sometimes
   - ☐ No, not much
   - ☐ No, not at all

*6. Things have been getting on top of me
   - ☐ Yes, most of the time I haven't been able to cope at all
   - ☐ Yes, sometimes I haven't been coping as well as usual
   - ☐ No, most of the time I have coped quite well
   - ☐ No, I have been coping as well as ever

*7 I have been so unhappy that I have had difficulty sleeping
   - ☐ Yes, most of the time
   - ☐ Yes, sometimes
   - ☐ Not very often
   - ☐ No, not at all

*8 I have felt sad or miserable
   - ☐ Yes, most of the time
   - ☐ Yes, quite often
   - ☐ Not very often
   - ☐ No, not at all

*9 I have been so unhappy that I have been crying
   - ☐ Yes, most of the time
   - ☐ Yes, quite often
   - ☐ Only occasionally
   - ☐ No, never

*10 The thought of harming myself has occurred to me
   - ☐ Yes, quite often
   - ☐ Sometimes
   - ☐ Hardly ever
   - ☐ Never

Administered/Reviewed by _____   Date _____

[1]Source: Cox, J.L., Holden, J.M., and Sagovsky, R. 1987. Detection of postnatal depression: Development of the 10-item Edinburgh Postnatal Depression Scale.   *British Journal of Psychiatry* 150:782-786 .

FIGURE 6-1.   Edinburgh Postnatal Depression Scale. (Reproduced, with permission, from Cox JL, Holden JM, Sagovsky R. Detection of postnatal depression: Development of the 10-item Edinburgh Postnatal Depression Scale. *Br J Psychiatry.* 1987;150(6):782-786).

TABLE 6-3.   Thyrotoxicosis Versus Hypothyroidism

	THYROTOXICOSIS	**HYPOTHYROIDISM**
Onset	1–4 months postpartum	4–8 months postpartum
Mechanism	Destruction-induced hormone release	Thyroid insufficiency
Symptoms	Small, painless goiter Palpitations, fatigue	Goiter, fatigue, inability to concentrate
Treatment	β-blocker	Thyroxine for 6–12 months
Sequela	Two-thirds euthyroid One-third hypothyroid	One-third permanent hypothyroidism

NOTES

CHAPTER 7

Medical Conditions in Pregnancy

WARD TIP

Women with pregestational diabetes have higher maternal and fetal complications when compared to those with gestational diabetes.

WARD TIP

Diabetic ketoacidosis may occur in patients with type 1 diabetes by:
- Corticosteroids (for lung maturity)
- β mimetics (for tocolysis)
- Hyperemesis gravidarum
- Infections

Pregestational Diabetes

- Diabetes that existed before pregnancy (see Table 7-1 and 7-2):
  - Type 1 diabetes: Insulin deficiency due to destruction of pancreatic beta cells
  - Type 2 diabetes: Insufficient insulin secretion or insulin resistance

T A B L E 7 - 1 .   Classification of Diabetes Complicating Pregnancy

		PLASMA GLUCOSE LEVEL		
CLASS	ONSET	FASTING	2-HOUR POST-PRANDIAL	THERAPY
A$_1$	Gestational	<105 mg/dL	<120 mg/dL	Diet controlled
A$_2$	Gestational	>105 mg/dL	>120 mg/dL	Insulin
CLASS	AGE OF ONSET	DURATION (YEAR)	VASCULAR DISEASE	THERAPY
B	Over 20	<10	None	Insulin
C	10–19	10–19	None	Insulin
D	Before 10	>20	Benign retinopathy	Insulin
F	Any	Any	Nephropathy	Insulin
R	Any	Any	proliferative retinopathy	Insulin
H	Any	Any	heart	Insulin

Reproduced, with permission, from Cunningham FG, Leveno KJ, Bloom SL, et al. *Williams Obstetrics.* 22nd ed. New York: McGraw-Hill: 2005:1171.

T A B L E 7 - 2 .   Complications Associated with Pre-existing Diabetes in Pregnancy

MATERNAL	FETAL	NEONATAL	OBSTETRIC
PP infections	Macrosomia	Hypoglycemia	Hypertensive disorders of pregnancy
Antepartum admission	Anomalies*	RDS	Caesarean delivery
	IUFD	NICU admission	Preterm delivery
	Polyhydramnios	Hyperbilirubinemia	

*Cardiac and spine anomalies are most common, risk proportional to A1c at conception.

IUFD. intrauterine fetal demise: NICU. neonatal intensive care unit: RDS.

MANAGEMENT

PRECONCEPTION	First trimester	Second trimester	Third trimester
• Optimize glycemic control • Goal HbA$_{1C}$ is <6 mg/dL. • HbA$_{1C}$ levels >10% significantly increase the risk of congenital malformations. • Folic acid 0.4 mg/day during preconception and early pregnancy to ↓ risk of NTDs. • Baseline 24-hr urine for total protein and creatinine clearance. • Ophthalmologic exam. • Electrocardiogram (ECG). • Thyroid-stimulating hormone (TSH).	• Start individualized insulin regimen. • Check fasting and 1-hr postprandial glucose. • Viability ultrasound. • Offer first trimester genetic screening (FTS or cfDNA). • Complete any remaining preconception evaluation	• 16–20 weeks: Offer quad screen if first trimester genetic screen not performed. • 18–20 weeks: Targeted ultrasound (US) to evaluate for anomalies, then US every 4 weeks for growth. • 20–22 weeks: Fetal echocardiogram looking for cardiac anomalies.	• Antenatal testing at 32–34 weeks or when poor glycemic control. • Monthly ultrasound to follow fetal growth • Consider delivery at 37–39 weeks depending on glycemic control • Recommend cesarean delivery if estimated fetal weight is >4500 g. • Start insulin drip in labor for glycemic control.

FIGURE 7-1. **Management of pre-existing diabetes in pregnancy.**

Thyroid Disease

Thyroid hormone is essential for the normal development of the fetal brain and mental function. The incidence of hyperthyroidism, hypothyroidism, and thyroiditis is each about 1%.

- Thyroid-stimulating hormone (TSH):
    - Essential for diagnosis of thyroid dysfunction in pregnancy
    - Unchanged in pregnancy
    - Does not cross the placenta
- Free thyroxine (T$_4$): Unchanged in pregnancy
- Thyroid-binding globulin (TBG) ↑ in pregnancy

HYPERTHYROIDISM

A 32-year-old G2P1001 patient at 16 weeks presents with symptoms of palpitations, nervousness, insomnia, and fatigue. Physical exam demonstrates a fine tremor in her hand, and pulse of 120 beats/min. What is the most likely diagnosis? What is the best treatment?
Answer: She has symptoms most consistent with hyperthyroidism. Although this patient has many symptoms that are normal for pregnancy, she should be screened for thyroid disorder with TSH and free T$_4$. Hyperthyroidism should be treated with propylthiouracil (PTU) or methimazole in pregnancy.

- Thyrotoxicosis complicates 1 in 2000 pregnancies.
- Graves' disease is the most common cause of thyrotoxicosis in pregnancy.

TREATMENT

- Ablation with radioactive iodine **contraindicated**.
- PTU:
    - Drug of choice for treatment during the first trimester of pregnancy.
    - Risk of liver failure has decreased use outside of T$_1$ (for first trimester).

EXAM TIP

Gestational diabetes causes macrosomia, especially when fasting glucose is high. Pregestational diabetes causes growth restriction especially due to concurrent maternal vascular disease.

WARD TIP

Insulin requirements ↑ during the second trimester due to the antagonistic effect of pregnancy hormones. Immediately following delivery, insulin requirements dramatically ↓.

WARD TIP

Patients in DKA will often have changes to the fetal heart rate tracing such as minimal variability and recurrent decelerations. In these settings, correcting maternal acidemia will correct the fetal acidemia.

WARD TIP

Free T$_4$ and TSH do not change in pregnancy and are the most sensitive markers to detect thyroid disease.

- Inhibits conversion of T_4 to T_3.
- Small amount transfers across the placenta.
- Methimazole:
  - Readily crosses placenta.
  - Associated with aplasia cutis and other teratogenic effects in fetus.
  - Currently used after T_1, (indicating first trimester) once organogenesis complete.
- Thyroidectomy:
  - Rarely necessary during pregnancy.
  - For patients who fail medical management.

COMPLICATIONS

- Patients who remain hyperthyroid despite treatment have higher incidence of preeclampsia, heart failure, and adverse perinatal outcomes (stillbirth, preterm labor).
- Neonatal thyrotoxicosis: 1% risk due to placental transfer of thyroid-stimulating antibodies.
- Fetal goiter/hypothyroid—from PTU.
- **Thyroid storm:** An acute, life-threatening, hypermetabolic state in patients with thyrotoxicosis. Often associated with heart failure. Treatment in intensive care unit (ICU) setting:
  - PTU orally or nasogastric tube.
  - β-blocker to control tachycardia.
  - Sodium iodide inhibits release of T_3 and T_4 (lithium if iodine allergic).
  - Dexamethasone blocks peripheral conversion of T_4 to T_3.

HYPOTHYROIDISM

- Hashimoto's thyroiditis is the most common cause of hypothyroidism during pregnancy.
- Subclinical hypothyroidism is more common than overt hypothyroidism.
  - Overt hypothyroidism is diagnosed by ↑ TSH and ↓ free T_4.
  - Subclinical hypothyroidism is an ↑ TSH with normal free T_4.
- Diagnosis may be difficult, as many of the symptoms of hypothyroidism (weight gain, fatigue, constipation, etc.) are also symptoms of pregnancy.
- The American College of Obstetricians and Gynecologists recommends **against** routine prenatal screening for subclinical hypothyroidism.

TREATMENT

Levothyroxine replacement:

- TSH is monitored every 4 weeks after the initiation of treatment or a change in dose.
- TSH is monitored every trimester if no change in medication is needed due to increased thyroxine requirements in advancing pregnancy.
- Usually requires 20% increase in dose once pregnancy is diagnosed (take extra done on Saturday and Sunday).

COMPLICATIONS OF UNTREATED HYPOTHYROIDISM

- Preeclampsia
- Placental abruption
- Cardiac dysfunction
- Low birth weight
- Still births

Chronic Hypertension

 A 37-year-old G3P2002 patient at 37 weeks presents to triage reporting a severe headache for 1 day that is unrelieved with acetaminophen. Her pregnancy has been complicated by chronic hypertension (HTN) that has been well controlled with methyldopa. Her blood pressures are normally 140/90. She had no proteinuria during her prenatal visits. She reports no visual changes, right upper quadrant pain, contractions, vaginal bleeding, or leakage of fluid. She reports good fetal movement. Her blood pressure is 180/110 and 175/100. She has 3+ proteinuria. Fetal heart rate is reassuring. What is the most likely diagnosis?

Answer: Chronic HTN with superimposed preeclampsia with severe features. Patients with chronic HTN are at high risk for developing preeclampsia; worsening blood pressure and new proteinuria can indicate the development of superimposed preeclampsia.

 WARD TIP

Poorly controlled HTN and presence of end organ damage = ↑ adverse outcomes in pregnancy

- HTN prior to 20th week of gestation.
- Prevalence is markedly ↑ in obese and diabetic patients.

PRECONCEPTION

Evaluate for renal and cardiac function:
- Echocardiography: Patients with left ventricular hypertrophy or cardiac dysrhythmias indicate long-standing or poorly controlled HTN leading to ↑ risk for congestive heart failure (CHF) in pregnancy.
- Serum creatinine and proteinuria: Abnormal results indicate risk for adverse pregnancy outcome.

 WARD TIP

Blood pressure is dynamic during pregnancy. It normally ↓ in T_2. If a patient with chronic HTN is seen for the first time in T_2, she may appear normotensive.

COMPLICATIONS

- Superimposed preeclampsia: Development of preeclampsia in the setting of chronic HTN. 25–50% of pregnancies with cHTN.
- Abruptio placenta: ↑ risk with severe HTN. Smoking compounds the risk.
- Fetal growth restriction: Directly related to the severity of HTN.
- Preterm delivery.

MANAGEMENT

- Fetus should undergo antenatal testing to assess for adequate placental perfusion.
- Fetus should receive ultrasounds to monitor growth.
- Unless other complications develop, patients with chronic HTN should deliver at term, 37–39 weeks.
- Vaginal delivery is preferred to cesarean.

 WARD TIP

In pregnancy, elevated blood pressure is defined as ≥140/90.

MEDICATIONS

- Labetalol: α- and β-adrenergic blocker
- α-Methyldopa: Generally not used outside obstetrics, not preferred
- Hydralazine: Vasodilator
- Nifedipine: Calcium channel blocker
- AVOID or DISCONTINUE Angiotensin-converting enzyme (ACE) inhibitors/angiotensin receptor blockers (ARBs) due to teratogenic potential (hypocalvaria and renal defects).

Cardiovascular Disease

- Pregnancy-induced hemodynamic changes have profound effects on underlying heart disease. Cardiac output ↑ by 50% in midpregnancy.
- Need to monitor for CHF.
- Some congenital heart lesions are inherited. There is a 4% risk of congenital heart disease in the infant of a patient with a particular defect.
- Pain control:
  - Essential during labor and delivery to decrease the cardiac workload.
  - Continuous epidural anesthesia is recommended.
  - General anesthesia can cause hypotension.
- Vaginal delivery (spontaneous, forceps, vacuum) desired over cesarean delivery.

MITRAL STENOSIS (MS)

- ↑ preload due to normal ↑ in blood volume results in left atrial overload. ↑ pressure in the left atrium is transmitted into the lungs, resulting in **pulmonary HTN**.
- Tachycardia associated with labor and delivery exacerbates the pulmonary HTN because of decreased filling time. May lead to pulmonary edema.
- Twenty-five percent of patients with mitral stenosis have cardiac failure for the first time during pregnancy.
- Fetus is at risk for growth restriction.
- **Peripartum period is the most hazardous time.**

MITRAL VALVE PROLAPSE

- Normally asymptomatic
- Systolic click on physical exam
- Generally safe pregnancy

AORTIC STENOSIS

- Similar problems with mitral stenosis
- Avoid tachycardia and fluid overload

EISENMENGER SYNDROME AND CONDITIONS WITH PULMONARY HYPERTENSION

- Extremely dangerous to the mother.
- This condition may justify the termination of pregnancy on medical grounds.
- Maternal mortality can be as high as **50%**, with death usually occurring postpartum.

Pulmonary Disease

The adaptations to the respiratory system during pregnancy must be able to satisfy the ↑ O_2 demands of the hyperdynamic circulation and the fetus.

Advanced pregnancy may worsen the pathophysiological effects of many acute and chronic lung diseases.

ASTHMA

- Asthmatics have a small but significant ↑ in pregnancy complications.
- Fetal growth restriction ↑ with the severity of asthma.
- Arterial blood gases analysis provides objective information as to severity of asthma.

EPIDEMIOLOGY

- One to four percent of pregnancies are complicated by asthma.
- The impact of pregnancy on asthma is variable; roughly 1/3 improve, 1/3 worsen, and 1/3 stay the same.

TREATMENT

- Generally, asthma is exacerbated by respiratory tract infections, so influenza vaccine should be given. Also, consider pneumococcal vaccine if the patient has not had recently.
- Pregnant asthmatics can be treated with β-agonists, epinephrine, and inhaled steroids (same medications used outside of pregnancy).

PNEUMONIA

The pathogens that cause pneumonia are in pregnancy at the same as they are outside of pregnancy. The diagnosis is also made the same way during pregnancy as in the nonpregnant patient. If anything, pregnant patients are at higher risk of pneumonia given the physiologic changes of pregnancy that makes them more susceptible to acute respiratory distress syndrome (ARDS). Respiratory viruses, including influenza and COVID are well known to be more severe when they infect pregnant patients, including higher risk of ICU admission, need for mechanical ventilation, and death. Patients with PNA are at high risk of preterm labor and preterm delivery. In a patient who is acidotic, there may be changes in the fetal heart rate tracing (decreased variability). This is a time where management should focus on stabilizing the patient, as this will correct the fetal academia and is safer for the patient than urgent delivery.

WARD TIP

Asthma follows the rule of 3rds: 1/3 of patients with asthma have improvement of symptoms during pregnancy, 1/3 have no change in disease severity, and 1/3 have worsening of symptoms during pregnancy.

WARD TIP

Pregnancy is associated with a physiologic respiratory alkalosis, thus a normal pH n pregnancy is higher than in the nonpregnant state.

WARD TIP

Severe pneumonia is a common cause of ARDS.

TABLE 7-3. Changes to ABG in Pregnancy

ARTERIAL BLOOD GAS MEASUREMENT	FIRST TRIMESTER	THIRD TRIMESTER	NONPREGNANT
pH	7.42–7.46	7.43	7.4
PaO_2 (mm Hg)	105–106	101–106	93
$PaCO_2$ (mm Hg)	28–29	26–30	37
Serum HCO_3 (mEq/L)	18	17	23

MANAGEMENT

- Any pregnant patient suspected of having pneumonia should undergo chest radiography (CXR) with an abdominal shield (indications are the same as in nonpregnant patients).
- Abnormalities seen on CXR may take up to 6 weeks to resolve.
- Pneumococcal vaccine is recommended in pregnant patients who are immunocompromised or have baseline cardiac/renal/pulmonary disease.
- Influenza vaccine is recommended for all patients in all trimesters.
- Antibiotics similar to nonpregnant patients. For uncomplicated community-acquired pneumonia, treat with a beta-lactam (ceftriaxone, cefotaxime, ampicillin-sulbactam) plus azithromycin.
- Vancomycin is added for community-acquired methicillin-resistant *Staphylococcus aureus* (MRSA).

WARD TIP

Pregnant patients with asymptomatic bacteriuria should be treated because of their ↑ risk of developing pyelonephritis.

Renal and Urinary Tract Disorders

Pregnancy causes hydronephrosis (dilatation of renal pelvis, calyces, and ureters; R > L):

- Pregnant uterus compresses the lower ureter.
- Hormonal milieu ↓ ureteral tone (progesterone).
- Urinary stasis and ↑ vesicoureteral reflux lead to increased risk of pyelonephritis.

WARD TIP

Hydronephrosis: Usually R > L

WARD TIP

High incidence of asymptomatic bacteriuria: patients with sickle-cell trait.

ASYMPTOMATIC BACTERIURIA

- Five percent incidence.
- If untreated, 25% will develop pyelonephritis.
- Routine screening at the first prenatal visit recommended.

PYELONEPHRITIS

 A 23-year-old G3P2002 patient at 25 weeks presents to triage with fever, nausea, and vomiting for 1 day. She reports back pain and lower abdominal pain. She has a fever of 101.2°F (38.4°C), clear lungs, and right costovertebral tenderness. Fetal heart rate is reassuring. The monitor shows contractions every 2 minutes. Cervix is closed/thick/high. Urine dip shows many bacteria, leukocytes, nitrites, and ketones. What is the most likely diagnosis? What is the next step in management?

Answer: The clinical presentation is most consistent with pyelonephritis. She should be admitted to the hospital and given IV hydration and IV antibiotics.

WARD TIP

Most common cause of septic shock in pregnancy: Urosepsis.

- Acute pyelonephritis is the most common serious medical complication of pregnancy and most common non-obstetric indication for antepartum admission.
- Unilateral, right-sided >50% of cases.
- *Escherichia coli* cultured 80% of cases.
- Bacteremia in 15–20% of patients with acute pyelonephritis.

COMPLICATIONS

- Renal dysfunction: ↑ creatinine
- Pulmonary edema: Endotoxin-induced alveolar injury

- ARDS
- Hemolysis
- Preterm labor

DIFFERENTIAL DIAGNOSIS

- Preterm labor
- Chorioamnionitis
- Appendicitis
- Placental abruption

MANAGEMENT

- Hospitalization
- IV antibiotics, usually cephalosporins (pending sensitivity studies)
- IV hydration for adequate urinary output
- Long-term antibiotic suppression for remainder of pregnancy is warranted

Gastrointestinal (GI) Disorders

During advanced pregnancy, gastrointestinal (GI) symptoms become difficult to assess, and physical findings are often obscured by the enlarged uterus.

APPENDICITIS

- Appendicitis is the most common surgical condition in pregnancy (occurs in 1 in 2000 births).
- Incidence is same throughout pregnancy, but rupture is more frequent in the third trimester (40%) than in the first trimester (10%).
- Symptoms of appendicitis, such as nausea, vomiting, and anorexia, may also be a part of normal pregnancy complaints, making diagnosis difficult.
- Uterus displaces the appendix superiorly and laterally. Pain may not be located at McBurney's point (RLQ).
- Physical exam may be obscured by the enlarging uterus.

COMPLICATIONS

- Preterm labor and Preterm delivery
- Maternal and fetal sepsis → neonatal neurologic injury

TREATMENT

- Appendectomy
- Laparoscopy (Ideally performed in the second trimester)
- Laparotomy in later pregnancy

CHOLELITHIASIS AND CHOLECYSTITIS

- Incidence of cholecystitis is 1 in 1000 pregnancies (more common than nonpregnant).
- Same clinical picture as nonpregnant.
- Medical management unless common bile duct obstruction or pancreatitis develops, in which case a cholecystectomy should be performed.
- High risk of preterm labor.

EXAM TIP

Most common cause of persistent pyelonephritis despite adequate therapy: Nephrolithiasis.

WARD TIP

Increased estrogen in pregnancy → increased cholesterol saturation in bile → increased biliary stasis and gallstones

WARD TIP

In pregnancy, the appendix is often displaced superiorly and laterally (i.e., not in right lower quadrant (RLQ)).

WARD TIP

Most common indications for surgery in pregnancy:
- Appendicitis
- Adnexal masses
- Cholecystitis/gallstones

WARD TIP

General anesthesia can be performed in any trimester without aberrant fetal effects. However, for nonemergent surgeries, the second trimester is preferred.

Seizure Disorder

COMPLICATIONS

- Patients with epilepsy taking anticonvulsants during pregnancy have higher risk of fetal malformations and preeclampsia.
- Pregnant patients with epilepsy are more prone to seizures due to the associated stress and fatigue of pregnancy, as well as the metabolic changes that often impact plasma levels of anti-epileptic medications.

TREATMENT

- Management of the epileptic patient should begin with pre-pregnancy counseling.
- Antiepileptic medications should be reduced to the minimum dose of the minimum number of antiepileptic medications that suppress seizure activity.
- Folic acid supplementation is recommended for those patients taking antiepileptic medications.
- Once pregnant, the fetus should be screened for NTDs and congenital anomalies.
- Blood levels of antiepileptic medications should be monitored throughout pregnancy to ensure the drug level is in the therapeutic range.

Thromboembolic Disorders

> A 27-year-old G1 patient at 26 weeks presents with swelling of the left leg and thigh since the previous night. She reports no trauma, dyspnea, or chest pain. She is afebrile and is in no apparent distress. Her left calf measures 4 cm more than the right and is tender to palpation. The fetal status is reassuring. What is the most likely diagnosis?
> **Answer:** Deep vein thrombosis.

DEEP VEIN THROMBOSIS (DVT)

SIGNS AND SYMPTOMS

- Calf/leg swelling
- Calf pain
- Palpable cord in calf

DIAGNOSIS (FIGURE 7-2)

- Venography: Gold standard; many complications, time consuming, cumbersome
- Impedance plethysmography: Better for larger veins
- Compression ultrasonography: Test most often used currently

COMPLICATIONS

Pulmonary embolism (PE) develops in about 25% of patients with untreated DVT.

TREATMENT

- Anticoagulation with unfractionated or low-molecular-weight heparin (LMWH) during pregnancy.
- Heparin and LMHW should be suspended during labor and delivery (ideally 12–24 hours before onset of labor if known) and restarted after 12–24 hours, depending on the degree of trauma to the genital tract.

WARD TIP

Contrast venography is the gold standard for diagnosis of lower-extremity DVT, but this is very rarely used. Diagnosis usually made with compression ultrasonography.

WARD TIP

Warfarin is a teratogen, so not used in pregnancy. Can breast-feed on it postpartum.

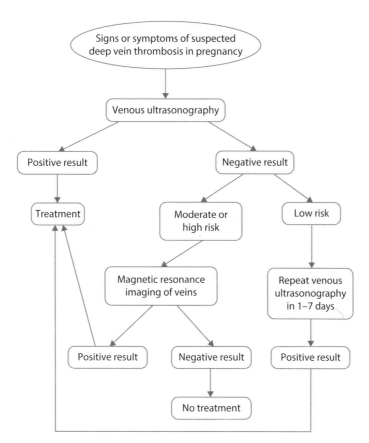

FIGURE 7-2. Diagnosis of deep venous thrombosis. (Reprinted with permission from American College of Obstetricians and Gynecologists. Robert Silver, MD and Charles Lockwood, MD, *Thrombosis, Thrombophilia, and Thromboembolism: Clinical Updates in Women's Health Care*, Volume XV, Number 3 Washington, DC: American College of Obstetricians and Gynecologists, May 2016.)

- Okay to convert to warfarin postpartum (do **not** use warfarin when pregnant), or continue LMWH.
- Anticoagulation ↓ the risk of PE to <5%.

PULMONARY EMBOLISM (PE)

- **Symptoms:** Dyspnea, chest pain, cough, syncope, hemoptysis.
- **Signs:** Tachypnea, tachycardia, apprehension, rales, hypoxemia.
- **Diagnosis:** CT pulmonary angiography or lung scintigraphy (ventilation/perfusion or V/Q scan).
- **Complications** Maternal death.
- **Treatment:** Anticoagulation with heparin/LMWH.
- Half of patients presenting with a DVT will have a "silent" PE.

THROMBOPHILIAS

- ↑ risk of thrombus formation and associated complications.
- **Antithrombin III deficiency:** The most thrombogenic of the heritable coagulopathies.
- **Protein C deficiency:** 6- to 12-fold ↑ risk of first venous thromboembolism (VTE) in pregnancy.
- **Protein S deficiency:** Two- to six-fold ↑ risk of first VTE in pregnancy.
- **Factor V Leiden mutation:**
  - Most common heritable thrombophilia; 5–8% of the general population.
  - Heterozygous inheritance.
  - Four- to eightfold ↑ risk of first VTE in pregnancy.

WARD TIP

Pulmonary embolus may originate in the iliac veins rather than the calf in pregnancy.

- **Antiphospholipid antibodies:** Commonly seen in patients with lupus. See section Antiphospholipid Syndrome.
- **Prothrombin G20210A mutation**.

COMPLICATIONS OF UNTREATED THROMBOPHILIA

- Preeclampsia/eclampsia
- HELLP syndrome (hemolysis, elevated liver enzymes, low platelets)
- Fetal growth restriction
- Placental abruption
- Recurrent abortion
- Intrauterine fetal demise

TREATMENT

Heparin or LMWH

Sickle Cell Disease

- Red cells with hemoglobin S undergo sickling with ↓ oxygen leading to cell membrane damage.
- One in 12 individuals of African descent are carriers.
- **Sickle-cell crisis:** Pain due to ischemia and infarction in various organs. Infarction of bone marrow causes severe bone pain.
- Crisis more common in pregnancy.
- Acute chest syndrome: Pleuritic chest pain, fever, cough, lung infiltrates, hypoxia.

PREGNANCY COMPLICATIONS

- Thromboses (cerebral vein thrombosis, DVT, PE)
- Pneumonia
- Pyelonephritis
- Gestational HTN, preeclampsia, or eclampsia

OBSTETRIC COMPLICATIONS

- Placental abruption
- Preterm delivery
- Fetal growth restriction
- Stillbirth

MANAGEMENT

- Supplementation with 4 mg/day of folic acid to accommodate for rapid cell turnover.
- IV hydration and pain control for crises.
- Prophylactic blood transfusions throughout pregnancy are **controversial**— though hemoglobin (Hgb) > 8 recommended at time of delivery.

Anemia

Physiologic anemia during pregnancy is due to a greater expansion of plasma volume relative to increase in RBC mass (hemodilution). Anemia during pregnancy also occurs due to iron deficiency. The CDC defines anemia during pregnancy as a hemoglobin <11 g/dL. Sixteen to twenty-nine percent of pregnant patients become anemic during T3. Anemia is associated with increased rates of preterm delivery, IUGR, and low birth weight. Patients with anemia should be evaluated for iron deficiency by checking folate, b12, ferritin, TIBC, and CBC. If there is evidence of iron deficiency, iron can be repleted orally or IV.

WARD TIP

The two most common causes of anemia during pregnancy and the puerperium are iron deficiency and acute blood loss.

Antiphospholipid Syndrome

DIAGNOSIS

Clinical Criteria
- Arterial or venous thrombosis
- Pregnancy morbidity (need one):
  - At least one otherwise unexplained fetal death at or beyond 10 weeks
  - At least one preterm birth before 34 weeks due to preeclampsia or severe growth restriction
  - At least three consecutive spontaneous abortions before 10 weeks

Laboratory Criteria
- Lupus anticoagulant.
- Anticardiolipin antibody.
- Anti-β_2 glycoprotein.
- At least one of these findings must be present in plasma, on at least two occasions >12 weeks apart.

MANAGEMENT
- Prophylactic anticoagulation in pregnancy
- Baby aspirin, baseline preeclampsia labs
- Assessment of fetal growth in the third trimester and antenatal testing

EXAM TIP

Antiphospholipid Syndrome is an acquired thrombophilia, thus it is not genetically inherited.

Systemic Lupus Erythematosus

COMPLICATIONS

Significant ↑ in maternal morbidity/mortality and other complications:
- Preeclampsia.
- Preterm labor.
- Fetal growth restriction.
- Anemia.
- Thrombophilia.
- Neonates may have symptoms of lupus for several months after birth.
- **Congenital heart block** may be seen in the offspring of patients with anti-Ro (SS-A) and anti-La (SS-B).

MANAGEMENT
- Patients should be counseled to get pregnant while their disease is in remission.
- Monitor for disease flares and hypertensive episodes.

EXAM TIP

Presence of anti-Ro (SS-A) and anti-La (SS-B) is associated with fetal congenital heart block.

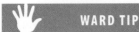

- Unless there is evidence of fetal compromise, the pregnancy should progress to term.
- High-dose methylprednisolone can be given for a lupus flare.
- Azathioprine is an immunosuppressant that can be used safely in pregnancy.
- Cyclophosphamide, methotrexate, and mycophenolate mofetil should be avoided, or at least not started until after 12 weeks' gestation. The risks and benefits should always be weighed.

Pruritic Urticarial Papules and Plaques of Pregnancy (PUPPP)

INCIDENCE

- The most common pruritic dermatosis in pregnancy.
- Incidence is 1/160–1/300 singleton pregnancies, 8- to 12-fold ↑ with multiples.
- Seldom occurs in subsequent pregnancies.

CLINICAL SIGNS AND SYMPTOMS

- Intensely pruritic cutaneous eruption that usually appears late in pregnancy.
- Usually starts as erythematous papules within stria with periumbilical sparing.
- Begins on the abdomen and spread to arms and legs. Coalesces to form urticarial plaques. The face, palms, and soles are usually spared.

TREATMENT

- Oral antihistamines and topical steroids are the mainstays of treatment.
- May require systemic corticosteroids for severe pruritus.
- Rash usually disappears shortly before or a few days after delivery.

Cancer Therapy During Pregnancy

SURGERY

As long as the reproductive organs are not involved, surgery is generally well tolerated by both the mother and fetus during pregnancy and should not be delayed.

RADIATION

- Therapeutic radiation can cause significant complications in the fetus, such as carcinogenesis, cell death, and brain damage.
- The most susceptible period is during organogenesis.
- The site of the tumor is important. Radiation to head and neck cancers can be done more safely than radiation to abdominal tumors.

CHEMOTHERAPY

- Risks to the fetus include malformations (if exposed in first trimester) and growth restriction.
- Risk is highest during organogenesis. Few adverse outcomes are seen if chemotherapeutic agents are used outside the first trimester.

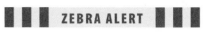 **ZEBRA ALERT**

A new cancer diagnosis in pregnancy is rare, but because symptoms (fatigue, anemia, malaise) often overlap with common pregnancy symptoms, diagnosis may be delayed.

NOTES

Obstetric Complications

WARD TIP

What is the treatment of choice for seizure prophylaxis in pregnant patient with preeclampsia? Magnesium sulfate (MgSO$_4$)
What is its antidote in case of mag toxicity? Calcium gluconate

WARD TIP

Chronic HTN:
- ↑ BP outside of pregnancy
- ↑ BP prior to 20 weeks' gestation
- ↑ BP persisting after 12 weeks post-partum

WARD TIP

BP in severe range should be treated within 30–60 minutes. Oral nifedipine or IV labetolol or IV hydralazine are all appropriate agents for lowering of severe range BPs.

Hypertension in Pregnancy

HYPERTENSIVE DISORDERS OF PREGNANCY

 A 28-year-old G2P1001 patient at 37 weeks complains of severe headaches and black spots in her vision. Her blood pressures (BP) are 165/95 and 163/96 and she has 4+ protein on urine dipstick. Her cervical exam is closed, thick, and high. The fetal heart tones are reassuring and she has no contractions. The ultrasound (US) shows a fetus that is appropriate for 37 weeks, with normal amniotic fluid index (AFI), and in cephalic position. What is the next best step?
Answer: This patient has signs and symptoms of preeclampsia with severe features and should be delivered immediately, especially when term. Induction of labor is a safe option in this care. Patients with preeclampsia can have a seizure at any point before, during, or after labor, so seizure prophylaxis with magnesium sulfate is indicated.

Hypertensive disorders of pregnancy include gestational hypertension (HTN), preeclampsia, preeclampsia with severe features, and chronic HTN with superimposed preeclampsia (with or without severe features) (Table 8-1). Eclampsia is the development of grand mal seizures in a pregnant or postpartum patient. HELLP (hemolysis, elevated liver enzymes, low platelets) is a manifestation of preeclampsia with severe features. Hypertensive disorders of pregnancy impact patients AFTER 20 weeks' gestation. Patients with elevated blood pressure (BP) prior to 20 weeks are considered to have chronic HTN.

There are four categories of HTN in pregnancy:
1. **Chronic HTN during pregnancy:**
   - Preexisting HTN begins prior to pregnancy or before 20 weeks.
   - Defined as a sustained systolic BP ≥ 140 mm Hg and/or diastolic BP ≥ 90 mm Hg documented on more than one occasion *prior* to the 20th week of gestation, HTN that existed before pregnancy, or HTN that persists >12 weeks after delivery.
   - Usually not associated with significant proteinuria or end-organ damage if well controlled.

TABLE 8-1. **Characteristics of Gestational Hypertensive Disorders**

	cHTN	gHTN	preX	sPREX
Onset of elevated BPs	Prior to pregnancy or <20 weeks	>20 weeks	>20 weeks	>20 weeks
BP criteria	>140/>90	>140/>90	>140/>90	>140/>90 with other s/sx OR >160/110 if only BP
Protienuria present	Yes or no	No	UPC > 0.3 24-hour urine 300 mg UA 1+ protein	May or may not be present
Associated symptoms	No	No	No	Can have HA, vision changes, right upper quadrant pain, nausea and vomiting
Lab abnormalities present	In severe cases can have elevated baseline Cr.	No	May have mildly low plts or mildly elevated LFTs	Plts < 100 Cr > 1.1 LFTs x2 normal

2. **Gestational HTN:**
   - HTN without proteinuria or other signs/symptoms of preeclampsia.
   - A sustained or transient systolic BP ≥ 140 mm Hg and/or diastolic BP ≥ 90 mm Hg occurs after 20 weeks.
3. **Preeclampsia:**
   - Defined as new onset HTN with either proteinuria or end-organ dysfunction (or both) after 20 weeks (proteinuria no longer required to diagnose preeclampsia with severe features).
   - **Criteria for diagnosis of preeclampsia:**
     - Systolic BP ≥140 mm Hg or diastolic BP ≥90 mm Hg twice at least 4 hour apart. AND
     - Proteinuria: 1+ on dipstick or ≥300 mg/24 hour or protein (mg/dL)/creatinine (mg/dL) ratio ≥0.3.
     - In pregnant patients with new onset HTN without proteinuria, a new finding of any of the following is diagnostic of preeclampsia: (though these would all be considered severe features)
       - Thrombocytopenia (platelet < 100,000/mL).
       - Serum creatinine >1.1 mg/dL or doubling of serum creatinine.
       - LFTs at least twice the normal concentration.
       - Pulmonary edema.
       - Cerebral or visual symptoms (headache, scotomata).
   - **Preeclampsia with severe features** is defined by the presence of one of the following:
     - Severe BP elevation: systolic BP ≥160 mmHg or diastolic BP ≥110 mmHg at least 4 hour apart. OR Systolic BP ≥140 mm Hg or diastolic BP ≥90 mm Hg twice at least 4 hour apart. AND
     - Neurologic dysfunction: headache, scotomata, altered mental status.
     - Renal abnormality: serum creatinine >1.1 mg/dL or doubling of serum creatinine.
     - Hepatic abnormality: Epigastric or right upper quadrant pain (hepatocellular ischemia and edema that stretches Glisson's capsule), ↑ aspartate transaminase (AST), alanine transaminase (ALT) ≥ twice the normal level, or both.
     - Pulmonary edema.
     - Thrombocytopenia (<100,000 platelets/μL).
4. **Superimposed preeclampsia:**
   - Preeclampsia in patients with chronic HTN in pregnancy—can be with or without severe features.
   - Defined by new onset of either proteinuria or end-organ dysfunction after 20 weeks in a patient with chronic HTN.
   - For patients with chronic HTN who have preexisting proteinuria, superimposed preeclampsia is defined by worsening HTN or development of severe features (see above).
   - Twenty-five percent of patients with chronic HTN in pregnancy develop preeclampsia.

PATHOPHYSIOLOGY

Vasospasm in various organs (brain, kidneys, lungs, uterus) causes most of the signs and symptoms of preeclampsia; however, the cause of the vasospasm is unknown.

The pathophysiology of preeclampsia has many factors that are poorly understood. However, one contributing factor is the method of development of placental vasculature in early pregnancy.

COMPLICATIONS

- Placental abruption
- Eclampsia

WARD TIP

Superimposed preeclampsia:
Preeclampsia in the presence of preexisting chronic HTN. Diagnosed with worsening BPs and new or worsening proteinuria. Patients with chronic HTN are at ↑ risk of developing superimposed preeclampsia.

WARD TIP

Though many patients have a lot of edema associated with preeclampsia, this is NOT part of the diagnostic criteria.

WARD TIP

Preeclampsia may be asymptomatic; it is critical to pick it up during routine prenatal visits.

WARD TIP

The only definitive treatment for preeclampsia is delivery.

WARD TIP

Magnesium toxicity (7–10 mEq/L) is associated with loss of patellar reflexes, respiratory depression, and cardiac arrest. Treat with calcium gluconate 10% solution 1 g IV.

WARD TIP

Eclampsia is considered a form of severe preeclampsia. More commonly it is NOT preceded by preeclampsia.

WARD TIP

Magnesium sulfate prevents seizures in preeclampsia; does not treat HTN.

- Coagulopathy
- Renal failure
- Hepatic subcapsular hematoma
- Uteroplacental insufficiency and fetal growth restriction

TREATMENT

- The only cure for preeclampsia and its variants is **delivery** of the fetus.
- Patients with any gestational hypertensive disorder >37 weeks → delivery.
- Patients with preeclampsia with severe features >34 weeks → delivery. (Table 8-2)
- **Magnesium sulfate (MgSO$_4$)** is given for **seizure prophylaxis** when the decision is made to deliver fetus or when expectantly managing a patient with severe preeclampsia. It is **not** a treatment for HTN.
- For patients with severe preeclampsia by BPs only—can start medications to maintain BPs <160/<110 and continue pregnancy if less than 34 weeks.
- **Preeclampsia management:**
  - Preterm: Close monitoring for worsening maternal or fetal disease (weekly BP checks and labs)
    - Antenatal testing: (non-stress tests [NSTs] and/or biophysical profiles [BPPs]) to ensure fetal well-being.
    - Bed rest is not necessary, although ↓ physical activity is recommended.
    - Administer steroids if indicated for fetal lung maturity.
    - Deliver based on gestational age (GA), and maternal and fetal condition.
- **Management of severe preeclampsia:**
  - Preterm: Close monitoring in hospital, and in general, deliver by 34 weeks or when the maternal or fetal condition is unstable.
    - Delivery may not be in the best interest of the preterm baby, but may be indicated to prevent worsening maternal disease.
    - Vaginal delivery is usually attempted via induction of labor; cesarean delivery for other obstetric indications.

WARD TIP

HTN may be absent in 20% of patients with HELLP syndrome and severe in 50%.

TABLE 8-2. Indications for Delivery in the Setting of Severe Preeclampsia

MATERNAL	OBSTETRIC	FETAL
Headache	Eclampsia	Reversed end diastolic flow in umbilical artery
Severe RUQ pain	Placental abruption	
LFTs > twice normal		Nonreasoning fetal heart rate tracing
Platelets <100K	HELLP	
Cr > 1.1 or twice patient's baseline	GA > 34 weeks	IUFD
Altered mental status or vision changes		Non-viable fetus
Stroke or MI		
Pulmonary edema		

GA, gestational age; HELLP, hemolysis, elevated liver enzymes, low platelets; IUFD, intrauterine fetal demise.

- Start MgSO₄ for seizure prophylaxis.
- Administer steroids for fetal lung maturity.
- Term patients with severe preeclampsia should be delivered.

HELLP SYNDROME

- HELLP syndrome is likely a manifestation of severe preeclampsia with:
  - **H**emolysis.
  - **E**levated **L**iver enzymes.
  - **L**ow **P**latelets.
- It is associated with high morbidity, and immediate delivery is indicated. It may occur with or without HTN.

ECLAMPSIA

Defined as seizure or coma without another cause in a patient with pre-eclampsia. Eclampsia → hemorrhagic stroke → death

TREATMENT

- Airway, breathing, and circulation (ABCs).
- Rule out other causes: Head trauma is a possible confounder; others include cerebral tumors, cerebral venous thrombosis, drug overdoses, epilepsy, and cerebrovascular accidents.
- Control seizures with magnesium sulfate (the only anticonvulsant used).
- Delivery is the only definitive treatment; expectant management is not appropriate.
  - Induction of labor may be appropriate to accomplish vaginal delivery, and factors such as GA, cervical exam, fetal position, and parity should be considered when deciding mode of delivery.
  - Control BP with antihypertensived.

RISK FACTORS FOR HYPERTENSIVE DISORDERS OF PREGNANCY

- Nulliparity
- Age <16 or >40 years
- Family history of preeclampsia in first degree relative
- Chronic HTN
- Chronic renal disease
- Antiphospholipid syndrome
- Diabetes mellitus
- Multiple gestation
- History of preeclampsia in prior pregnancy

ANTIHYPERTENSIVE AGENTS USED IN PREGNANCY

Short-Term Control

- **Hydralazine:** IV or PO, direct vasodilator. Side effects: systemic lupus erythematosus (SLE)-like syndrome, headache, palpitations.
- **Labetalol:** IV or PO, nonselective β₁ and α₁ blocker. Side effects: headache and tremor.
- **Nifedipine:** PO, calcium channel blocker. Side effects: edema, dizziness.

Long-Term Control

- **Nifedipine:** PO, calcium channel blocker. Side effects: edema, dizziness.
- **Labetalol:** PO, nonselective β₁ and α₁ blocker. Side effects: headache and tremor, can exacerbate asthma.

Gestational Diabetes Mellitus (GDM)

 A 33-year-old G4P3003 patient at 26 weeks undergoes the 50-g glucose challenge test (GCT). The result is 160 mg/dL. What is the next step in management?
Answer: She should undergo the 3-hour glucose tolerance test (GTT) since her 1-hour result was >140 mg/dL.

- **Pregestational diabetes (DM):** Patient diagnosed with DM prior to pregnancy.
- **Gestational diabetes (GDM):** Patient develops diabetes only during pregnancy.
    - Prevalence in 6–7% of population.
    - A1: Controlled with diet.
    - A2: Requires insulin or oral agents.

Screening

When obtaining a patient's history, look for risk factors for gestational diabetes or undiagnosed type 2 diabetes. This will direct screening. If patient is suspected of having type 2 diabetes, order HbA1c at first visit.
- See Chapter 7 regarding Pregestational Diabetes.
- **Risk factors for GDM:**
    - Age >35.
    - Prior pregnancy with gestational diabetes.
    - Family history of diabetes in a first degree relative.
    - Obesity (BMI >30).
    - Previous infant >4000 g (8¾ lb).
- Screening for GDM:
    - Two-step approach:
        - Most widely used.
        - First step is GCT to identify patients at high risk—i.e., screening test.
        - Second step is GTT—i.e., diagnostic test.

TWO-STEP APPROACH

- **GCT** at 24–28 weeks or at new OB in patients with risk factors:
    - Give 50-g glucose load (nonfasting state).
    - Draw glucose blood level 1 hour later.
    - If ≥140, a 3-hour GTT is then administered to diagnose GDM.
    - If >200, patient is diagnosed with GDM and a diabetic diet is initiated.
- **3-hour GTT**—if GCT is ≥140 and <200:
    - Fast at least 8 hour.
    - Draw fasting glucose level.
    - Give 100-g glucose load.
    - Draw glucose levels at 1 hour, 2 hour, and 3 hour.
    - Diagnosis of GDM made if two or more values are equal to or greater than those listed. Either criterion can be used to make the diagnosis.

Management

The key factors involved in successful management of pregnancies complicated by GDM:
- Nutrition counseling and glucose log should be reviewed on a regular basis.
- Goal blood glucoses: fasting <95 and 2-hour postprandial (breakfast, lunch, dinner) glucose <120.

EXAM TIP

What is a major fetal complication of GDM? Macrosomia

EXAM TIP

Gestational diabetes results from human placental lactogen secreted during pregnancy, which has large glucagon-like effects.

WARD TIP

If a pregnant patient has an abnormal 1-hour GCT, then check a 3-hour GTT.

WARD TIP

Fasting glucose is the most important for fetal and maternal outcomes.

WARD TIP

Thirty percent of patients with GDM develop diabetes mellitus in later life.

TABLE 8-3. Complications of GDM

MATERNAL	OBSTETRIC	FETAL/NEONATAL
Increased risk of third/fourth degree laceration	Increased risk of caesarean delivery or operative vaginal delivery	Macrosomia and large for gestational age Hyperbilirubinemia
↑ lifetime risk of type 2 diabetes.	Shoulder dystocia	Hypoglycemia NICU admission

NICU; neonatal intensive care unit.

- If A1 with continued ↑ in glucose, start insulin (metformin can be used as well).
- If A2 with continued ↑ in glucose, increase insulin.
- If A2 on oral agent with continued ↑ in glucose, switch to insulin.
- **At 32–34 weeks for A2 gestational diabetics:**
  - Fetal testing and monthly assessment for fetal growth.
  - For A1 well-controlled GDM:
    - US for growth 36–39 weeks.
    - Antenatal testing is not indicated.
- **Delivery:**
  - A1 GDM: Await labor. Deliver no later than 41 weeks.
  - A2 GDM:
    - If glucose is well controlled, deliver at 39 weeks to decrease risk of stillbirth.
    - If glucose is poorly controlled, deliver as clinically indicated before 37–39 weeks.
  - Maintain euglycemia during labor (insulin drip).
  - Recommend cesarean delivery (to avoid birth trauma or shoulder dystocia) if estimated fetal weight ≥4500 g.

 EXAM TIP

Fetal anomalies are NOT increased with GDM, because the onset is after organogenesis

Shoulder Dystocia

A 25-year-old G1P0 patient presents in labor. She has a protracted labor course and pushes for 3 hours. The head delivers and then retracts into the perineum (i.e., turtle sign). The infant's anterior shoulder does not deliver with gentle downward traction. What is the diagnosis? What is the next step in management?

Answer: Shoulder dystocia. The next step is to call for help (nursing, anesthesia, pediatrics) and prepare to perform additional maneuvers.

Shoulder dystocia is diagnosed when the anterior fetal shoulder is lodged behind the pubic symphysis after the fetal head has been delivered, and gentle downward traction fails to accomplish delivery. The fetal head retracts against the perineum, forming the "turtle sign." The incidence is 0.2–3% of births, and it is considered to be an obstetric emergency. If infant is not delivered quickly, it may suffer neurologic injury or death from hypoxia. A patient with a history of a severe shoulder dystocia is offered primary cesarean in subsequent pregnancies.

 WARD TIP

Shoulder dystocia = Obstetric emergency

WARD TIP

Shoulder dystocia management:
Call for Help
Hyper flexion of hips (McRoberts maneuver)
Suprapubic pressure
Attempt shoulder rotation (Woods screw or Rubin maneuver)
Delivery of the posterior arm
Return head into vagina for cesarean delivery (Zavanelli)—LAST RESORT

RISK FACTORS

- Shoulder dystocia cannot accurately be predicted by either risk factors or imaging studies predicting fetal weight.
- Maternal factors:
  - History of shoulder dystocia
  - Obesity
  - Multiparity
  - Gestational and preexisting diabetes
- Fetal factors:
  - Postterm pregnancy (>42 weeks)
  - Macrosomia
- Intrapartum factors:
  - Prolonged first and/or second stage of labor
  - Operative vaginal delivery

COMPLICATIONS

- Brachial plexus nerve injuries
- Fetal humeral/clavicular fracture
- Hypoxia/death

TREATMENT

Several maneuvers can be performed to dislodge the shoulder:

- **McRoberts maneuver:** Maternal thighs are sharply flexed against maternal abdomen. This flattens the sacrum and the pubic symphysis and may allow the delivery of the fetal shoulder. Performed at the same time as suprapubic pressure. (See Figure 8-1.)
- **Suprapubic pressure** slightly superior to the pubic symphysis and at a 45 degree angle in the direction of the desired shoulder rotation. (NOTE: NOT fundal pressure!)
- **Woods screw maneuver:** Pressure is applied to the anterior surface of the posterior shoulder to rotate the posterior shoulder and "unscrew" the anterior shoulder. (See Figure 8-2.)
- **Rubin maneuver:** Pressure is applied to the most accessible part of the fetal shoulder and rotated toward the chest. (See Figure 8-3.)
- **Posterior arm delivery:** Hand is inserted into vagina and posterior arm is pulled across chest, delivering posterior arm and shoulder. This creates a shorter distance between the anterior shoulder and posterior axilla, allowing the anterior shoulder to be delivered.
- Episiotomy does not unlodge/clear a shoulder dystocia. However, it may create more room for the provider to attempt maneuvers.
- **Zavanelli maneuver:** If the above measures do not work, the fetal head can be returned to the uterus by reversing the cardinal movements of labor. At this point, a cesarean delivery can be performed. (See Figure 8-4.) (LAST RESORT)
- Maneuvers that do not require direct contact with the fetus should be done first because they have lower morbidity for the fetus.
- Delivery of the posterior shoulder has been shown to be most effective internal maneuver—thus is often attempted if McRoberts and suprapubic fail.

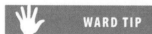

WARD TIP

Do not apply fundal pressure in shoulder dystocia. It causes further impaction of the shoulder behind the pubic symphysis

WARD TIP

Shoulder dystocia is a boney problem. Episiotomy only creates more soft tissue space for providers to attempt maneuvers, it in itself does not relieve the impacted shoulder.

Hyperemesis Gravidarum

Many patients have nausea and vomiting in early pregnancy. Hyperemesis Gravidarum is diagnosed when patients have moderate to severe weight loss and metabolic derangements. It requires inpatient admission often for correction of electrolyte disturbances and titrations of medications.

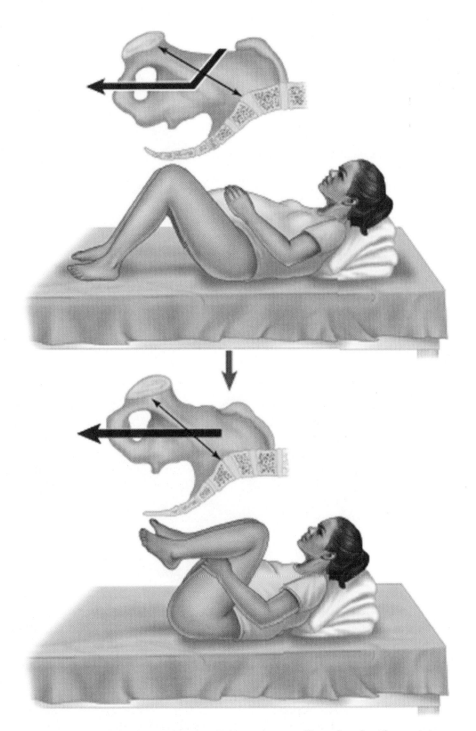

FIGURE 8-1. **McRoberts maneuver for shoulder dystocia.** (Reproduced, with permission, from Ganti L. *Atlas of Emergency Medicine Procedures*. New York, NY: Springer Nature; 2016.)

- Severe vomiting in early pregnancy that results in:
  - Moderate to severe weight loss
  - Dehydration
  - Metabolic derangements
- Due to high levels of human chorionic gonadotropin (hCG), estrogen, progesterone, or a combination

RISK FACTORS

- History of hyperemesis in prior pregnancy
- Multiple gestations

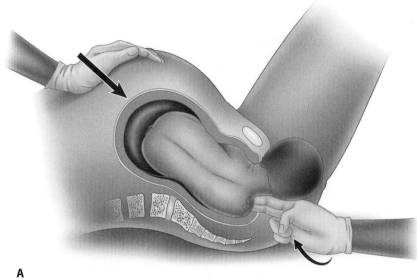

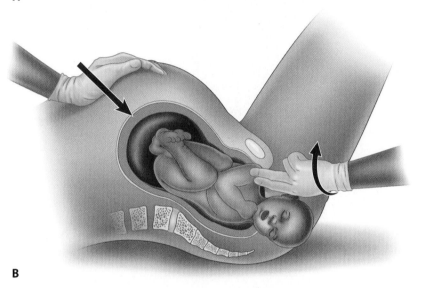

FIGURE 8-2. **Woods corkscrew maneuver for shoulder dystocia. (A) pressure is applied to the clavicle of the posterior arm and (B) enabling rotation and dislodgement of the anterior shoulder.** (Reproduced, with permission, from Ganti L. *Atlas of Emergency Medicine Procedures*. New York, NY: Springer Nature; 2016.)

A

B

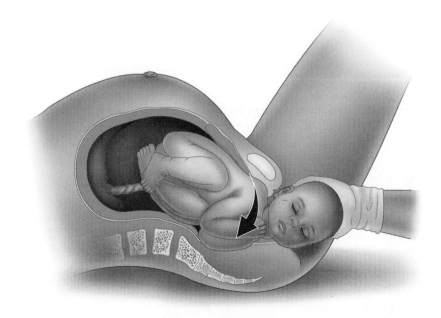

FIGURE 8-3. **Ruben maneuver for shoulder dystocia: pressure is applied to the most accessible part of the fetal shoulder and rotated toward the chest.** (Reproduced, with permission, from Ganti L. *Atlas of Emergency Medicine Procedures*. New York, NY: Springer Nature; 2016.)

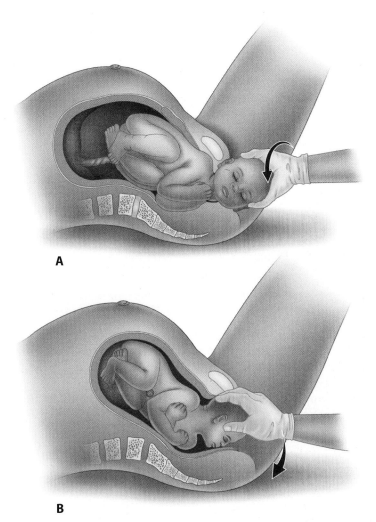

FIGURE 8-4.   Zavanelli maneuver. (A) The fetal head is rotated into the direct occiput anterior position, flexed and (B) pushed back into the birth canal. (Reproduced, with permission, from Ganti L. *Atlas of Emergency Medicine Procedures.* New York, NY: Springer Nature; 2016.)

MANAGEMENT

- Rule out other causes (molar pregnancy, thyrotoxicosis, GI etiology)
- First line: Vitamin B$_6$ with doxylamine
- IV hydration, thiamine/electrolyte replacement, acid reducing medications, antiemetics
- Parenteral nutrition if needed

Isoimmunization

 A 29-year-old G2P1001 patient at 16 weeks presents for prenatal care. Her blood type is A negative and she has a positive antibody screen. What is the next step in management?
Answer: Identify the antibody. Some can be dangerous for the fetus and some are benign.

WARD TIP

Maternal antibodies: **K**ell **K**ills, **D**uffy **D**ies, **L**ewis **L**ives.

- In each pregnancy, every patient should have her blood type, Rh status, and antibody screen evaluated at the initial prenatal visit. If the antibody screen is positive, the next step is to identify the antibody. Some antibodies pose no harm to the fetus (i.e., anti-Lewis), while others can cause hemolytic disease of the newborn (HDN) and can be fatal (i.e., anti-D, anti-Kell, anti-Duffy).

■ Along with antibodies to antigens on fetal red blood cells (RBCs), antibodies may be directed against fetal platelets.

■ If the antibodies are not harmful to the fetus, no further workup needs to be done at this time, but patient may need type and cross at delivery because often matching blood in case of transfusion can be challenging.

■ If antibodies are known to cause harm to the fetus, next step is to determine the titer of the antibodies and assess paternal antigen status. A **critical titer**, usually 1:16 at most institutions, is the titer associated with a significant risk for HDN. Fetal surveillance with possible therapeutic interventions may be needed if the partner is not antigen negative (and paternity is assured). (See Figure 8-5.)

ANTI-D ISOIMMUNIZATION

An understanding of D (or Rho) RBC antigen compatibility is a crucial part of prenatal care. If a mother and developing child are incompatible, very serious complications can cause fetal death. This section will review the appropriate screening and therapy for anti-D isoimmunization. Of note, we use RhD as an example here—but this process can occur with any RBC antigen that causes HDN.

What Is Rh or D?

■ The surface of the human RBC may or may not have a Rho (Rh) antigen. If a patient with blood type A has a Rho antigen, the blood type is A+. If that person has no Rho antigen, the blood type is A–. In the following discussion, the Rh antigen will be referred to as D.

■ Half of all antigens on fetal RBCs come from the father, and half come from the mother. That means that the fetus may have antigens to which the mother's immune system is unfamiliar.

The Problem with D Sensitization

■ If the mother is D negative and the father is D positive, there may be a chance that the baby may be D positive.

■ If the mother is D negative and her fetus is D positive, she may become sensitized to the D antigen and develop antibodies against the baby's RBCs.

■ In her next pregnancy, if the baby is D positive, these antibodies cross the placenta and attack the fetal RBCs, resulting in fetal RBC hemolysis. The hemolysis results in significant fetal anemia, resulting in fetal heart failure, hydrops, and death. This disease process is known as HDN.

■ Sensitization is the development of maternal antibodies against D antigens on the fetus RBC. Sensitization may occur whenever fetal blood enters the maternal circulation. The fetus of the pregnancy when sensitization occurred usually suffers no harm because the maternal antibody titers are low. The subsequent pregnancies with a D-positive fetus are at significantly higher risk of HDN because the mother has already developed memory cells that quickly produce anti-D antibodies against the fetus RBCs.

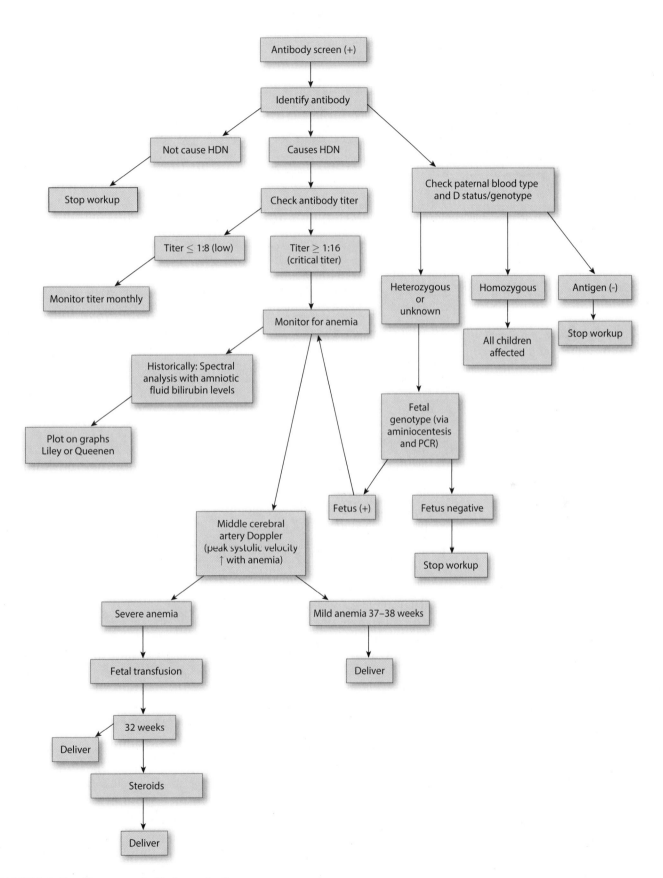

FIGURE 8-5. Management of isoimmunization.

Kleihauer-Betke test determines the number of fetal RBCs in the maternal circulation (see section on RhoGAM).

The standard dose of RhoGAM is 300 μg. It is sufficient for 15 mL of D-positive fetal RBCs (30 mL of whole fetal blood). Kleihauer-Betke (KB) test estimates the number of fetal RBCs that are present in the maternal circulation. The dose of anti-D IgG is based on the results of the KB test.

- The following conditions can cause fetal-maternal bleeding, and lead to sensitization:
  - Chorionic villus sampling
  - Amniocentesis
  - Spontaneous/induced abortion
  - Threatened/incomplete abortion
  - Ectopic pregnancies
  - Placental abruption/bleeding placenta previa
  - Vaginal or cesarean delivery
  - Abdominal trauma
  - External cephalic version

Anti-D Immune Globulins (IgG) (Brand Name: RhoGAM)

Anti-D immune globulins are collected from donated human plasma. When a patient is given a dose of anti-D IgG, the antibodies bind to the fetal RBCs that have the D antigen on them and clear them from the maternal circulation. The goal is to prevent the patient's immune system from recognizing the presence of the D antigen and forming antibodies against it.

- Give to D-negative patients, who have <u>not</u> formed antibodies against D antigen.
- **Not** indicated for patients who already have anti-D antibodies and are sensitized.
- Indicated for patients who might be sensitized to other blood group antigens.

Management of the Unsensitized D-Negative Patient (The D-Negative Patient with a Negative Antibody Screen)

1. Antibody screen should be done at the initial prenatal visit and again at 28 weeks.
2. If antibody screen negative, the fetus is presumed to be D positive, and one dose of anti-D IgG immune globulin is given to the mother at 28 weeks to prevent development of maternal antibodies. Anti-D immune globulins last for ~12 weeks, and the highest risk of sensitization is in the third trimester.
3. At birth, the infant's D status is tested. If the infant is D negative, no anti-D IgG is given to the mother. If the infant is D positive, anti-D IgG is given to the mother within 72 hour of delivery. The dose of anti-D IgG is determined using a KB test.
4. Administration of anti-D IgG at 28 weeks' gestation and within 72 hour of birth reduces sensitization to 0.2%.

   *If there is any maternal trauma during the pregnancy, an additional dose of RhoGAM can be considered, and in this case a KB test can help assist with dosing.

Hemolytic Disease of the Newborn
HDN/fetal hydrops occurs when the mother lacks an antigen present on the fetal RBC → fetal RBCs in maternal circulation trigger an immune response → maternal antibodies lyse fetal RBCs → fetal anemia → fetal hyperbilirubinemia + kernicterus + heart failure, edema, ascites, pericardial effusion → death.

Management of the Sensitized D-Negative Patient (Antibody Screen Positive for Anti-D Antibody)

A 35-year-old G4P2012 patient at 26 weeks is diagnosed with anti-Kell antibodies with the titer of 1:32. Amniocentesis shows that the fetus is positive for the Kell antigen. In addition to antenatal (i.e., biophysical profile), what other testing is critical for this fetus?

Answer: The fetus should be monitored with middle cerebral artery (MCA) Dopplers, which indicate the severity of anemia.

1. If antibody screen at initial prenatal visit is positive, and is identified as anti-D.
2. Check the antibody titer. Critical titer is 1:16.

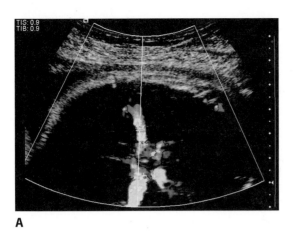
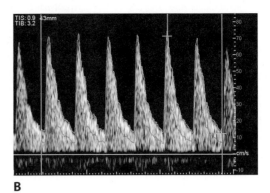

A   **B**

FIGURE 8-6. **Middle cerebral artery. (A) Doppler. (B) Waveform.** (Reproduced, with permission, from Cunningham FG, Leveno KJ, Bloom SL, et al. *Williams Obstetrics.* 23rd ed. New York, NY: McGraw-Hill; 2010:365.)

- If titer remains stable at <1:16, the likelihood of HDN is low. Follow the antibody titer every 4 weeks.
- If the titer is ≥1:16 and/or rising, the likelihood of HDN is high. Amniocentesis is recommended.
3. If the patient undergoes amniocentesis:
    - Fetal cells are analyzed for D status—if the fetus is D+ it is as risk of HDN—and monitor as below. If D− then no further US indicated.
    - If the patient declines amniocentesis, the fetus is assumed to be D+ and monitored as below.
4. Serial US monitoring for fetal anemia with MCA Dopplers (see Figure 8-6).
5. If evidence of anemia on MCA Dopplers, proceed with inutero blood transfusion (IUT). At this time, assessment of fetal antigen status can be performed if not done previously. If close to term, consider delivery.

✋ WARD TIP

Fetal hydrops = Collection of fluid in two or more body cavities:
- Scalp edema
- Pleural effusion
- Pericardial effusion
- Ascites

KELL ISOIMMUNIZATION

With the use of anti-D immune globulin, there is an ↑ of isoimmunization caused by minor antigens acquired by incompatible blood transfusion. Some minor antigens cause HDN, and some do not. Those that do cause HDN are managed the same way as anti-D isoimmunized mothers. Kell isoimmunization is an exception because:
- It results in more severe anemia than alloimunization due to other erythrocyte antigens because it also causes fetal marrow suppression in addition to hemolysis.
- Maternal Kell antibody titers are not predictive of the severity of fetal anemia in the same way that titers are with anti-D sensitization.
- MCA Dopplers are accurate in predicting severe anemia with Kell isoimmunization.

Preterm Labor

DIAGNOSTIC CRITERIA

GA < 37 weeks with regular uterine contractions and cervical change.

RISK FACTORS

- Previous history of preterm delivery.
- Polyhydramnios.

- Multiple gestations.
- Substance abuse.
- Systemic infection (pyelonephritis, appendicitis, etc.)
- Vaginal infections (bacterial vaginosis (BV), chlamydia)
- Placental abruption
- PPROM

ASSESSMENT

- Evaluate for causes such as infection (gonococcus, BV, urinary tract infection), abruption, and drug use
- Predictors of preterm labor:
  - Transvaginal cervical length measurement:
    - >30 mm: Low risk of preterm delivery
    - <20 mm (especially with funneling): High risk of preterm delivery
  - Fetal fibronectin assay:
    - Vaginal swab of posterior fornix prior to digital exam
    - If negative, 99% predictability for no preterm delivery within 1 week
    - Can be especially helpful predicting risk of preterm delivery in patients with cervical length <30 mm but >20 mm

MANAGEMENT OF PRETERM LABOR

Hydration

Not proven to reduce preterm labor or preterm delivery, but hydration may decrease uterine irritability. Dehydration causes antidiuretic hormone (ADH) secretion, and ADH mimics oxytocin, which causes uterine contractions.

Tocolytic Therapy

Tocolysis is the pharmacologic inhibition of uterine contractions. Tocolytic drugs have not been shown to decrease neonatal morbidity or mortality, but may prolong gestation for 2–7 days to allow time for administration of steroids and transfer to a facility with a neonatal ICU. Tocolysis is contraindicated in patients with intra-amniotic infection, PPROM, abruption, or IUFD.

Tocolytic Agents

- **Magnesium sulfate:** Suppresses uterine contractions (not commonly used).
  - Unknown mechanism of action: Competes with calcium, inhibits myosin light chain.
  - Maternal side effects: Flushing, lethargy, headache, muscle weakness, diplopia, dry mouth, pulmonary edema, cardiac arrest. Toxicity is treated with calcium gluconate.
  - Fetal side effects: Lethargy, hypotonia, respiratory depression.
  - Contraindications: Myasthenia gravis.
- **Nifedipine:** Oral calcium channel blocker.
  - Maternal side effects: Flushing, headache, dizziness, nausea, transient hypotension.
  - Fetal side effects: None yet noted.
  - Contraindications: Maternal hypotension, cardiac disease; use with caution with renal disease. Avoid concomitant use with magnesium sulfate.
- **Ritodrine, terbutaline:** β-agonist: β_2-receptor stimulation on myometrial cells →↑ cyclic adenosine monophosphate (cAMP) →↓ intracellular Ca →↓ contractions (good for acute tocolysis).
  - Maternal side effects: Pulmonary edema, tachycardia, headaches.
  - Fetal side effect: Tachycardia.
  - Contraindications: Cardiovascular disease, hyperthyroidism, uncontrolled diabetes mellitus.

- **Indomethacin:** Prostaglandin inhibitors: For <32 weeks. Good first line agent.
  - Maternal side effects: Nausea, heartburn.
  - Fetal side effects: Premature constriction of ductus arteriosus, pulmonary HTN, reversible ↓ in amniotic fluid.
  - Contraindications: Renal or hepatic impairment, peptic ulcer disease.

Corticosteroids

- Indicated for patients at high risk of preterm delivery from 24 to 37 weeks
- Actions: Accelerate fetal lung maturity (↓ RDS), and reduce intraventricular hemorrhage

Neuroprotection

If at high risk for imminent delivery, administer magnesium sulfate for neuroprotection between 24 and 32 weeks. The dosing regimen is different than that given for tocolysis. Give 4 g bolus followed by 1 g/hr maintenance. This decreases risk for cerebral palsy and death.

Prevention of Preterm Labor

Progesterone supplementation has been shown to decrease the risk of preterm birth in women with:
- A history of term singleton preterm delivery
- A shortened cervix on ultrasound (US) during current pregnancy

Progesterone relaxes the myometrium and suppresses cytokine production. It may be started between 16 and 20 weeks and continued through 36 weeks. Preparations include:
- 17α-hydroxyprogesterone caproate 250 mg IM every week
- Micronized progesterone tablet 100–200 mg per vagina each evening

Prelabor Rupture of Membranes (PROM)

A 24-year-old G3P1102 patient at 38 weeks presents to triage with a report of leakage of fluid from the vagina. She reports good fetal movement, no vaginal bleeding, and no contractions. She is afebrile. Sterile speculum exam demonstrated a pool of fluid in the vagina which is nitrazine positive and shows ferning on glass slide exam. On exam, her cervix is 1 cm and long. Fetal heart rate (FHR) tracing is reassuring, and no contractions are noted. What is the diagnosis?

Answer: Prelabor rupture of membranes (PROM) is diagnosed when the membranes rupture prior to the onset of labor. Rupture of membranes is confirmed by the sterile speculum exam. Based on the cervical exam and the absence of contractions, the patient is not in labor. Considering that the fetus is term, the next step should be induction of labor in order to prevent chorioamnionitis.

Prelabor rupture denotes spontaneous rupture of fetal membranes before the onset of labor. This can occur at term (PROM) or preterm (PPROM).
- **ROM:** Rupture of membranes
- **PROM:** Prelabor rupture of membranes (ROM before the onset of labor)
- **PPROM:** Preterm (<37 weeks) prelabor rupture of membranes
- **Prolonged rupture of membranes:** Rupture of membranes present for >18 hour

WARD TIP

Contraindications to tocolysis:
BAD CUP
- **B**leeding (severe) from any cause
- **A**bruptio placentae
- **D**eath of fetus
- **C**horioamnionitis
- **U**nstable **P**atient hemodynamics

WARD TIP

Maternal corticosteroid administration with:
- Preterm labor likely to deliver in next 7 days
- Preterm prelabor rupture of membranes (PPROM)
- Severe preeclampsia
- Severe IUGR with umbilical artery Dopplers with absent or reversed end diastolic flow
- Patient at <37 weeks with high risk of delivery in next 7 days

WARD TIP

Fetal benefits:
- ↓ respiratory distress syndrome (RDS)
- ↓ intraventricular hemorrhage

WARD TIP

PPROM: Most common diagnosis associated with preterm delivery

ETIOLOGY

- Unknown but hypothesized:
  - Vaginal and cervical infections
  - Cervical insufficiency → premature cervical dilation

COMPLICATIONS

- Preterm delivery: If PROM occurs at <37 weeks, the fetus is at risk of being born prematurely with its associated complications.
- Pulmonary hypoplasia: If PROM occurs at <22 weeks (*also known as previable PPROM*) → anhydramnios/oligohydramnios → **pulmonary hypoplasia**.
- Chorioamnionitis.
- Placental abruption.
- Neonatal infection/sepsis.
- Umbilical cord prolapse.
- Preterm labor.
- IUFD

MANAGEMENT OF ALL PROM PATIENTS

- Avoid vaginal exams if possible to ↓ risk of chorioamnionitis.
- Evaluate patient for chorioamnionitis: Fever >100.4°F (38°C), leukocytosis, maternal/fetal tachycardia, uterine tenderness, malodorous vaginal discharge.
- If chorioamnionitis present, delivery is performed regardless of GA, and broad-spectrum antibiotics (ampicillin, gentamicin) are initiated.

SPECIFIC MANAGEMENT FOR PROM AT TERM

Ninety percent of term patients go into spontaneous labor within 24 hour after rupture:

- Patients in active labor should be allowed to progress.
- If labor is not spontaneous, it should be induced. Cesarean delivery should be performed for obstetric indications.

SPECIFIC MANAGEMENT OF PPROM

An 18-year-old G1P0 patient at 30 weeks presents to triage with a report of clear fluid leaking from her vagina. Her exam is positive for pooling, ferning, and nitrazine. The cervix is visually closed on sterile speculum exam. FHR is reassuring, and no contractions are noted. The US shows a breech singleton fetus. What is the next step in management?

Answer: The patient has PPROM. She should be admitted to the hospital. Steroids should be administered to ↓ the risk of RDS in the fetus, and antibiotics should be given to ↑ the latency period.

- Fifty percent of PPROM patients go into labor within 24 hours after rupture.
- Management strategy balances the risks of preterm birth against the risks of complications such as infection, abruption, and cord accident.
- US to assess GA, anomalies, presentation, and AFI.
- Monitor in hospital for infection, abruption, fetal distress, and preterm labor.
- If <37 weeks' gestation, give steroids to ↓ the incidence of RDS.
- If delivery is thought to be imminent and <32 weeks, administer magnesium sulfate for neuroprotection.
- Antibiotic coverage to prolong latency period (time between ROM and onset of labor) if >34 weeks.

TABLE 8-4.   **PROM Management by GA**

	>37	34/0–36/6	23/0–33/6	<23/0
Expectant management?	No—delivery indicated	Consider with shared decision making	Yes	Consider with shared decision making
Steroids	No	Yes	Yes	No
Antibiotics for latency	No	No	Yes	Consider with shared decision making
Magnesium for neuroprotection?	No	No	Yes if <32 weeks	No

- Fetal testing to ensure fetal well-being.
- Delivery:
  - If infection, abruption, fetal distress noted.
  - Usually recommended at 34 weeks' gestation. At this GA, most babies have low risk of RDS, and risks of complications such as infection outweigh risks of prematurity. However, in some cases with shared decision making, expectant management until 37 weeks can be considered.

WARD TIP

Never do a digital vaginal exam in third-trimester bleeding until placenta previa is ruled out.

Third-Trimester Bleeding

INCIDENCE

Occurs in 2–5% of pregnancies

WORKUP

- History, including trauma.
- Vitals: Signs of hypovolemia include hypotension and tachycardia.
- Labs: Complete blood count (CBC), coagulation profile, type and crossmatch, urinalysis, drug screen.
- US to look for placenta previa, as well as monitoring for fetal well-being.
- Determine whether blood is maternal, fetal, or both:
  - **Kleihauer-Betke test:** Take blood from mother's arm and determine percentage of fetal RBCs in maternal circulation: >1% = Fetal bleeding. Maternal cells are washed out (ghost cells); fetal cells are bright red (due to fetal hemoglobin). This is the test most commonly used.

DIFFERENTIAL

- **Obstetric causes:**
  - Placental abruption
  - Placenta previa
  - Vasa previa/velamentous insertion
  - Uterine rupture
  - Extrusion of cervical mucus ("bloody show")
- **Nonobstetric causes:**
  - Cervicitis
  - Neoplasm
  - Vaginal laceration
  - Post-coital bleeding

WARD TIP

Kleihauer-Betke test determines if blood is fetal, maternal, or both.

EXAM TIP

Whose blood is lost with a ruptured vasa previa? Fetal!!

WARD TIP

Two most common causes of third-trimester bleeding = Placenta previa and abruption

WARD TIP

Most nonobstetric causes of vaginal bleeding result in relatively little blood loss and minimal threat to the mother and fetus.

PLACENTAL ABRUPTION (ABRUPTIO PLACENTAE)

> 👤 A 32-year-old G2P1001 patient at 34 weeks is brought to triage after a motor vehicle accident. She was a restrained driver who was rear-ended while going 65 miles per hour on the freeway. The airbags were deployed. She has dark-red vaginal bleeding and severe abdominal pain. Her vitals are stable. On exam, her abdomen is firm and tender. FHR shows a baseline of 130, ↓ variability, no accelerations, and late decelerations. Contractions are seen on the monitor. What is the most likely diagnosis?
> **Answer:** Placental abruption.

WARD TIP

Pregnant patient + vaginal bleeding + pain = Abruption until proven otherwise

Premature separation of placenta from uterine wall before the delivery of baby (see Figure 8-7).

INCIDENCE

0.5–1.3%; severe abruption can lead to death (0.12%).

RISK FACTORS

- Trauma (motor vehicle accident, domestic violence)
- Previous history of abruption
- Preeclampsia (and chronic HTN)
- Smoking
- Cocaine abuse

CLINICAL PRESENTATION

> 👤 A 28-year-old patient at 35 weeks' gestation is brought in by ambulance following a car accident. She reports severe abdominal pain, and on exam, she is found to have vaginal bleeding. An US shows a fundal placenta and a fetus in the cephalic presentation. FHT shows minimal variability and late decelerations. What is most likely the cause?
> **Answer:** Placental abruption. What is the next step? Expedite delivery. Type and cross the patient—in case of massive maternal hemorrhage.

- Vaginal bleeding (can be mild or life-threatening)
- Constant and severe abdominal pain
- Irritable, tender, and typically hypertonic uterus
- Evidence of fetal distress (if severe)

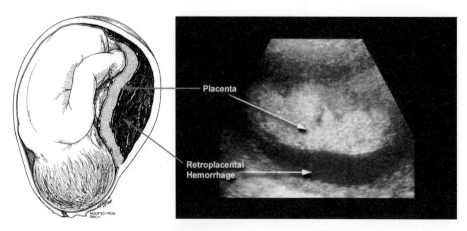

FIGURE 8-7. **Placental abruption.** (Courtesy of SUNY at Buffalo School of Medicine, Residency Program in Emergency Medicine.)

- Maternal shock
- Disseminated intravascular coagulation

DIAGNOSIS

- Retroplacental hematoma on US supports diagnosis, but is not rarely seen.
- Clinical findings most important.

MANAGEMENT

- Correct shock (IV fluids, packed RBCs, fresh frozen plasma, cryoprecipitate, platelets).
- Maternal oxygen administration.
- Expectant management or delivery depending on GA and maternal and fetal status: Close observation of mother and fetus with ability to intervene immediately.
- If there is fetal distress, perform cesarean delivery. Otherwise may be candidate for vaginal delivery.

ZEBRA ALERT

Retroplacental hematoma on US is diagnostic of abruption, but rarely seen.

- - - - - - - - - - - -

 WARD TIP

Up to 20% of placental abruptions can present without vaginal bleeding because bleeding is concealed.

PLACENTA PREVIA

A condition in which the placenta is implanted in the immediate vicinity of the cervical os.

- **Placenta previa:** The placenta covers the entire internal cervical os or part of the os (see Figure 8-8).
- **Low-lying placenta:** Within 2 cm of the internal cervical os.

INCIDENCE

0.5–1%

ETIOLOGY

Associated with:

- Multiparity
- Advanced maternal age.

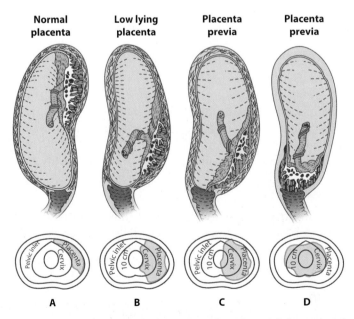

FIGURE 8-8. **(A) Normal placenta. (B) Low implantation. (C) Partial placenta previa. (D) Complete placenta previa.** (Modified, with permission, from DeCherney AH, Nathan L. *Current Obstetric & Gynecologic Diagnosis & Treatment.* 9th ed. New York, NY: McGraw-Hill; 2003.)

- Previous history of placenta previa
- Multiple gestation
- Previous cesarean delivery
- Infertility treatment

CLINICAL PRESENTATION

- **Painless** vaginal bleeding in second or third trimester.
- If patient has not had a second-trimester US, do not perform digital vaginal exam until US demonstrates placental location.

DIAGNOSIS

- **Transabdominal US** (95% accurate). **Transvaginal US** helps to further define placental location.

MANAGEMENT

Asymptomatic placenta previa:
- If diagnosed at routine second-trimester US:
    - Recommend avoid intercourse and vigorous exercise.
    - Repeat US around 28–32 weeks to see if resolved as the lower uterine segment develops.
    - If unresolved, repeat US around 34–36 weeks to see if resolved as the lower uterine segment develops.
- Delivery by cesarean between 36 and 37 weeks if not resolved.

Bleeding placenta previa:
- Most patients who present with bleeding due to placenta previa can be managed conservatively and do not require delivery. However, they should be consented for cesarean delivery, 2 large-bore IVs, and type and screen obtained. Betamethasone should be given if >37 weeks.
- Severe bleeding should be managed by correcting shock and stabilizing mother, and cesarean delivery.

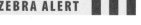

FETAL VESSEL RUPTURE

Two conditions cause third-trimester bleeding resulting from fetal vessel rupture: (1) vasa previa and (2) velamentous cord insertion. These two conditions often occur together and can cause fetal hemorrhage and death very quickly.

Vasa Previa

- A condition in which the unprotected fetal cord vessels pass over the internal cervical os, making them susceptible to rupture when membranes are ruptured or if dilation occurs
- **Prevalence:** 1/2500 deliveries and higher with use of fertility treatments

Velamentous Cord Insertion

- Fetal vessels insert in the membranes and travel unprotected to the placenta, with no protection from Wharton's jelly. This leaves them susceptible to tearing when the amniotic sac ruptures.
- **Prevalence:** 1% of singletons, 10% of twins.

CLINICAL PRESENTATION

Vaginal bleeding with fetal distress.

MANAGEMENT

Immediate cesarean delivery.

UTERINE RUPTURE

The disruption of the uterine musculature through all of its layers, usually with part of the fetus protruding through the opening.

COMPLICATIONS

- Maternal: Hemorrhage, hysterectomy, death
- Fetal: Permanent neurologic impairment, cerebral palsy, death

RISK FACTORS

Prior uterine scar from a cesarean delivery is the most important risk factor:
- Vertical scar: 3–10% risk due to scarring of the active, contractile portion of the uterus.
- Low transverse scar: <1% risk.
- Can occur in the setting of trauma.

PRESENTATION AND DIAGNOSIS

- Nonreassuring fetal heart tones or bradycardia: Most suggestive of uterine rupture.
- Sudden cessation of uterine contractions.
- "Tearing" sensation in abdomen.
- Presenting fetal part moves higher in the pelvis (i.e., loss of station).
- Vaginal bleeding.
- Maternal hypovolemia from concealed hemorrhage.

MANAGEMENT

- Immediate laparotomy and delivery
- May require a cesarean hysterectomy if uterus cannot be reconstructed — though this is uncommon

EXAM TIP

The biggest risk for uterine rupture is a prior cesarean delivery.

OTHER OBSTETRIC CAUSES OF THIRD-TRIMESTER BLEEDING

Extrusion of cervical mucus ("bloody show"): A consequence of effacement and dilation of the cervix, with tearing of the small vessels leading to small amount of bleeding that is mixed with the cervical mucus. Benign finding. Often used as a marker for the onset of labor.

Abnormalities of the Third Stage of Labor

A 37-year-old G6P6006 patient with a history of asthma and chronic HTN undergoes a spontaneous vaginal delivery of a 4500-g infant. After the placenta delivers spontaneously, profuse vaginal bleeding was noted from the vagina. Pitocin is given, fundal massage is performed, and large clots are removed from the uterus. No lacerations are noted. Estimated blood loss is 1100 cc. What is the most likely cause of the bleeding? What is the next step in management?

Answer: Uterine atony is the most likely cause for this patient's postpartum hemorrhage (PPH). Prostaglandin F2α (asthma) and methergine (HTN) are contraindicated due to her medical conditions. The next best agent is TXA and misoprostol.

EXAM TIP

One unit of packed red blood cells (PRBCs) contains ≈ 250 mL/unit.

EXAM TIP

Incidence of excessive blood loss following vaginal delivery is 5–8%.

POSTPARTUM HEMORRHAGE (PPH)

- Excessive bleeding that makes patient symptomatic and/or results in signs of hypovolemia.
- Blood loss >1000 mL for delivery (difficult to quantify).

- During first 24 hour: "**Early**" PPH.
- Between 24 hour and 6 weeks after delivery: "**Late**" PPH.
- The most common cause of early PPH is uterine atony (the uterus does not contract as expected). Normally when the uterus contracts, it compresses blood vessels and prevents bleeding. Other causes of PPH are: retained placenta, cervical or vaginal lacerations, and coagulopathy.

RISK FACTORS

- Blood transfusion/hemorrhage during a previous pregnancy
- Prolonged labor
- Retained placenta/membranes
- Multiparity
- Overdistended uterus: macrosomia/twins/polyhydramnios
- Operative vaginal delivery (vacuum, forceps)
- Chorioamnionitis

MANAGEMENT

1. Manually compress and massage the uterus, empty the bladder—controls most cases of hemorrhage due to atony.
2. Start two large-bore IVs and infuse isotonic crystalloids. Type and cross blood. Monitor vitals, including ins and outs.
3. Carefully inspect the placenta to ensure it is intact (Consider bedside ultrasound if not).
4. Inspect the cervix and vagina for trauma/lacerations.
5. If uterus is boggy, suspect atony:
   - Give additional oxytocin.
   - Methergine—contraindicated: HTN.
   - Prostaglandin F2α—contraindicated: Moderate to severe asthma.
   - Misoprostol.
   - Tranexamic Acid (TXA)
   - Intrauterine balloon tamponade.
   - ↓ uterine pulse pressure:
     - Uterine artery embolization.
     - Surgical exploration: Hypogastric artery ligation, uterine artery ligation, ligation of utero-ovarian ligament, uterine compression suture (B-Lynch stitch).
   - Hysterectomy.
6. Consider coagulopathy if persistent bleeding with above management.
   - Red top tube for clot retraction test. Normal coags if clot forms <8 minutes. Coagulopathy if no clot >12 minutes.
   - Uterine balloon tamponade until fresh frozen plasma and/or cryoprecipitate available.
   - Hysterectomy (additional surgery) should be avoided in setting of coagulopathy.

PLACENTAL ACCRETA SPECTRUM

Abnormal implantation of the placenta in the uterus can cause retention of the placenta after delivery and heavy bleeding.

TYPES

- **Placenta accreta:** Placental villi attach directly to the myometrium rather than to the decidua basalis (see Figure 8-9).
- **Placenta increta:** Placental villi invade the myometrium.
- **Placenta percreta:** Placental villi penetrate through the myometrium. May invade the bladder.

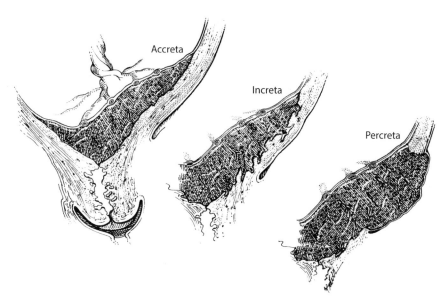

FIGURE 8-9. Placenta accreta, increta, and percreta. (Reproduced, with permission, from Cunningham FG, Leveno KJ, Bloom SL, et al. *Williams Obstetrics*. 22nd ed. New York, NY: McGraw-Hill; 2005:831.)

ETIOLOGY

Placenta accreta, increta, and percreta are associated with:
- Placenta previa
- Previous cesarean delivery (↑ number, ↑ risk)
- Previous dilation and curettage (D&C)
- Grand multiparity

MANAGEMENT

All of these conditions result in hemorrhage in the third stage of labor. Treatment of choice: cesarean hysterectomy. Patients with suspected placenta accreta spectrum disorders should delivery at a tertiary care center with experienced surgeons. If unrecognized, EBL is higher, a morbidity markedly worse.

UTERINE INVERSION

This medical emergency may result from excessive cord traction during placental delivery, and can also be a result of abnormal placental implantation. Morbidity results from shock and sepsis.

INCIDENCE

One in 2200 deliveries.

MANAGEMENT

- Call for help.
- Ensure adequate anesthesia.
- Large-bore IV.
- Do not remove placenta until the uterus has been replaced.
- Stop uterotonic medications and give uterine relaxants.
- Immediately try to replace inverted uterus by pushing on the fundus toward the vagina.
- Oxytocin is given after uterus is restored to normal configuration and anesthesia is stopped.

WARD TIP

If a mass is palpated in the vagina immediately after the placenta delivers, suspect uterine inversion.

WARD TIP

Never pull excessively on the cord to deliver the placenta. Gentle traction will be sufficient in a normally implanted placenta.

NOTES

CHAPTER 9

Infections in Pregnancy

Immune System in the Developing Embryo, Fetus, and Newborn

EXAM TIP

IgG "goes" across the placenta.

Infant cell-mediated and humoral immunity begins to develop at 9–15 weeks. The initial fetal response to infection is the production of immunoglobulin M (IgM). Passive immunity is provided by transplacental crossing of IgG from the mother. After birth, breast-feeding provides some protection that wanes after 2 months. IgA is the antibody present in breast milk. Infections diagnosed in neonates less than 72 hours of age are usually acquired in utero or during delivery. Infections after this time are acquired after birth (see Table 9-1).

TABLE 9-1. Perinatal Infections

INTRAUTERINE[a]	VIRAL	BACTERIAL	PROTOZOAN
Transplacental	Varicella-zoster	*Listeria*	Toxoplasmosis
	Coxsackievirus	Syphilis	Malaria
	Parvovirus		
	Rubella		
	CMV		
	HIV		
	Hepatitis		
	HSV		
Ascending infection	HSV	GBS	
		Coliforms, GC/	
		chlamydia	

Intrapartum[b]

Maternal exposure	HSV	Gonorrhea	
	Papillomavirus	*Chlamydia*	
	HIV	GBS	
	HBV	TB	
	HCV		
External contamination	HSV	*Staphylococcus*	
		coliforms	

Neonatal

Human transmission	HSV	*Staphylococcus*	
Respirators and		*Staphylococcus*	
catheters		coliforms	

[a]Bacteria, viruses, or parasites may gain access transplacentally or cross the intact membranes.

[b]Organisms may colonize and infect the fetus during L&D.

GBS, group B Streptococcus; GC, gonococcus; HBV, hepatitis B virus; HCV, hepatitis C virus; HIV, human immunodeficiency virus; HSV, herpes simplex virus; TB, tuberculosis.

Varicella-Zoster

 A 25-year-old G1P0 patient at 15 weeks' gestation reports that she came in contact with a child that had chickenpox 2 days ago. She does not recall ever having chickenpox or the vaccine. What is the next step?

Answer: She should be tested for the presence of varicella antibodies. Many people are immune to chickenpox, but do not recall ever having it or being vaccinated. If testing indicates that she lacks the antibodies, she should receive the varicella immunoglobulin within 96 hours. If she has the varicella antibodies, nothing further needs to be done.

- Infection is more severe in adults; even more severe in pregnancy.
- Can cause **pneumonia**; treat with IV acyclovir.
- Varicella vaccine introduced in 1995 has decreased the incidence of the disease.
- The presence of antibodies should be assessed as part of the new OB labs. Patients who are not immune or equivocal should get the vaccine postpartum.
- Post-exposure prophylaxis with **VZIG** (varicella-zoster immune globulin) within 10 days of exposure is indicated for those who are exposed <u>and</u> susceptible.
- Shingles outbreak in pregnancy does not put the fetus at risk for fetal infection.

 WARD TIP

Varicella vaccine is a live vaccine, so cannot be used in pregnancy.

 ZEBRA ALERT

Varicella infection can cause severe maternal pneumonia in pregnancy.

FETAL EFFECTS

- Early pregnancy: Transplacental infection causes congenital malformations.
  - Chorioretinitis.
  - Cerebral cortical atrophy.
  - Hydronephrosis.
  - Cutaneous and bony leg defects.
- Late pregnancy: Lower risk of congenital varicella infection.
- Before/during labor:
  - Much higher risk to infant due to absence of protective maternal antibodies.
  - Neonates develop disseminated disease that can be fatal.
  - If maternal infection 5 days before or after delivery, give infant VZIG for passive immunity.

VACCINE

- Live attenuated: **Not** recommended for pregnant patients or newborn.
- Not secreted in breast milk, so can give postpartum.

Influenza

Pregnant patients with influenza are more likely to develop severe illness, to be hospitalized, to require ICU admission, and die. Severe influenza is associated with increased risk of growth restriction. Though, it is unclear if this is due to the virus itself or a sequalae of being severely ill. This virus does not cause fetal infection.

TREATMENT

- Neuraminidase inhibitors oseltamivir or zanamivir are recommended for treatment and prophylaxis.

 WARD TIP

Any pregnant patient exposed to influenza should receive prophylaxis with a neuraminidase inhibitor.

 WARD TIP

Influenza vaccine should be given to all pregnant patients at any GA.

- Inactivated vaccine recommended for all pregnant patients at any gestational age (GA) during flu season.
- Live attenuated intranasal vaccine not recommended for pregnant patients.

Parvovirus (B19)

 A 30-year-old G2P1001 patient at 24 weeks' gestation presents with a bright red rash on both of her cheeks that started yesterday. She reports a 2-day history of fever of 100.4°F (38°C) and lethargy. On physical exam, she is afebrile and has a fine erythematous, lacelike rash on her arms. What is the most likely diagnosis? What is the risk to the fetus?

Answer: Flulike symptoms, slapped cheek rash, and fine reticular rash (erythema infectiosum) are a classic presentation for parvovirus infection. The fetus is at risk for aplastic anemia, which can cause nonimmune hydrops and fetal death.

- Causes **erythema infectiosum** or **fifth disease**.
- Transmitted via respiratory or hand-to-mouth contact.
- Infectivity highest before clinical illness.
- Highest infection in patients with school-aged children and day-care workers (not teachers).
- Flulike symptoms are followed by bright red rash on the face—**slapped-cheek** appearance. Rash may become lacelike, spreading to trunk and extremities.
- Twenty to thirty percent of adults are asymptomatic.
- IgM is produced 10–12 days after infection and persists for 3–6 months.
- IgG present several days after IgM appears. IgG persists for life and offers natural immunity against subsequent infections.

FETAL EFFECTS

- Fetal death
- Nonimmune hydrops: 1% of infected patients, due to fetal aplastic anemia

MANAGEMENT

- After exposure, check IgM and IgG.
- If IgM+, then perform ultrasound (US) for hydrops and middle cerebral artery Doppler to assess for anemia.
- If IgG positive, no further assessment needed.

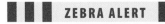
ZEBRA ALERT

Hydrops in a fetus after parvovirus infection is due to aplastic anemia.

- - - - - - - - - - - -

ZEBRA ALERT

Most common finding in congenital rubella syndrome: Neonatal hearing loss

- - - - - - - - - - - -

Rubella (German Measles)

Mild infection in adults caused by an RNA virus. All patients should be screened for rubella immunity at the time of their first obstetrics (OB) visit.

FETAL EFFECTS

- One of the most teratogenic infections, worse during organogenesis.
- Congenital rubella syndrome:
  - Cataracts, congenital glaucoma (blindness).
  - **Hearing loss:** Most common single defect.

- Central nervous system (CNS) defects: Microcephaly, intellectual disability.
- Newborns shed virus for many months.

PRENATAL DIAGNOSIS

Rubella RNA in chorionic villi, amniotic fluid, and fetal blood can confirm fetal infection for a patient with exposure and nonimmune/equivocal immune status.

VACCINE

Live attenuated vaccine should be avoided 1 month before and during pregnancy. Should be given postpartum to patients who are nonimmune or equivocal.

Cytomegalovirus (CMV)

- Most common cause of perinatal infection in the developed world.
- Spread via body fluids and person-to-person contact.
- Fetal infection via intrauterine, intrapartum, or postpartum infection (breast-feeding).
- Day-care centers are common source of infection.

EXAM TIP

Most common cause of perinatal infection: CMV.

MATERNAL INFECTION

- Most asymptomatic.
- Fifteen percent of adults have mononucleosis-type symptoms (fever, pharyngitis, lymphadenopathy, polyarthritis).
- Primary infection → virus latent → periodic reactivation and shedding.
  - Primary infections cause severe fetal morbidity in fetus.
  - Infections from reactivation have few sequelae.
- Maternal immunity does not prevent:
  - Recurrence.
  - Reactivation.
  - Exogenous infection.
  - Congenital infection.
  - Infection from a different strain.

CONGENITAL INFECTION

Five percent of infected infants have this syndrome:

- **Intracranial calcifications**
- **Chorioretinitis**
- Microcephaly
- Intellectual disability and motor retardation
- Hemolytic anemia
- Sensorineural deficits

WARD TIP

Previous CMV infection does **not** confer immunity.

PRENATAL DIAGNOSIS

- US can show microcephaly, ventriculomegaly, and intracranial calcifications.
- Polymerase chain reaction (PCR) detects and quantifies viral DNA in amniotic fluid and fetal blood.

MANAGEMENT

- Routine maternal serologic screen is not recommended.
- Measurement of maternal serum IgM and IgG can be used to confirm maternal primary infection. Though amniocentesis is the gold standard for fetal infection.

TREATMENT

No maternal treatment exists. No fetal treatment or prophylaxis has been shown to be beneficial.

Group B *Streptococcus* (GBS)

 A 27-year-old patient at 37 weeks' gestation presents with a 2-day history of fever of 101°F (38.3°C), loss of fluid from the vagina, and diffuse abdominal tenderness. What is the most likely diagnosis? What is the gold standard for diagnosis? What is the most common cause? How is it treated?

Answer: Intra-amniotic infection (IAI) (infection of the amniotic fluid, membranes, placenta or decidua—also known as chorioamnionitis). Amniotic fluid culture is the gold standard for diagnosis, though this is rarely used. Most common cause is polymicrobial. It is treated with IV antibiotics: ampicillin + gentamicin.

Asymptomatic carrier state of GBS (*Streptococcus agalactiae*) in vagina and rectum is common. The vast majority patients have no sequalae.

COMPLICATIONS

- Preterm labor
- Premature rupture of membranes (PROM)
- Chorioamnionitis
- Fetal/neonatal infections
- Pyelonephritis
- Endometritis
- Urinary tract infection

NEONATAL SEPSIS

- Low-birth-weight and premature infants have worse outcome than term infants.
- **Early-onset disease:**
  - Neonatal infection <7 days after birth.
  - Can be prevented with intrapartum prophylaxis.
  - Results from vertical transmission.
  - Sepsis, pneumonia, and meningitis are most common manifestations.
- **Late-onset disease:**
  - Infection 1 week to 3 months after birth.
  - Usually meningitis or bacteremia.
  - Not preventable with intrapartum prophylaxis.
  - Infection is community acquired or nosocomial.

PREVENTION

- Culture-based approach [recommended by Centers for Disease Control and Prevention (CDC)]:
  - Culture all patients for GBS at 35–37 weeks.
  - Intrapartum prophylaxis if GBS positive.
- Risk-based approach: For unknown GBS at the time of labor, treat if rupture for >18 hours, prior infant with GBS sepsis, or preterm status
  - **Penicillin:** First-line agent.
  - Penicillin allergy: Cefazolin if anaphylaxis risk low.
  - If anaphylaxis risk is high, perform sensitivities for erythromycin and clindamycin.
  - If resistant to above, give vancomycin.

Toxoplasmosis

- Toxoplasma gondii transmitted by:
  - Eating infected raw or undercooked meat.
  - Infected cat feces.
- Maternal infections are usually asymptomatic.
- Infection confers immunity; pre-pregnancy infection almost eliminates vertical transmission.
- Infected fetus clears the infection from organs, but it may be localized to CNS.
- Severity of fetal infection depends on the GA at the time of the maternal primary infection.
- **Classic triad** of newborn complications:
  - Chorioretinitis
  - Intracranial calcifications.
  - Hydrocephalus.
  - Can also cause intellectual disability and vision loss.

MANAGEMENT

- Routine screening not recommended.
- Confirm diagnosis:
  - By seroconversion of IgG and IgM or >4-fold rise in paired specimen.
  - Avidity IgG testing: If high-avidity IgG is found, infection in the preceding 3–5 months is excluded.
  - PCR for *Toxoplasma gondii* in amniotic fluid.

TREATMENT

- Prevents and reduces congenital infection. Does not eliminate the risk.
- Sulfadiazine + pyrimethamine: Presumptive treatment in late pregnancy. Higher potential toxicity.
- Spiramycin.

PREVENTION

- No vaccine available.
- Practice good hygiene when handling raw meat and contaminated utensils.
- Clean and peel fruits and vegetables.
- Wear gloves when cleaning cat litter or delegate the duty. Keep cats indoors.

  ZEBRA ALERT

Congenital toxoplasmosis presents with: **Classic triad** of neonatal chorioretinitis, intracranial calcifications, and hydrocephalus.

Bacterial Vaginosis (BV)

 A 32-year-old G2P1001 patient at 32 weeks' gestation presents with a 4-day history of vaginal discharge. She does not report itching, burning, or pain. On physical exam, a homogenous white discharge is noted to coat the vaginal side walls. A wet mount of the discharge shows clue cells, and a fishy odor is noted when KOH is added to the discharge. What is the most likely diagnosis? What is the best treatment?

Answer: Symptoms and diagnosis based on Amsel's criteria is consistent with bacterial vaginosis. The treatment of choice in pregnancy is oral metronidazole.

Clinical syndrome that results from replacement of normal *Lactobacillus* in the vagina with anaerobic bacteria, *Gardnerella vaginalis*, and *Mycoplasma hominis*. Occurs at any time in a patient's life, including pregnancy.

DIAGNOSIS

- **Amsel clinical criteria:**
  - Homogenous, white discharge that coats vaginal walls.
  - Clue cells on microscopy.
  - Vaginal pH > 4.5.
  - Whiff test positive: Fishy odor when KOH added to vaginal discharge.
- Nugent criteria: Gram stain for the diagnosis.
- Pap tests have low sensitivity for the diagnosis of BV and thus are not routinely used.
- Increased risk of antepartum complications:
  - Preterm birth.
  - PROM.
  - Chorioamnionitis.

TREATMENT

- Does not improve perinatal outcome.
- Oral metronidazole or vaginal clindamycin for symptoms.
- Treatment of partners not routinely recommended.

Candidiasis

Yeast infection on the vulva and in the vagina usually caused by *Candida albicans*.

DIAGNOSIS

Pseudohyphae seen on microscopy.

TREATMENT

- Topical treatment with antifungals preferred.
- Treat with topical (vaginal) azole therapy for 7–14 days.

Sexually Transmitted Infections (STIs)

See Chapter 31 for additional information on STIs.

SYPHILIS

- *Treponema pallidum* spirochetes cross the placenta and cause congenital infection.
  - Any stage of maternal syphilis may result in fetal infection.
- Newborns can have jaundice, hepatosplenomegaly, skin lesions, rhinitis, pneumonia, myocarditis, nephrosis.
- One screening test should be followed by one confirmatory test:
  - Screening tests:
    - Rapid plasma reagin (RPR).
    - Venereal Disease Research Laboratory (VDRL).
  - Confirmatory tests:
    - Fluorescent treponemal antibody absorption test (FTA-ABS).
    - Microhemagglutination assay (MHA-TP).
- US findings: Fetal edema, ascites, hydrops, thickened placenta.

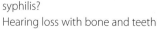

ZEBRA ALERT

What are late manifestations of congenital syphilis?
Hearing loss with bone and teeth abnormalities:

- Frontal bossing
- Short maxilla
- High palatal arch
- Saddle nose deformity
- Malformed teeth

- **Penicillin** is the treatment of choice for all stages of syphilis (same as nonpregnant patients). If patient is penicillin allergic, then she must be desensitized and still treated with penicillin.
- **Jarisch–Herxheimer reaction** may occur with penicillin treatment. The reaction occurs due the maternal inflammatory response to rupturing spirochetes after treatment with penicillin. It involves uterine contractions and late decelerations in the fetal heart rate as the dead spirochetes occlude the placental circulation.

GONORRHEA

- The patient will often have concomitant *Chlamydia* infection.
- In pregnancy, usually limited to lower genital tract (cervix, urethra, periurethral glands, and vestibular glands). Acute salpingitis or PID is rare in pregnancy.
- Prenatal screen should be done at the first prenatal visit. Repeat later in pregnancy if high risk or if required by state law.
- Diagnosed with nucleic acid PCR.
- Treat with ceftriaxone.
- Gonorrhea can cause conjunctivitis and vision loss in neonates. All newborns are given prophylaxis against conjunctivitis.

CHLAMYDIA

- Most pregnant patients are asymptomatic.
- Can cause delayed postpartum uterine infection.
- Diagnosed with nucleic acid PCR.
- **Neonatal infections:**
  - Ophthalmia neonatorum: Conjunctivitis, blindness.
  - Pneumonia.
- Prenatal screen: Screen at the first prenatal visit. Repeat in T3 if at high risk or if required by state law.
- Treatment: Azithromycin.

HERPES SIMPLEX VIRUS

- **Signs and symptoms:** Numbness, tingling, pain (prodromal symptoms), vesicles with erythematous base that heal without scarring.
- **Treatment:** Acyclovir and valacyclovir can shorten the length of symptoms and amount of viral shedding. Shedding not completely eliminated.
  - Safe in pregnancy.
  - Suppression with acyclovir starting at 36 weeks is indicated for those with a history of herpes.
- Neonatal infections can occur via intrauterine (5%), peripartum (85%), and postnatal (10%).
- Newborn infection with three forms:
  - Skin, eye, mouth with localized involvement.
  - CNS disease with encephalitis.
  - Disseminated disease with multiple organ involvement.
- When patient with history of HSV presents in labor:
  - Ask about prodromal symptoms.
  - Examine perineum, vagina, cervix for lesions.
  - If prodromal symptoms or lesions are present, patient should be offered a cesarean delivery to ↓ the risk of vertical transmission.
- Can breast-feed, even when on antivirals. Avoid breast-feeding if herpes lesions on breast that can come in contact with infant.

EXAM TIP

Penicillin is the only syphilis therapy that prevents congenital syphilis.

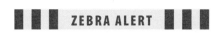

ZEBRA ALERT

Jarisch–Herxheimer reaction is a maternal immune response to lysing Treponema.

EXAM TIP

Most common cause of ophthalmia neonatorum: *Chlamydia trachomatis*

EXAM TIP

If herpes lesions or prodromal symptoms are present at the time of labor, a cesarean delivery should be performed to ↓ the risk of vertical transmission.

HEPATITIS B VIRUS (HBV)

A 30-year-old G1P0 patient at 39 weeks' gestation is admitted for active labor. Her prenatal course is complicated by an infection with chronic hepatitis B. How should the infant be treated once the delivery takes place?

Answer: The infant should receive the first dose of the hepatitis vaccine series and hepatitis immune globulin soon after birth.

- Chronic infection occurs in 70–90% of acutely infected infants leading to:
  - Cirrhosis.
  - Hepatocellular carcinoma.
- Screen at first prenatal visit and at delivery with hepatitis B surface antigen (HBsAg).
- Antiviral treatment recommended in pregnancy (first line: tenofovir; second line: lamivudine or telbivudine): indications are the same outside of pregnancy.
  - For women who do not meet these criteria, recheck viral load at 26–28 weeks, if $>10^6 \rightarrow$ initiate treatment to decrease risk of vertical transmission.
- Small amount of transplacental passage.
- Most neonatal infection due to ingestion of infected fluid in the peripartum or with breast-feeding.
- ↑ risk of infectivity with ↑ levels of hepatitis B early antigen (HBeAg).
- Vaccine can be given during pregnancy.
- **Prevention** of neonatal infection: If mother with hepatitis B:
  - Give hepatitis B immunoglobulin (HBIG) to infant upon delivery.
  - Give first of three hepatitis B vaccines upon delivery.
  - Can breast-feed if infant given prophylaxis.

HUMAN IMMUNODEFICIENCY VIRUS (HIV)

- HIV screening recommended at first prenatal visit. Some states require a repeat test in T3.
  - **Screening:** Enzyme-linked immunosorbent assay (ELISA).
  - **Confirmatory:** Western blot and/or PCR.
  - If available, currently the preferred algorithm uses a fourth-generation antigen/antibody combination HIV-1/2 immunoassay plus a confirmatory HIV-1/HIV-2 antibody differentiation immunoassay.
- The vast majority of cases of pediatric AIDS are secondary to vertical transmission from mother to fetus.
- Risk of perinatal transmission ~25%. If zidovudine (ZDV) is given during antepartum, intrapartum, and to neonate, risk of transmission is reduced to 8%.
- Combination antiretroviral therapy should be started in the antenatal period if not previously taking and can reduce risk of vertical transmission to 2%.
- Reduce maternal viral load:
  - Antiretroviral therapy should be recommended in **all** HIV-infected pregnant patients regardless of CD4+ count and viral load in order to reduce vertical transmission.
  - In pregnancy, antiretroviral treatment usually consists of nucleoside reverse transcriptase inhibitor (NTRI) zidovudine-lamivudine because of its safety profile in pregnancy, combined with a protease inhibitor such as atazanavir-ritonavir.

- CD4+ counts and viral loads should be monitored at regular intervals.
- Blood counts and liver functions should be monitored monthly while patient is on antiretroviral therapy.
- Reduce vertical transmission:
  - Give maternal IV ZDV intrapartum.
  - Reduce duration of ruptured membranes.
  - Recommend cesarean delivery before labor or rupture of membranes if viral load >1000 copies.
  - Avoid breast-feeding.
  - Give infant post-exposure prophylaxis with ZDV for 6 weeks.

HUMAN PAPILLOMAVIRUS (HPV)

Chronic viral infection that can cause genital condyloma, cervical, vaginal, and vulvar cancer.
- Clearance of virus slower during pregnancy.
- Condyloma acuminata, external genital warts, ↑ in number and size in pregnancy.
- If size and location of lesions obstruct vaginal delivery, may need to perform a cesarean delivery.
- Lesions often regress spontaneously after delivery.

TREATMENT

- Trichloroacetic or bichloroacetic acid applied weekly for external warts.
- Cryotherapy.
- Laser.
- **Not** recommended for pregnancy:
  - Podophyllin resin.
  - Podofilox.
  - 5-fluorouracil.
  - Imiquimod.
  - Interferon.

TRICHOMONIASIS

- Diagnosis is made when **flagellated organisms** seen on **wet prep**.
- **Complications:**
  - Preterm delivery.
  - Preterm premature ruptured membranes.
- Treat with oral metronidazole.

EXAM TIP

Two main strategies to ↓ vertical transmission of HIV:
- Antiretroviral therapy
- Cesarean delivery if high viral load

WARD TIP

Breast-feeding is contraindicated in patients with HIV, even if viral load is undetectable.

ZEBRA ALERT

HPV can cause laryngeal papillomatosis in fetus.

NOTES

Twin Gestation

By 25 weeks, a uterus with twins is the same size as a 40-week singleton uterus.

Zygosity is the number of eggs fertilized; chorionicity is the number of placentas.

Chorionicity is important to determine early in the pregnancy—can be done with ultrasound (US).

Number of twin pregnancies is on the rise due to ↑ use of assisted reproductive technologies.

Multiple gestation pregnancy has a high incidence of preterm labor, preterm premature rupture of the membranes (PPROM), and preterm birth.

Serial US assessments are the only reliable way to document adequate fetal growth and fetal growth restriction.

In the setting of Di/Di twins, if they have discordant genders, then they are dizygotic. However, if the gender is the same in both twins, zygosity can only be determined with genetic testing.

Twin pregnancy continues to ↑ in the United States secondary to assisted reproductive technologies and an advancing maternal age. Maternal and perinatal morbidity are ↑ in multiple gestations. Twin pregnancies have higher rates of almost every potential pregnancy complication, including preterm delivery, growth restriction, and congenital anomalies. Prenatal visits are more frequent with multiple gestations, since they are at increased risk for complications. Normal physiologic changes are increased, and there is an increase in cardiac output, iron requirements, plasma volume, blood volume, glomerular filtration rate, and caloric requirements.

Maternal Adaptations

Maternal physiologic changes are more exaggerated compared to a singleton pregnancy.
- **Cardiac:**
  - ↑ heart rate, ↑ stroke volume, ↑ cardiac output is more secondary to the ↑ myometrial contractility and blood volume.
  - ↑ in uterine volume/weight.
- **Respiratory:** Further ↑ in tidal volume and oxygen consumption.
- **Renal:** ↑ GFR and ↑ in renal size.
- **Nutrition:**
  - Calories: Increase intake by 300 kcal/day above that for singleton pregnancy, or 600 kcal/day above that of a nonpregnant patient.
  - Weight gain: Avg/week is 1–1.75 pounds; total gain: 37–54 pounds for a normal weight patient.

Types of Twins

A 22-year-old P2012 patient at 15 weeks' gestation presents for her first prenatal visit. On physical exam, her fundal height is 20 cm, at the level of the umbilicus. A bedside US reveals a twin gestation. Management of her prenatal care should include which important tests/procedures?

Answer: A formal US to determine chorionicity and serial USs to check for fetal growth restriction/discrepancy. Further monitoring may be needed depending on the type of chorionicity and amnionicity. The patient will also need baseline preeclampsia labs.

A **zygote** is the result of fertilization of an ovum with a spermatozoan.
- **Dizygotic twins** are the result of two ova fertilized by two different sperm. Risk factors include fertility drugs, ancestry, advanced maternal age, and parity. These are fraternal or non-identical twins.
- **Monozygotic twins** are the result of a single ovum fertilized by one sperm which subsequently divides. The frequency is 1 in 250 pregnancies (see Figure 10-1). These are identical twins.
- The timing of cell division within the monozygotic twin determines the amnionicity and chorionicity of twins, as well as the number of sacs and placentas (see Table 10-1.)
  - Division of the ovum between days 0 and 3: Dichorionic, Diamniotic monozygotic twins (aka Di/Di twins).
  - Division between 4 and 8 days: Monochorionic, Diamniotic monozygotic twins (aka Mo/Di twins).

Incidence: 1:250 pregnancies

Fetal Sex: same (except meiotic non-disjunction, eg., xo, xy)

Fertilization: 1 sperm, 1 egg

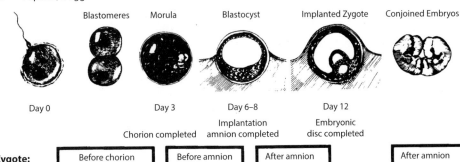

FIGURE 10-1. **Mechanism of monozygous twinning.** (Reproduced, with permission, from Cunningham FG, Leveno KJ, Bloom SL, et al. *Williams Obstetrics.* 22nd ed. New York: McGraw-Hill; 2005:914.)

TABLE 10-1. **Differences Between Monozygotic Twin Types**

	DI/DI TWINS	MONO/DI TWINS	MONO/MONO TWINS
Number of eggs	1	1	1
Number of placentas	2	1	1
Number of sacs	2	2	1

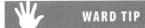

- Division between 9 and 12 days: Monochorionic, Monoamniotic monozygotic twins (aka Mo/Mo twins).
- Division after 13 days: Conjoined twins.
- Twin gestation complications are higher than singleton pregnancies. The associated risks and management are determined by the amnionicity and chorionicity (see Table 10-2).
    - Monochorionic twins have more complications than dichorionic.
    - Monoamniotic twins have more complications than diamniotic.

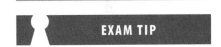

Prenatal Diagnosis

- Diagnosis and genetic counseling is important because of the ↑ risk of congenital anomalies.
- Both monozygotic and dizygotic twins are at ↑ risk for structural anomalies.
- Multiple gestation has an increased risk of aneuploidy.

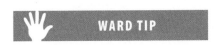

Differential diagnoses for a size/date discrepancy in pregnancy include:

- Twins
- Fibroids
- Distended bladder
- Fetal macrosomia
- Polyhydramnios
- Maternal obesity
- Uncertain last menstrual period (LMP) (wrong dates)
- Molar pregnancy

TABLE 10-2.   Twin Complications and Management

	DI/DI TWINS	MONO/DI TWINS	MONO/MONO TWINS
At increased risk for anomalies?	Yes	Yes	Yes
At risk for TTTS	No	Yes	No
At risk for cord entanglement	No	No	Yes
At risk for preterm birth	Yes	Yes—high	Yes—very high
Additional surveillance needed	No	TTTS checks every 2 weeks from 16 weeks' gestation	Admission at viability with frequent fetal monitoring
Delivery timing in uncomplicated cases	38–38/6 weeks	34–37/6 weeks	32–34/0 weeks

TTTS, twin-twin transfusion syndrome

Diagnosis and Management of Twins

- **Physical exam** may show a uterine size/gestational age (GA) difference with size greater than expected from GA.
- **US** is used for the following in multiple gestations:
    - Confirm diagnosis.
    - Determine chorionicity.
    - Detect fetal anomalies.
    - Evaluate for fetal growth.
    - Confirm fetal well-being.
- Determining chorionicity is important:
    - Chorionicity can best be determined in the first or early second trimester by US.
    - Di/Di twins can be diagnosed by the "Lambda sign"—the thickened area where the membrane comes off the placenta/uterine wall (Figure 10-2).
    - Mo/Di Twins have a "T" sign (and thinner membrane) (Figure 10-3).
    - Mo/Mo twins have no membrane between them.
    - All twins should undergo US examination to follow fetal growth every 4 weeks starting at 28 weeks (fundal height is not reliable in twins).
    - Growth restriction rates are higher among the monochorionic in comparison to the dichorionic twin gestation.
    - Monochorionic twins may also be at risk for twin-twin transfusion syndrome (TTTS).
- Preterm delivery is very common—either due to preterm labor, PPROM, or preeclampsia. Delivery timing for twins varies by twin type.
- Determining the route of delivery (vaginal versus cesarean) should be based on the experience of the obstetrician, other obstetric indications (i.e., placenta previa), and the presentation of both twins:
    - Trial of vaginal delivery is appropriate in situations where both twins are cephalic.
    - Cephalic presentation of Twin A and breech presentation of Twin B should be managed based on the experience of the obstetrician.

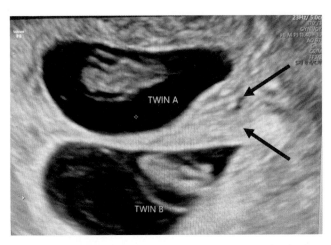

FIGURE 10-2. Lambda sign in Di/Di twins. Black arrows point to the thick intertwin membrane and "Lambda sign."

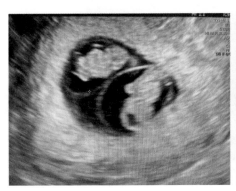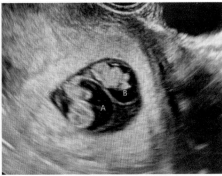

FIGURE 10-3. MO/DI TWINS T SIGN. Note the lack of the lambda sign and thin intertwin membrane in these two images of mono/di twins.

Vaginal delivery may be appropriate, with a plan for an internal podalic version or breech extraction of the second twin after delivery of the first twin.
- Breech presentation of Twin A requires delivery by cesarean.

Twin-Twin Transfusion Syndrome (TTTS)

- A **serious complication** of monochorionic twin gestation in which blood/intravascular volume is shunted from one twin to another across the shared placenta.
- The major risk is intrauterine fetal demise, in which one twin develops complications due to underperfusion (donor twin) and the other due to overperfusion (recipient twin).
- The cause is unbalanced vascular anastomoses between the two sides of the placenta.
- US is needed for diagnosis—and usually manifests first as oligohydramnios in the donor twin and polyhydramnios in the recipient twin.
- The severity and the stage are determined by US findings (see Table 10-3).
- **Treatment** is laser coagulation of the anastomoses when severe.

 ZEBRA ALERT

With dizygotic twins, one twin may be genetically and structurally normal, while the other may have genetic or structural anomalies.

 EXAM TIP

Multiple gestation pregnancies are at increased risk for complications such as gestational diabetes, gestational hypertensive disorders, congenital anomalies, and growth restriction.

 WARD TIP

Dizygotic twins are more common than monozygotic twins.

 EXAM TIP

Monochorionic twins have higher complication rates than dichorionic twins and require more frequent surveillance.

 ZEBRA ALERT

In the setting of TTTS, the donor twin has oligohydramnios and intrauterine growth restriction (IUGR), while the recipient twin has polyhydramnios and is at risk for fluid overload.

 EXAM TIP

TTTS: Serious complication in monochorionic diamniotic twin gestations due to aterio-venous anastomosis between two sides of the placentas.

EXAM TIP

The biggest risk in monochorionic monoamniotic twin gestations is cord entanglement (Figure 10-4).

TABLE 10-3. **TTTS Stages**

STAGE	ULTRASOUND FINDINGS
Stage 1	Oligohydramnios and polyhydramnios
Stage 2	Absent bladder on donor twin
Stage 3	Abnormal umbilical artery Dopplers
Stage 4	Hydrops noted in one or both twins
Stage 5	Death of one or both twins

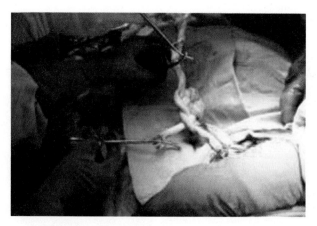

FIGURE 10-4. **Cord knots.**

Higher Order Multiples

Though much less common, higher order multiples pose very high risk for both the patient and the fetuses. Maternal physiologic adaptations are even further increased in these settings as are obstetric risks, such as extreme prematurity, gestational diabetes and preeclampsia. As a sense, over 90% of triplets deliver preterm and more than 1 in 3 set of triplets deliver prior to 32 weeks. Zygosity can vary in triplets and quadruplets as can chorionicity and amnionicity. Thus, early ultrasound is recommended. Given the extremely high risk associated with higher order multiples, selective reduction (termination of one or more fetuses) should be offered to all patients in these settings to reduce maternal risk and risk of prematurity for the remaining fetuses.

Early Pregnancy Loss and Fetal Demise

Approximately 30% of pregnancies end with spontaneous abortion.

WARD TIP

Always check blood type and Rh on all pregnant patients with vaginal bleeding. Give anti-D immunoglobulin if Rh negative.

WARD TIP

An anti-D antibody injection should be given to all pregnant patients in the first trimester that have:
- Vaginal bleeding
- D (Rh) antigen negative
- D (Rh) antibody screen negative

First-Trimester Bleeding

Bleeding in the first trimester can be from many causes that may or may not be related to the pregnancy.

DIFFERENTIAL DIAGNOSIS

- Spontaneous abortion (including threatened abortion)
- Ectopic pregnancy
- Hydatidiform mole
- Benign and malignant lesions (i.e., cervical polyp, cervical cancer)
- Trauma
- Infection
- Implantation bleeding

WORKUP

- History: Vaginal bleeding +/− abdominal pain.
- Physical:
  - Vital signs (rule out shock/sepsis).
  - Pelvic exam (note the source of bleeding and cervical dilation).
- Diagnostic tests:
  - Quantitative β-human chorionic gonadotropin (hCG) level.
  - Complete blood count (CBC).
  - Blood type and Rh. An anti-D immunoglobulin injection should be given to all D (Rh) antigen negative pregnant patients that have vaginal bleeding and a negative D (Rh) antibody screen.
    - Prevents maternal isoimmunization (generation of antibodies against fetal red blood cells in current or future pregnancies).
  - Ultrasound (US) assesses location of pregnancy, fetal viability, and contents of the uterus. See Table 11-1.

Spontaneous Abortion

Spontaneous abortion (or miscarriage) is a clinically recognized pregnancy loss before 20 weeks' gestation. It is also known as "early pregnancy loss" or EPL. There are many risk factors, including advanced maternal age, maternal smoking, and history of previous spontaneous abortion.

- **Abortion** = Intentional or unintentional termination of a pregnancy <20 weeks' gestation. In the media and non-medical world, the term

TABLE 11-1. Ultrasound Findings Based on Gestational Age in Setting of a Normal Singleton Pregnancy

GESTATIONAL AGE	ULTRASOUND FINDING
4.5–5 weeks	Gestational sac in the uterus
5–6 weeks	Gestational sac with a yolk sac in the uterus
5.5–6 weeks	Fetal pole
6+ weeks	Cardiac activity in the fetal pole

"abortion" is used to refer to intentional/elective termination of pregnancy, but in medicine, it is used to describe *any and all* pregnancies that end prior to 20 weeks' gestation.
- Completed spontaneous abortion is the spontaneous expulsion of all fetal and placental tissue from the uterine cavity before 20 weeks' gestation.
- Occurs in 8–20% of all recognized pregnancies.
- Most spontaneous abortions are clinically unrecognized because they occur before or at the time of the next expected menses (13–26%).
- Diagnostic criteria for a failed pregnancy are determined by US findings (see Table 11-2).

ETIOLOGIES

The causes of fetal demise vary by trimester. See Table 11-3.

Chromosomal Abnormalities
- Most common cause of spontaneous abortion and accounts for 50% of all miscarriages. The majority of abnormal karyotypes are numeric abnormalities as a result of errors during gametogenesis, fertilization, or the first division of the fertilized ovum.
- Frequency:
  - Aneuploidy (abnormal number of chromosomes): 85%.
  - Triploidy: 10%.
  - Tetraploidy: 4%.

Maternal Structural Anomalies
- Uterine anomaly
- Cervical insufficiency

TABLE 11-2. Diagnostic Criteria for Failed Pregnancy

A gestational sac ≥25 mm in mean diameter that does not contain a yolk sac or embryo
An embryo with a crown-rump length (CRL) ≥7 mm that does not have cardiac activity
After a pelvic ultrasound showed a gestational sac without a yolk sac, absence of an embryo with a heartbeat in ≥2 weeks
After a pelvic ultrasound showed a gestational sac with a yolk sac, absence of an embryo with a heartbeat in ≥11 days

TABLE 11-3. Causes of Fetal Demise by Trimester

FIRST TRIMESTER	SECOND TRIMESTER	THIRD TRIMESTER	ANY TRIMESTER
Chromosomal abnormalities	Placental insufficiency	Placental abruption	Trauma, including intimate partner violence
Environmental factors (i.e., medications, smoking, toxins)	Antiphospholipid antibody syndrome	Infections (e.g., toxoplasmosis, CMV, parvovirus)	Cord accident
Maternal anatomic defects (i.e., Müllerian defects)	Chromosomal or genetic abnormalities	Placental insufficiency	Maternal systemic disease (e.g., diabetes, hypertension)
Endocrine factors (i.e., thyroid dysfunction, diabetes)	Anatomic anomalies of uterus and cervix	Hypertensive disorders of pregnancy	Maternal infection (e.g., chorioamnionitis)
		Antiphospholipid antibody syndrome	Substance abuse (e.g., cocaine)

CMV, cytomegalovirus

- Leiomyomas (especially submucosal)
- Intrauterine adhesions (i.e., from previous curettage or surgery)

Maternal Physiologic Factors
- Thrombophilias
- Uncontrolled diabetes (type 1 or type 2)

Environmental Factors
- Tobacco: ≥14 cigarettes/day ↑ spontaneous abortion rates
- Alcohol
- Irradiation
- Environmental toxin exposure
- Trauma (more common in the second trimester)

Types of Spontaneous Abortion

See Table 11-4.

THREATENED ABORTION

 A 34-year-old G1P0 patient at 8 weeks' gestation presents to the emergency department with vaginal bleeding. She reports no cramping, trauma, or intercourse. She is afebrile and hemodynamically stable. Physical exam reveals a nontender abdomen. Sterile speculum shows 5 cc of dark blood in the vagina with no active bleeding. The cervix is closed and thick. US shows an 8-week intrauterine pregnancy with cardiac activity. What is the most likely diagnosis? What is the best treatment for her condition?
Answer: Threatened abortion. The patient should be managed expectantly. Many patients will go on to have a normal pregnancy course.

Threatened abortion is uterine bleeding from a gestation that is <20 weeks without cervical dilation or passage of tissue.

TABLE 11-4. Types of Abortions

	THREATENED	INEVITABLE	INCOMPLETE	COMPLETE	MISSED	SEPTIC
Clinical presentation	Vaginal bleeding	Cramping, bleeding	Cramping, bleeding (ongoing)	Cramping, bleeding (resolved)	Asymptomatic	Fever, abdominal/ pelvic pain, ruptured membranes
Passage of tissue	No	No	Some but not all tissue passed	All tissue passed (done)	No	Variable
Cervical Os	Closed	Open	Open	Closed	Closed	Variable
Pregnancy viable	~50% will miscarry	100% will miscarry	No	No	No	Variable
Management	Confirm intrauterine gestation, then expectant management	Surgical, medical, or expectant management	Surgical, medical, or expectant management	Follow hCG levels to negative	Surgical, medical, or expectant management	IV antibiotics, D&C

- Pregnancy may continue, but there is an increased risk of pregnancy loss.
- It increases the risk of preterm labor and delivery and other adverse pregnancy outcomes.

DIAGNOSIS

- Speculum exam reveals blood coming from a closed cervical os, without amniotic fluid or products of conception (POC) in the endocervical canal.
- US will vary depending on gestational age.

MANAGEMENT

Once intrauterine gestation is proven, then observation and support can be offered to the patient. Can consider follow-up US in 7–10 days for confirmation of viability. If a yolk sac (or more) is not seen in the uterus, then the pregnancy is considered to be a "pregnancy of unknown location" (PUL), and close patient follow-up with serial assessment of β-hCG and follow-up US is indicated.

In some cases, a patient will present with a threatened abortion but the US will be nondiagnostic for viable intrauterine pregnancy. In other words, the US will show a gestational sac without a yolk sac, or a yolk sac without a fetal pole. These findings are suggestive of an intrauterine pregnancy, but not necessarily a *viable* intrauterine pregnancy. In these cases, a β-hCG should be trended and a follow-up US should occur 10–14 days later. If the below criteria are met, a missed abortion can be diagnosed.

INEVITABLE ABORTION

An 18-year-old G1P0 patient at 8 weeks' gestation presents to the emergency department reporting cramping and vaginal spotting. She reports no passage of tissue. Physical exam shows bleeding from the cervical os, which is open. US shows an intrauterine pregnancy with cardiac activity. What is the most likely diagnosis?

Answer: Vaginal bleeding before 20 weeks' gestation, open cervical os, and no expulsion of POC is an inevitable abortion.

Inevitable abortion is vaginal bleeding, cramps, and cervical dilation at <20 weeks' gestation without expulsion of POC. Expulsion of POC is imminent. This term is usually only used in the first trimester.

DIAGNOSIS

- Presence of menstrual-like cramps.
- Speculum exam reveals blood coming from an **open** cervical os.
- Fetal cardiac activity may or may not be present on US.

MANAGEMENT

Any of these three are options—though patients should be counseled on the risks and benefits of each one:
- Surgical evacuation of the uterus with dilation and curettage (D&C)
- Medical uterine evacuation with misoprostol (prostaglandin E1)
- Expectant management

INCOMPLETE ABORTION

Incomplete abortion is the **passage of some, but not all, POC** from the uterine cavity before 20 weeks' gestation. (Again, this term is usually used in the first trimester).

Increased risk of:
- Ongoing bleeding requiring a blood transfusion
- Ascending infection, septic abortion

DIAGNOSIS

- Cramping and bleeding.
- Enlarged, boggy uterus, dilated internal os.
- POC present in the endocervical canal or vagina.
- POC retained in the uterus may be seen with US.

MANAGEMENT

- Assess hemodynamic status and stabilize (IV fluids, blood transfusion).
- If unstable, surgical management (via suction D&C) to remove the POC from the uterus.
- If stable, expectant management, medical management (with misoprostol), or surgical management are options. If the individual elects expectant or medical management, follow-up in 1–2 weeks should be arranged.
- Consider sending POC for karyotype if recurrent abortion.

EXAM TIP

Dilated cervix is seen with inevitable and incomplete abortions.

COMPLETE ABORTION

 A 24-year-old patient at 9 weeks' gestation presents to the emergency department with vaginal bleeding and cramping that is now decreased. She reports that she had an US 3 days prior showing a viable fetus. Vitals are normal. On physical exam there is no abdominal tenderness, there is 5 cc of dark blood in the vagina, and the cervix is closed. An US shows an empty uterus. What is the most likely diagnosis?
Answer: Complete abortion.

Complete abortion is the **complete passage of POC**. The **cervical os is closed** after the abortion is completed.

DIAGNOSIS

- Pain has ceased.
- Uterus is well contracted. Cervical os may be closed.
- US shows empty uterus.

MANAGEMENT

- If possible, send POC to pathology to verify intrauterine pregnancy. (Note: This is usually not possible.)
- Observe patient for further bleeding and signs of infection.
- D&C usually reserved for patients with excessive bleeding or unstable vitals.

MISSED ABORTION

Missed abortion is **fetal demise** before 20 weeks' gestation **without expulsion of any POC.**

DIAGNOSIS

- The pregnant uterus fails to grow, and symptoms of pregnancy have disappeared.
- Intermittent vaginal bleeding/spotting/brown discharge and a closed cervix.
- Quantitative β-hCG may decline, plateau, or continue to ↑.

- US confirms absent fetal cardiac activity or empty gestational sac.

In this setting, it is important to document if there is an embryo present or not, as this may help future physicians to better counsel patients.

Embryonic demise: Early first-trimester loss with an embryo present (fetal pole, embryo, or fetus without cardiac activity).

Anembryonic demise: Early first-trimester loss without an embryo present (empty gestational sac).

MANAGEMENT

- Expectant management.
  - Most patients will spontaneously deliver a missed abortion within 2 weeks.
  - Risk of incomplete or septic abortion that may require a D&C (very rare).
  - Concern for coagulopathy if dead fetus is not evacuated, higher risk in T2 and T3.
- Surgical management: Suction D&C.
- Medical management: Using misoprostol (PG E_1) with or without mifepristone.

SEPTIC ABORTION

> A 25-year-old G3P1011 patient presents to the emergency department with fever, lower abdominal pain, and foul-smelling discharge. She reported having a medical termination of pregnancy 6 days prior. Her temperature is 101.1°F (38.3°C), blood pressure 110/70, pulse 100, and respiratory rate 18. On physical exam, she appears lethargic and ill. She has lower abdominal tenderness, and sterile speculum exam shows a copious amount of foul-smelling discharge in the vagina. Bimanual exam reveals uterine tenderness and no adnexal masses. The cervix is dilated 1 cm and thick. Complete blood count (CBC) shows a white blood cell count (WBC) of 20,000K. US shows a large amount of heterogeneous tissue in the uterus. What is the most likely diagnosis? What is the best treatment for her condition?
>
> **Answer:** The patient has a septic abortion and should receive broad-spectrum IV antibiotics and a D&C.

- **Infected POC are present.**
- Rare with spontaneous abortion, and more likely to occur after surgical procedure.
- The infection is usually polymicrobial.
- Infection can spread from endometrium, through myometrium, to parametrium and sometimes to peritoneum.
- Septic shock may occur.

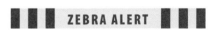

ZEBRA ALERT

If POC are not removed in a septic abortion, severe sepsis may occur.

DIAGNOSIS

- Fever, hypotension, tachycardia, generalized pelvic discomfort, uterine tenderness, signs of peritonitis.
- Speculum exam: Malodorous vaginal and cervical discharge, Bimanual with cervical motion tenderness
- Leukocytosis.
- US shows retained POC.

MANAGEMENT

- Check CBC, urinalysis (UA), serum electrolytes, liver function tests (LFTs), blood urea nitrogen (BUN), creatinine, and coagulation panel. For patients in florid sepsis, consider blood cultures.
- Broad-spectrum IV antibiotics with excellent anaerobic bacteria coverage.

EXAM TIP

RPL is three or more pregnancy losses before 20 weeks.

EXAM TIP

After two miscarriages, patients have a 25–30% risk of recurrence.

EXAM TIP

Testing for antiphospholipid antibody syndrome includes beta-2 glycoprotein, anti-cardiolipin antibody, and lupus anticoagulant.

- D&C promptly after starting antibiotics and stabilizing patient.
- Hysterectomy if unable to evacuate the infected uterine contents or it patient does not clinically improve after evacuation.

RECURRENT PREGNANCY LOSS (RPL)

- Three or more successive clinically recognized pregnancy losses prior to 20 weeks' gestation.
- Patients with two successive spontaneous abortions have a recurrence risk of 25–30%.

ETIOLOGY

- Chromosome abnormalities: Aneuploidy, parental chromosome rearrangements (balanced translocation is the most common).
- Anatomic uterine abnormalities: Congenital uterine anomalies such as uterine didelphys, septate uterus, and bicornuate uterus. Septate uterus is the most common anomaly associated with RPL.
- Acquired uterine defects: Intrauterine synechiae (Asherman syndrome), submucous leiomyomas.
- Cervical insufficiency: Painless cervical dilation leads to second-trimester pregnancy loss. Treat with cervical cerclage.
- Endocrine abnormalities: Diabetes mellitus, thyroid disorders.
- Autoimmune conditions: Antiphospholipid syndrome (thrombosis results in fetal demise).
- Unexplained in a majority of cases.

MANAGEMENT

Investigate possible etiologies. Potentially useful tests include:
- Karyotyping of POC.
- Parental karyotypes: Balanced translocation in parents may result in unbalanced translocation in the fetus.
- Sonohysterogram, hysteroscopy: Evaluate uterine cavity (high yield especially for losses >12 weeks).
- Immunologic workup: Anti-cardiolipin antibodies, beta-2 glycoprotien, and lupus anticoagulant.
- Thyroid function tests.

Induced Abortion (Pregnancy Termination)

DEFINITIONS

- Induced abortion: Intentional termination of pregnancy also known as elective termination of pregnancy or therapeutic abortion.

ASSESSMENT OF THE PATIENT

- **Confirm gestation age.**
  - US most reliable method and most commonly used.
  - Definitive LMP date and pelvic exam consistent with suspected dates is acceptable in T1.
  - Adequate dating helps determine legality of the procedure—states usually set gestational age limits.

- **Blood type and Rh type:** If patient is Rh negative, anti-D immunoglobulins should be administered prophylactically.
- Some states have mandatory requirements for waiting times, counseling scripts, and parental notification for minors.

INDICATIONS FOR THERAPEUTIC ABORTION (NOT AN EXHAUSTIVE LIST)

Maternal

Severe maternal disease where continuation of pregnancy may be life-threatening: Severe cardiovascular disease, early severe preeclampsia (after 20 weeks), maternal malignancy requiring prompt chemotherapy, preterm premature rupture of the membranes (PPROM) with maternal sepsis. Unplanned and undesired pregnancy is another indication. Rape and incest are other scenarios where termination is often pursued. Major fetal anomalies are another indication where patients may consider termination—anencephaly, holoprosencephaly, skeletal dysplasias, or hypoplastic left heart syndrome (among others). Families may also pursue termination in the setting of life limiting genetic conditions such as spinal muscular atrophy or trisomy 13.

WARD TIP

Differential diagnosis for T1 bleeding:
- Spontaneous abortion
- Ectopic pregnancy
- Molar pregnancy
- Vaginal/cervical lesions/lacerations

METHODS OF PREGNANCY TERMINATION

- Pharmacologic agents.
- Surgical methods.

Pharmacologic Agents

- Abortions in T1 and T2 can be performed with pharmacologic agents.
- **Prostaglandin E_2, E_1, $F_2\alpha$:**
  - Typically used for T2 pregnancy terminations.
  - Can be administered orally or vaginally, depending on the type of prostaglandin.
  - Given every 2–6 hour until uterus evacuated.
  - **Advantages:** Easy to use, can be safely used in patients with prior cesarean delivery in the first and second trimesters.
  - **Disadvantages:** Diarrhea, fever.
- **Mifepristone (RU 486) and misoprostol:**
  - Primarily used for T1 abortion.
  - Antiprogestin mifepristone 200 mg orally is followed by 800 μg buccal or oral misoprotol 24–48 hours later.
  - Ninety-two percent successful for pregnancy <49 days' gestation (7 weeks).
  - Seventy-seven percent successful for pregnancy 57–63 days' gestation (8–9 weeks).

All of these can be used in the setting of a missed abortion as well.

WARD TIP

Differential diagnosis for T3 bleeding:
- Placental abruption
- Placenta previa
- Rupture of vasa previa
- Uterine rupture

EXAM TIP

Ninety percent of all pregnancy terminations are performed in the first trimester.

Surgical Method

- May be used in T1 or T2.
- **D&C:** Involves dilation of cervix and curettage of uterine contents (usually used in the first and early second trimesters).
- **Manual Vacuum Aspiration (MVA):** Involves dilation of cervix and aspiration of uterine contents using suction curettage.
- **Dilation and evacuation (D&E):** Involves dilation of cervix (osmotic, mechanical, pharmacologic) and extraction of fetal parts using various instruments.

- **Advantages:** Can be done urgently or acutely (i.e., don't have to wait), in T1 can be done in the office.
  - **Disadvantages:** Need technical expertise for second trimester.
- Hysterotomy: Rarely performed unless contraindications to other methods.

COMPLICATIONS OF SURGICAL PREGNANCY TERMINATIONS

- Infection: Most common complication (though risk quite decreased with routine pre-op antibiotics, less than 1%)
- Incomplete removal of POC (also a risk in the setting of medical management or expectant management)
- Hemorrhage (also a risk in the setting of medical management or expectant management)
- Cervical laceration
- Uterine perforation/rupture (less than 1%)

Fetal Demise (Intrauterine Fetal Demise—IUFD)

Death of the fetus >20 weeks' gestation, **while still in utero.**

ETIOLOGY/RISK FACTORS

The risk factors are grouped into three main classes: fetal, placental, and maternal.

Fetal

- Fetal growth restriction: Significant ↑ in the risk of IUFD. It is associated with:
  - Fetal aneuploidies.
  - Fetal infection.
  - Placental insufficiency.
- Chromosomal and genetic abnormalities: Found in up to 8–13% of fetal demise.
- Multiple gestation.

Placental

- Placental abruption is a common cause of fetal demise (10–20% of all IUFDs).
- Causes of abruption include:
  - Maternal cocaine and other illicit drug use.
  - Smoking.
  - Chronic hypertension.
  - Preeclampsia.
- Placental infarction.
- Placental or membrane infection.
- Twin-twin transfusion syndrome (Mo/Di twins) or cord entanglement (Mo/Mo twins).

Maternal

- Advanced maternal age
- Obesity
- Drugs, alcohol, smoking
- Medical comorbidities:
  - Hypertension
  - Diabetes
  - Autoimmune disease

CAUSES OF INTRAUTERINE FETAL DEMISE BASED ON TRIMESTER

Diagnosis

- In late pregnancy, absent fetal movement detected by the mother is usually the first sign.
- Absent fetal heart tones by Doppler.
- Real-time US showing absence of fetal cardiac activity is the diagnostic method of choice.

Management

- D&E may be used if fetal demise occurs in T2. D&E has ↓ maternal mortality compared to PGE_2 labor induction, but also has the risk of uterine perforation. Depending on when in the second trimester, many families desire to hold the infant after delivery, which is not possible after D&E.
- Labor induction is usually offered if fetal demise occurs >18–20 weeks. Induction of labor with vaginal misoprostol is safe and effective even in patients with a prior cesarean delivery.
- Every attempt should be made to avoid a hysterotomy.
- The patient should be encouraged to seek counseling due to emotional stress caused by diagnosis of fetal demise. Pregnancy loss support groups are helpful for some patients. Low dose selective serotonin reuptake inhibitors (SSRIs) can be considered as well. Close follow up with a care provider 1–2 weeks after the loss is also important to assess maternal mental health.

EXAM TIP

The frequency of chromosomal abnormalities in IUFDs is 10 times higher than that in live births.

EXAM TIP

A carefully performed autopsy is the single most useful step in identifying the cause of fetal demise.

WARD TIP

Intimate partner violence is one of the leading causes of maternal and fetal demise in pregnancy.

WARD TIP

Up to 35% of IUFDs are associated with the presence of congenital malformation.

NOTES

Ectopic Pregnancy

ZEBRA ALERT

Heterotopic pregnancy is a coexisting intrauterine pregnancy (IUP) and ectopic pregnancy.

WARD TIP

Ectopic pregnancy is the leading cause of pregnancy-related maternal death during T1. Diagnose and treat *before* rupture occurs to ↓ the risk of death!

EXAM TIP

Most common site of ectopic pregnancy: Ampulla of fallopian tube

ZEBRA ALERT

Pregnancy after tubal ligation or with intrauterine device (IUD) in place is very rare, but when it does occur, the risk of ectopic pregnancy is high.

Ectopic pregnancy is a pregnancy that is located outside the uterine cavity. The most common site is the **fallopian tubes** (97%), followed by the abdominal cavity, ovary, and cervix. In rare cases, a pregnancy can implant in the cesarean scar—this is also a form of ectopic pregnancy. Within the fallopian tubes, the **ampulla** is the most common site, followed by the isthmus and fimbria. Cornual pregnancies that occur in the intramural portion of the fallopian tube are the most dangerous due to ↑ risk of uterine rupture (see Figure 12-1). Rupture of the ectopic pregnancy can lead to rapid bleeding and death.

Epidemiology

- Incidence: 20/1000 reported pregnancies.
- Increased risk of recurrence.
- Three to four times more common in patients over age 35 compared to those in the 15- to 24-year-old age group.

Risk Factors

 A 20-year-old G1P1001 patient presents to the emergency department (ED) with right lower quadrant (RLQ) pain and vaginal spotting. She reports that her menses have been regular, except that she is currently 3 weeks late and her last menstrual period (LMP) was 7 weeks ago. She has a history of pelvic inflammatory disease (PID), and she smokes one pack of cigarettes per day. Review of systems is positive for nausea and vomiting. Physical exam shows blood pressure 100/70, heart rate 90, and temperature 98.8°F (37.1°C). She has RLQ tenderness without rebound or guarding. Pelvic exam shows 5 cc of dark blood in the vault and right adnexal tenderness. Quantitative β-human chorionic gonadotropin (β-hCG) is 3000 mIU/mL. Ultrasound (US) shows an empty uterus. What is the most likely diagnosis?

Answer: Ectopic pregnancy. All reproductive-age patients who present with abdominal pain and vaginal bleeding should have a β-hCG performed. In this case, the quantitative β-hCG is at a level where an intrauterine pregnancy (IUP) should be visualized in the uterus. Since the uterus is empty, the pregnancy must be in an ectopic location.

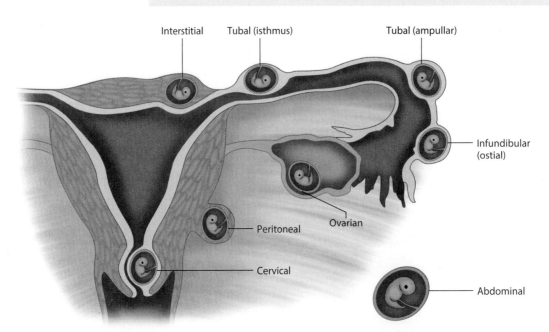

FIGURE 12-1. **Sites of ectopic pregnancy.** (Reproduced, with permission, from Ganti L. *Atlas of Emergency Medicine Procedures.* New York: Springer Nature; 2016.)

- PID and/or history of sexually transmitted infections (STIs) are major risk factors. This can create scarring of the fallopian tubes.
- Previous ectopic pregnancy.
- Tubal scarring from prior surgery (tubal reanastamosis or sterilization).
- Current tobacco use.
- Assisted reproductive technology: Ovulation-inducing drugs and in vitro fertilization.
- In utero diethylstilbestrol (DES) exposure.

Exam

- Pelvic exam may reveal normal or slightly enlarged uterus.
- Vaginal bleeding.
- Pelvic pain.
- Palpable adnexal mass may or may not be present.
- Signs of **ruptured** ectopic:
  - Hypotension.
  - Tachycardia.
  - Abdominal exam with rebound and guarding.

Differential Diagnosis

Think of anything that can cause abdominal pain, adnexal pain, or bleeding in a premenopausal patient:

- Threatened abortion
- Ovarian torsion
- PID
- Acute appendicitis
- Ruptured ovarian cyst
- Tubo-ovarian abscess
- Degenerating uterine leiomyoma

Diagnostic Studies

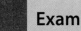 A 26-year-old G2P0010 patient at 6 weeks' gestation by LMP presents to the ED with left-sided abdominal pain and vaginal bleeding. She reports no chest pain, dizziness, or shortness of breath. She had a positive home pregnancy test 2 weeks ago, but has not received prenatal care yet. She was treated for PID 1 year ago. The serum β-hCG is 2000 mIU/mL. What is the next step in the evaluation of this patient?
Answer: Transvaginal ultrasound (TVUS) should be done next and is the imaging modality of choice. The presence of an IUP makes the risk of ectopic very low (not zero). The TVUS may show an empty uterus, an early IUP, or findings consistent with an ectopic pregnancy.

- **Urine pregnancy test (UPT)** to confirm pregnancy: The UPT will be positive, with β-hCG levels >25 mIU/mL, approximately 1 week after conception.
- **Quantitative serum β-hCG:**
  - Should ↑ by at least 66% every 48 hours in the first 6–7 weeks of gestation after day 9.
  - Value of serial β-hCGs: Stable reliable patients can be followed with serial β-hCG levels. Inadequate rise in β-hCG is suggestive of ectopic or nonviable pregnancy.

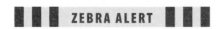

WARD TIP

β-hCG levels **do not** correlate with:
- Size of ectopic
- Potential for rupture
- Location of ectopic
- Gestational age of ectopic

EXAM TIP

If the quantitative β-hCG is >3500 mIU/mL, and there is no evidence of an IUP, suspect ectopic pregnancy.

EXAM TIP

- β-hCG of 25 will have a positive urine pregnancy test.
- β-hCG of 3500: IUP detectable with TVUS.
- β-hCG of 5000: IUP detectable with abdominal US.

- Once that quantitative β-hCG is >2000 mIU/mL, 91% of pregnancies will have a visible gestational sac on TVUS. At >3500, 99% will. Thus, most centers use a value of >3500 mIU/mL to expect to see an IUP.
- **Progesterone:** Not used routinely. Higher with viable IUP.
  - >25 ng/mL: Suggests normal IUP.
  - <5 ng/mL: Suggests abnormal pregnancy (either ectopic or nonviable pregnancy).
  - 5–25 ng/mL: Unclear. Unfortunately, many results fall in this range and are not helpful.
- **US: Diagnostic modality of choice:**
  - TVUS is more sensitive than transabdominal approach.
  - Ectopic pregnancy is suspected if a gestational sac is not seen within the uterine cavity with a serum β-hCG at a threshold value. Threshold for detecting an IUP on TVUS is β-hCG = 3500. This is called the **discriminatory zone**.
    - The **discriminatory zone** is the serum β-hCG level above which a gestational sac should be visualized by TVUS if an IUP is present (see Figure 12-2).
  - US findings suggestive of ectopic pregnancy:
    - **Absence of intrauterine gestational sac.**
    - Gestational sac or cardiac activity seen outside the uterus.
    - Complex adnexal mass.
    - Fluid in the cul-de-sac: Fluid in the dependent portion of the pelvis can represent blood from the ruptured ectopic pregnancy.

Management

A 30-year-old G3P1011 patient at 6 weeks' gestation presents to the ED with vaginal spotting and right lower quadrant (RLQ) pain. She reports no medical problems, and her only surgical history is a left salpingectomy for ectopic pregnancy 2 years ago. She is afebrile with stable vital signs. Physical exam demonstrates RLQ tenderness without rebound or guarding. Serum β-hCG is 4000 mIU/mL. TVUS shows an empty uterus with a 2.5-cm hyperechoic ring in the right adnexa consistent with an ectopic pregnancy. There is a small amount of fluid in the cul-de-sac. What is the best treatment for this patient?

Answer: This hemodynamically stable patient has findings consistent with an ectopic pregnancy. The patient can be counseled on pros and cons of medical versus surgical management. In this case, treatment with methotrexate (MTX) will allow the patient to avoid the risks of surgery and preserve the remaining fallopian tube.

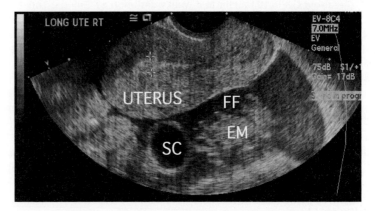

FIGURE 12-2. **Transvaginal ultrasound demonstrating an ectopic pregnancy.** Note the large amount of free fluid (FF) in the pelvis. No intrauterine pregnancy was seen. A large complex echogenic mass (EM) was seen in the left adnexa, consistent with an ectopic pregnancy. A simple cyst (SC) is also seen, in the right adnexa.

GENERAL MANAGEMENT

Determine if the patient is hemodynamically stable → if not, the patient needs emergent surgery.

Determine if the ectopic pregnancy is ruptured → if so, the patient needs emergent surgery.

Administer anti-D immunoglobulin if patient is D negative.

MEDICAL MANAGEMENT

MTX is an option for treatment of an unruptured early ectopic pregnancy.
- Antimetabolite.
- Inhibits dihydrofolic acid reductase.
- Interferes with DNA synthesis.
- Treatment of certain neoplastic diseases, rheumatoid arthritis, psoriasis, and ectopic pregnancies.
- Indications:
  - Hemodynamically stable patient.
  - Ectopic pregnancy <3.5 cm.
  - Patient reliable for follow-up.
  - IUP ruled out.
  - β-hCG ≤ 5000 mIU/mL.
  - No fetal cardiac activity.
- Relative and/or absolute contraindications:
  - Fetal cardiac activity of ectopic pregnancy.
  - Quantitative β-hCG >15,000 mIU/mL.
  - Ectopic pregnancy >3.5 cm.
  - Hemodynamically unstable patient: MTX requires time to work.
  - Leukopenia: MTX can further suppress immune system.
  - Thrombocytopenia (<100,000).
  - Active renal/hepatic disease (MTX is renally cleared and can be hepatotoxic).
  - Active peptic ulcer disease (MTX may worsen).
  - Possibility of concurrent viable IUP.
  - Presence of ruptured ectopic pregnancy.
  - Breast-feeding.

> ✋ **WARD TIP**
>
> Do not co-administer a nonsteroidal anti-inflammatory drug (NSAID) with MTX, as it can potentiate nephrotoxicity.

SURGICAL MANAGEMENT

Place two large-bore IVs to administer normal saline and type and cross for blood.
- **Surgical approach varies:** Laparoscopy or laparotomy depending on surgeon preference and urgency.
  - **Laparoscopy:** Entry into peritoneal cavity via small incisions and visualization of abdominal and pelvic organs with a small camera.
  - **Laparotomy:** Enter into the peritoneal cavity via a large incision on abdominal wall.
  - Can be diagnostic (only visualize) or operative (perform surgical procedures).
- **Salpingectomy:** Removal of the affected fallopian tube.
  - Performed to treat ruptured ectopic pregnancy or severely damaged tube.
- **Salpingostomy:**
  - Incision on the antimesenteric portion of the tube.
  - Used for unruptured distal tubal ectopic pregnancy.
  - Allows pregnancy to be removed while sparing the tube.

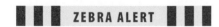

A patient is able to get pregnant from one ovary and one contralateral tube, e.g., ovulate from the right ovary, and conceive in the left fallopian tube.

 WARD TIP

In cases where the β-hCG is abnormally rising but pregnancy location is unclear, obstetrics/gynecologists (OB/GYNs) may perform a dilation and curettage (D&C) first. After D&C, the specimen is sent to pathology immediately to assess for presence of chorionic villi. Presence of villi confirms a diagnosis of abnormal IUP. Absence of villi suggests a diagnosis of ectopic pregnancy.

EXAM TIP

Patients who desire sterilization may have bilateral salpingectomies at the time of their surgery for ectopic pregnancy.

■ Should follow the β-hCG down to zero as some pregnancy tissue may be left behind and continue to grow, which can cause a chronic ectopic.

After medical or surgical management of ectopic pregnancy, the β-HCG should be followed back down to zero, especially in cases of medical management to ensure the ectopic was completely treated.

High-Yield Facts in Gynecology

CHAPTER 13

Contraception and Sterilization

Contraception

Contraception is a way to prevent pregnancy using medications, devices, or abstinence. Contraceptives can be used regularly prior to intercourse, at the time of intercourse, or after intercourse. A patient's choice of contraceptive method will be influenced by personal considerations, co-morbid medical conditions, non-contraceptive benefits, efficacy, safety, cost, and contraceptive method (see Table 13-1).

TABLE 13-1. **Contraception Agents Compared Including Best-Suited Patients**

CATEGORY	AGENTS	MECHANISM	BEST SUITED FOR	DISADVANTAGES AND CONTRAINDICATIONS
Barrier	Diaphragm Cervical caps Condoms (male and female)	Mechanical obstruction	Breast-feeding Not desiring hormones **Decrease STIs (male condom provides the best protection against STI)**	Patient discomfort with placing devices on genitals **Lack of spontaneity** Allergies to material Diaphragm may be associated with more UTIs and risk of toxic shock syndrome
Combined hormonal (estrogen and progestin)	Combined oral contraceptives Contraception patch Vaginal ring	Inhibits ovulation Thickens cervical mucous to inhibit sperm penetration Alters motility of uterus and fallopian tubes Thins endometrium	Iron-deficiency anemia Dysmenorrhea Ovarian cysts Endometriosis **OCP**—take pill each day **PATCH**—less to remember **RING**–less to remember, vaginal irritation, and discharge	Known thrombogenic mutations Prior thromboembolic event Cerebrovascular or coronary artery disease (current or remote) Cigarette smoking (>15 cigarettes/day) at or over the age of 35 Uncontrolled hypertension Diabetic retinopathy, nephropathy, peripheral vascular disease Known or suspected breast or endometrial cancer Undiagnosed vaginal bleeding Migraines with aura Benign or malignant liver tumors, active liver disease, liver failure Known or suspected pregnancy
Progestin-only pill	Minipill	Thickens cervical mucus to inhibit sperm penetration Inhibits ovulation Alters motility of uterus and fallopian tubes Thins the endometrium	**Breast-feeding**	Very dependent on taking pill each day at same time Patient needs to remember to take pill
Injectables	Depot medroxy progesterone acetate	Inhibits ovulation Thins endometrium Alters cervical mucus to inhibit sperm penetration	Breast-feeding Iron-deficiency anemia **Sickle cell disease** **Epilepsy** Dysmenorrhea Ovarian cysts Endometriosis	Depression Osteopenia/osteoporosis Weight gain

(Continued)

TABLE 13-1. **Contraception Agents Compared Including Best-Suited Patients** (*Continued*)

CATEGORY	AGENTS	MECHANISM	BEST SUITED FOR	DISADVANTAGES AND CONTRAINDICATIONS
Implants (subdermal in arm)	Etonogestrel implant (Nexplanon)	Inhibits ovulation Thins endometrium Thickens cervical mucus to inhibit sperm penetration	Breast-feeding Desires long-term contraception (lasts for 3 years) Iron-deficiency anemia Dysmenorrhea Ovarian cysts Endometriosis	Hepatic tumors (benign or malignant), active liver disease Undiagnosed abnormal vaginal bleeding Known or suspected carcinoma of the breast or personal history of breast cancer Hypersensitivity to any of the components of etonogestrel implant **May lead to irregular vaginal bleeding**
IUD	Levonorgestrel intrauterine device	Thickens cervical mucus to inhibit sperm penetration Thins endometrium	Breast-feeding Desires long-term, reversible contraception Stable-mutually monogamous relationship Menorrhagia Dysmenorrhea (NOTE: decreased bleeding and dysmenorrhea)	**Current STI or PID** Unexplained vaginal bleeding Malignant gestational trophoblastic disease Untreated cervical or endometrial cancer Current breast cancer Anatomical abnormalities distorting the uterine cavity Uterine fibroids distorting endometrial cavity
IUD	Copper	Inhibits sperm migration and viability Changes transport speed of ovum Damages ovum	Desires long-term reversible contraception (10 years) Stable, mutually monogamous relationship Contraindication to hormonal steroids	Current STI Current or PID within the past 3 months Unexplained vaginal bleeding Malignant gestational trophoblastic disease Untreated cervical or endometrial cancer Anatomical abnormalities distorting the uterine cavity Uterine fibroids distorting endometrial cavity **Wilson disease** **May cause more bleeding or dysmenorrhea**
Permanent sterilization	Bilateral tubal occlusion	Mechanical obstruction or removal of tubes	Does not desire future fertility	Contraindications to surgery Risk of regret

Reproduced, with permission, from Toy EC, Ross PJ, Baker B, Jennings JC. *Case Files: Obstetrics and Gynecology.* 5th ed. New York: McGraw-Hill Education; 2016:Table 44-2.

IUD, intrauterine device; PID, pelvic inflammatory disease; STI, sexually transmitted infection; UTI, urinary tract infection

General methods of preventing pregnancy include:
- Barrier
- Hormonal (including oral, injectable, implants)
- Intrauterine device (IUD)
- Sterilization
- Abstinence

BARRIER METHODS

Female Condom

- Rarely used because of expense and inconvenience.
- It offers labial protection, unlike the male condom.

  Consists of an outer ring, middle sheath that lines the vagina, and inner ring/sponge that covers the cervix.

- Efficacy: 79%.

Male Condom

TYPES

- Latex: Most common, inexpensive, protects against sexually transmitted infections (STIs), some women have allergy/sensitivity.
- Synthetic (polyurethane): Expensive, protects against STIs, non-allergenic.
- Natural membrane (lamb skin): Least protection against STIs.

EFFICACY

86–97%, depending on proper and consistent use

DRAWBACKS

- Must be placed properly before genital contact.
- Requires partner cooperation.
- ↓ sensation for some people.
- May rupture.

Diaphragm

A reusable flexible ring with a rubber dome that must be fitted by a gynecologist. It creates a barrier between the cervix and the lower portion of the vagina. It must be inserted with spermicide and left in place after intercourse for 6–8 hours. Does not protect against STIs.

EFFICACY

80–94%

COMPLICATIONS

- If left in for too long (>24 hours), in rare cases, may result in *Staphylococcus aureus* infection (which may cause **toxic shock syndrome**).
- May ↑ risk of urinary tract infection (UTI).

Cervical Cap

A reusable silicone cup that fits directly over the cervix. Holds spermicide against the cervix to kill sperm. It is more popular in Europe than in the United States. Size selection and efficacy impacted by parity due to changes in the size and shape of the cervix in parous women.

EFFICACY

- In women who have not given birth: 80–90%
- In women who have given birth: 60–70%

Spermicide

Foams, gels, creams, films, and tablets inserted into the vagina up to 30 minutes before intercourse designed to kill or immobilize sperm. Does not protect against STIs. Most effective when used in combination with barrier methods such as a condom or diaphragm.

TYPES

Nonoxynol-9 (most common) and octoxynol-3 are active ingredients of spermicide, which disrupt the sperm cell membrane; effective for only about 1 hour.

EFFICACY

74–94%

Sponge

A polyurethane sponge containing nonoxynol-9 that is placed over the cervix. It must be moistened with at least 2 tablespoons of tap water before insertion in order to activate the spermicide. It can be inserted up to 24 hours before intercourse and should be left in place for 6 hours after intercourse. Available over-the-counter.

EFFICACY

84%

RISK

Toxic shock syndrome (rare)

HORMONAL AGENTS

A 37-year-old G2P2 patient desires a reversible form of contraception. Her history is significant for migraines with visual aura, uncontrolled hypertension (HTN), and family history of breast cancer in her mother. She smokes two packs of cigarettes daily. She requests combination oral contraceptives (COCs). How should this patient be counseled?

Answer: The patient is not a candidate for COCs because she has several contraindications that put her at an increased risk for developing venous thromboembolism and stroke. Contraindications for COC use include age >35 years old and smoking, history of venous thromboembolism, uncontrolled HTN, diabetes with vascular disease, migraines with visual aura, and benign or malignant liver tumors, cirrhosis, and personal history of breast cancer.

Combination Oral Contraceptives (COCs)
EFFICACY

- 92–99.9% (variability due to compliance)
- Contain estrogen and progestin; types include monophasic dosing and multiphasic dosing:
  - **Monophasic:** Contains the same dose of estrogen and progestin in each of the hormonally active pills
  - **Multiphasic dosing:** Gradual ↑ in the dose of either or both hormones

MECHANISM OF ACTION

- **Estrogen** suppresses follicle-stimulating hormone (FSH) and therefore prevents follicular development. Maintains stability of endometrium.
- **Progesterone** prevents luteinizing hormone (LH) surge and therefore inhibits ovulation.
  - Thickens cervical mucus to pose as a barrier for sperm.
  - Alters motility of fallopian tube and uterus.
  - Causes endometrial atrophy.

EXAM TIP

P450 inducers will decrease the efficacy of oral contraceptives (OCPs) (e.g., phenytoin, rifampin, griseofulvin, carbamazepine, barbiturates) due to accelerated metabolism of OCPs.

EXAM TIP

Hormonal patch may be less effective in obese (≥200 lb) women.

WARD TIP

Types of endogenous estrogens:
  Estradiol: Reproductive life
  Estriol: Pregnancy
  Estrone: Menopause

EXAM TIP

Tension headaches are **not** a contraindication for COCs. Migraine headaches with visual aura can ↑ risk of stroke in patients who take combination hormonal contraception.

SIDE EFFECTS

- Nausea
- Headache
- Bloating

BENEFITS

- ↓ risk of ovarian cancer by 75%
- ↓ risk of endometrial cancer by 50%
- ↓ bleeding and dysmenorrhea
- Regulates menses
- Reduces the risk of pelvic inflammatory disease (PID) (thicker mucus), fibrocystic breast change, ovarian cysts, ectopic pregnancy, osteoporosis, acne, and hirsutism
- ↓ risk of anemia

RISKS

- ↑ risk of venous thromboembolism/stroke
- ↑ risk of myocardial infarction (in smokers >35 years old)
- Mood changes
- Migraines

CONTRAINDICATIONS

- Known thrombophilias
- Prior thromboembolic events
- Cerebrovascular or coronary artery disease (current or remote)
- Cigarette smoking and age over 35
- Uncontrolled HTN
- Diabetic retinopathy, nephropathy, peripheral vascular disease
- Known or suspected breast or endometrial cancer
- Undiagnosed vaginal bleeding
- Migraines with visual aura
- Benign or malignant liver tumors, active liver disease, liver failure
- Known or suspected pregnancy

Progestin-Only Oral Contraceptives

EFFICACY

Slightly higher failure rate when compared to COCs (91–97% effective), but must be taken at same time each day (within 3 hours).

MECHANISM OF ACTION

- Thickens mucus to prevent sperm penetration.
- Alters motility of uterus and fallopian tubes.
- Causes thinning of endometrial glands.
- Contain only progestin: There is LH suppression and therefore no ovulation. The main differences from combination pills are:
  - A mature follicle is formed (but not released).
  - No placebo is used.
- Progestin-only pills are best for:
  - Lactating women (progestin, unlike estrogen, does *not* impact breast milk supply).
  - Women for whom estrogen is contraindicated (e.g., migraine with aura, history of VTE).

SIDE EFFECTS

- Breakthrough bleeding
- Nausea (10–30% of women)

Transdermal Contraceptive Patch

- Contains estrogen and progesterone.
- Efficacy similar to COCs (combined estrogen/progesterone).
- Apply and change patch once a week for 3 weeks. Remove for one patch-free week to have withdrawal bleed, then place new patch.
- May have reduced efficacy in obese women.
- May have better compliance.
- May come off and need replacement.
- Possible ↑ risk of thromboembolic events compared to COC users.

Hormonal Contraceptive Vaginal Ring

- Contains estrogen and progesterone.
- Efficacy similar to COCs (combined estrogen/progesterone).
- Insert and leave in place for 3 weeks. Remove for one ring-free week to have withdrawal bleed, then replace on the same day of the week the old ring was removed.
- May have reduced efficacy in obese women.
- May have better compliance.

Injectable Hormonal Agents

> A 20-year-old G0 patient desires long-acting reversible contraception. She has a history of epilepsy for which she takes an anticonvulsant. She still has seizures once about every 6 months. She is also wary of anything that goes 'in her body'. What is the best contraceptive method for her?
>
> **Answer:** Medroxyprogesterone acetate (DMPA) injection can ↑ the seizure threshold and ↓ the number of seizures. It also ↓ the number of sickle cell crises in patients with sickle cell disease. It improves anemia, ↓ dysmenorrhea and ovarian cysts, and improves symptoms of endometriosis.

DMPA IM injection given every 3 months. Patients have a window within which they must return to the clinic for the subsequent injection.

EFFICACY

99.7%

MECHANISM OF ACTION

Sustained high progesterone level to block LH surge (and hence ovulation). Thicker mucus and endometrial atrophy also contribute. There is no FSH suppression.

INDICATIONS

- Especially suitable for women who cannot tolerate COCs, who are unable to take COCs as prescribed, or for whom estrogen is contraindicated.
- DMPA can provide non-contraceptive benefits in:
  - Seizure disorder: ↓ the number of seizure episodes
  - Sickle cell disease: ↓ the number of sickle cell crises

SIDE EFFECTS

- Bleeding irregularity/spotting
- Unknown when menstruation/fertility will resume after treatment cessation (can impact menstrual cycle regularity for up to 9 months after last shot)
- ↑ hair shedding
- Mood changes
- ↓ high-density lipoprotein (HDL)
- ↓ libido

WARD TIP

Estrogen can impact breast milk supply and production, so combination pills are not recommended for nursing mothers until milk supply is stable. Progestin-only pills are recommended until that time.

WARD TIP

There is no proven link between OCP use and ↑ in breast cancer.

EXAM TIP

Side effects of estrogen:
- Breast tenderness
- Nausea
- Headache

EXAM TIP

Side effects of progestin:
- Depression
- Acne
- Weight gain
- Irregular bleeding

- Weight gain!! (most common complaint / reason for stopping)
- Osteopenia/osteoporosis. Reverses when stop using DMPA.

CONTRAINDICATIONS

- Known/suspected pregnancy
- Undiagnosed vaginal bleeding
- Breast cancer
- Liver disease
- Osteoporosis/osteopenia

Implantable Hormonal Agents

Etonogestrel (progestin) containing single rod inserted in the subcutaneous tissue of the inner upper arm. It is replaced every 3 years.

EFFICACY

99.8%

MECHANISM OF ACTION

- Suppression of LH surge and inhibition of ovulation
- Thickened mucus
- Endometrial atrophy

INDICATIONS

- Contraindication/intolerance to oral contraceptives
  - Smokers >35 years old
  - Women with diabetes mellitus, HTN, coronary artery disease (CAD)
- Or patient preference in those who do not have contraindication to estrogen

SIDE EFFECTS

- Irregular bleeding
- Acne
- Weight gain
- Headache
- Possible difficult removal

CONTRAINDICATIONS

- Thrombophlebitis/embolism
- Known/suspected pregnancy
- Liver disease/cancer
- Breast cancer
- Undiagnosed genital bleeding

INTRAUTERINE DEVICE (IUD)

A 25-year-old G1P1patient, who delivered a full-term infant 6 months previously, presents for IUD insertion. She reports that she is in a long-term, monogamous relationship. She reports no history of STIs or other medical conditions. She undergoes the insertion of an IUD without any apparent complications. The patient presents 4 days later with abdominal pain, nausea, vomiting, and fever. Speculum exam reveals malodorous discharge and IUD strings at the cervical os. What is the most likely cause for the patient's symptoms?

Answer: Endometritis due to contamination during insertion. Infections that occur near the time of IUD insertion are usually due to ascending infection from vaginal flora. Infections, months to years, after the IUD placement may be due to STIs.

EFFICACY

97–99.1%

MECHANISM OF ACTION

- Copper IUD:
  - Copper causes a sterile inflammatory reaction, creating a hostile environment.
  - Inhibits sperm migration and viability.
  - Damages ovum, changes ovum transport speed.
  - Used for 10 years.
- Levonorgestrel IUD:
  - Thickens cervical mucus.
  - Thins endometrium.
  - Used for 5 years.
  - Can be placed immediately after placental delivery (higher expulsion rates), at the postpartum visit, or at the time of any gynecology visit.

INDICATIONS

- Contraindication to estrogen:
  - Oral contraceptives contraindicated/not tolerated.
  - Smokers >35 years old.
- Levonorgestrel IUD can be used to treat heavy menstrual bleeding.
- Patient preference.

CONTRAINDICATIONS

- Severe distortion of uterine cavity
- Acute pelvic infection
- Active liver disease (Levonorgestrel IUD only)
- Known/suspected pregnancy
- Wilson disease or copper allergy (Copper IUD only)
- Unexplained abnormal uterine bleeding
- Current breast cancer (Levonorgestrel IUD only)

COMPLICATIONS

- Infection (endometritis or PID—very rare)
- Uterine perforation
- Ectopic pregnancy
- Irregular bleeding
- IUD expulsion
- *Actinomyces* infection

WARD TIP

Non-user-dependent methods like the IUD, subdermal implant, and injections have lower failure rates than OCPs.

WARD TIP

Contraindication for IUD placement: Severe distortion of uterine cavity (e.g., bicornuate uterus or large obstructive fibroids), due to increased difficulty with insertion, increased risk of IUD expulsion/embedment/perforation, and decreased efficacy.

WARD TIP

The absolute risk of ectopic pregnancy is lower for women using an IUD compared with women not using contraception or using other reversible methods of contraception. However, should a pregnancy occur in a patient using and IUD, the risk of ectopic pregnancy is higher, ranging from 10 to 30%.

POSTCOITAL/EMERGENCY CONTRACEPTION

A 19-year-old G0P0 patient presents to the office concerned that she may have an undesired pregnancy after engaging in unprotected sex with her boyfriend 2 days ago. The patient does not remember the date of her last menstrual period. What therapy may be offered to this patient?

Answer: Emergency contraception is effective when initiated within 120 hours (5 days) of intercourse. It consists of high-dose progestin, high-dose OCPs, or insertion of a copper IUD.

Up to 5 Days After Intercourse

Levonorgestrel: One 1.5 mg tablet taken within 120 hours of intercourse. Available over-the-counter without age restriction. Efficacy: 97%. Efficacy better within 72 hours, but can use up to 120 hours or 5 days. Mechanism of action is to inhibit or delay ovulation. Will not interrupt an existing pregnancy.

Up to 5 Days After Intercourse

Copper IUD or levonorgestrel IUD: Can be left in the uterine cavity and provide contraception for up several years. Efficacy: >99%.

Ulipristal acetate: 30 mg single dose of antiprogestin. Efficacy: 98%. Mechanism of action: Progestin receptor modulator prevents progestin/progesterone from binding to receptor; thus, it postpones follicular rupture if administered prior to ovulation, and/or alters endometrium, impairs implantation.

Sterilization

Sterilization is an elective surgery that leaves a male or female unable to reproduce. Female sterilization is the most popular form of birth control in the United States, with approximately 22% of women choosing this method. The failure rate for both male and female sterilization is about 1%.

- Male type: Vasectomy.
- Female type: Tubal occlusion or bilateral salpingectomy (tubal removal).
- It is estimated that 10–12% of men and 13–25% of women who undergo permanent sterilization may experience regret. Risk factors for regret include women younger than age 30, non-white race, women not married at the time of their sterilization procedure, or women whose tubal procedure was performed less than a year after delivery.
- Sterilization is intended to be a permanent, non-reversible procedure. Patients should be counseled about this as part of the consent process. Patients interested in potential reversibility should be counseled to avoid sterilization and instead consider long-acting reversible methods. Although some methods of tubal sterilization may be reversed surgically, these methods are not guaranteed, are very expensive, and are often not covered by insurance.

MALE STERILIZATION: VASECTOMY

- Excision of a small section of both vas deferens, followed by sealing of the proximal and distal cut ends (office procedure done under local anesthesia). Ejaculation still occurs.
- Sperm can still be found proximal to the surgical site, so to ensure sterility one must use contraception for 12 weeks or 20 ejaculations and then have two consecutive negative sperm counts.

FEMALE STERILIZATION

There are several methods of female sterilization.

Procedures can be performed (Figure 13-1) either immediately postpartum (during cesarean delivery or after vaginal delivery) or interval (remote from a pregnancy). An interval tubal occlusion should be performed in the follicular phase of the menstrual cycle in order to avoid the time of ovulation and possible pregnancy, unless the patient is on reliable contraception at the time of surgery. Tubal occlusion methods should be performed on the mid-isthmic section of the tube. The proximal isthmus, which is immediately adjacent to the cornua, should be avoided to reduce the risk of fistula formation between

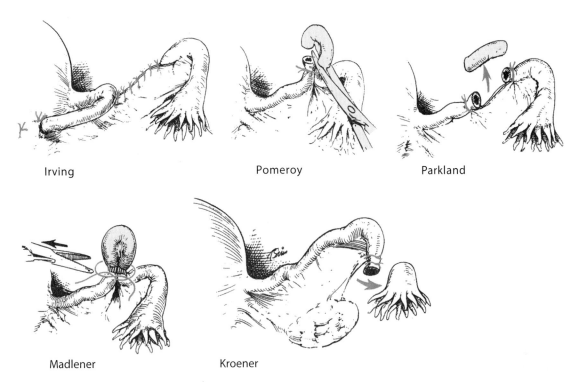

Irving   Pomeroy   Parkland

Madlener   Kroener

FIGURE 13-1.   Various techniques for tubal sterility. (Reproduced, with permission, from Cunningham FG, Gant NF, Leveno KJ, et al. *Williams Obstetrics.* 21st ed. New York: McGraw-Hill; 2001:1556.)

the interstitial portion of the tube and the peritoneal cavity. The distal portion of the tube should be avoided as it may increase the risk of injuring adjacent structures, and distal fimbriectomy is not ideal as it has been associated with a higher risk of sterilization failure.

Laparoscopic Tubal Occlusion

Eighty to ninety percent of tubal occlusions are done laparoscopically. All methods occlude the fallopian tubes bilaterally and are comparably safe and effective.

Electrocautery

This involves the cauterization of a 3-cm zone of the isthmus, resulting in destruction of the tubal lumen. It is the most popular method as it is lower cost (employs reusable instruments and is readily available), but may have a higher risk of ectopic pregnancy.

Clipping

The Hulka clip (spring clip) or Filshie clip (titanium clip) are applied at a 90-degree angle on the isthmus. This method may have the highest failure rate.

Banding

A length of isthmus is drawn up into the end of the trocar, and a silicone band, or Fallope ring, is placed around the base of the drawn-up portion of fallopian tube. This method is associated with the highest rate of postoperative pain.

Bilateral Salpingectomy

This method is increasingly being offered as a method of tubal sterilization. Removal of the entire fallopian tubes increases the effectiveness of the

---

WARD TIP

Tubal sterilization facts:
- It is the most frequent indication for laparoscopy in the United States.
- Electrocautery method is most popular and most difficult to reverse.
- Clipping method is most easily reversed, but also the most likely to fail.
- Hysteroscopic occlusion (Essure®) methods are no longer manufactured or sold in the United States.

WARD TIP

Be sure to follow-up on pathology report after tubal excision to ensure that tissue excised was fallopian tubes.

WARD TIP

Important parts of the history to consider when selecting patients for tubal sterilization include:

- Assess surgical risks (e.g., risk of presence of pelvic adhesions) and medical comorbidities (e.g., obesity).
- Assess risk of regret.
- Ensure reversible methods have been discussed.
- Ensure patient understands this procedure is considered permanent and not reversible.
- Ensure the patient is using reliable contraception or abstinence before the procedure.

WARD TIP

NFP has a 75–99% success rate in preventing pregnancy, depending on patient compliance.

procedure and reduces the risk of needing subsequent surgery for ectopic pregnancy. In addition, bilateral salpingectomy has been associated with up to a 65% reduction in the lifetime risk of serous epithelial ovarian cancers.

Postpartum Tubal Sterilization

These methods involve removal of a segment of fallopian tube, resulting in scarring and closure of the tubal remnants. Care should be taken to remove at least a 2-cm segment of the mid-isthmic section of the tube. The segments of tube removed should be sent for pathology evaluation to confirm excision of the full thickness of the tube. The Pomeroy and Parkland methods (partial salpingectomy) are the most common. The Irving and Uchida methods both require more extensive dissection, increased operative time, and have a greater risk of bleeding when compared to partial salpingectomy methods. These methods are not commonly used in the United States. They both involve burying a tubal stump in a nearby structure, and were developed to minimize the risk of tuboperitoneal fistula formation and contraceptive failure.

- **Pomeroy method:** A segment of isthmus is lifted and a suture is tied around the approximated base. The resulting loop is excised, leaving a gap between the proximal and distal ends.
- **Parkland method:** A window is made in the mesosalpinx and a segment of isthmus is tied proximally and distally and then excised.
- **Irving method:** The isthmus is cut, with the proximal end buried in the myometrium and the distal end buried in the mesosalpinx.
- **Uchida method:** Epinephrine is injected beneath the serosa of the isthmus. The mesosalpinx is reflected off the tube, and the proximal end of the tube is ligated and excised and pulled into the mesosalpinx. The distal end is not excised. The mesosalpinx is reattached to the excised proximal stump, while the long distal end is left to "dangle" outside of the mesosalpinx.

Bilateral Salpingectomy

Removal of all of the fallopian tube, as described above.

Luteal-Phase Pregnancy

A luteal-phase pregnancy is a *pregnancy diagnosed after tubal sterilization but conceived before*. It occurs in around 2–3/1000 sterilizations. It is prevented by either performing sensitive pregnancy tests prior to the procedure or performing the procedure during the follicular phase.

Complications of Tubal Occlusion

- Failure of procedure (1–3%, depending on method) and subsequent increased risk of ectopic pregnancy
- **Ectopic pregnancy:** Up to 1/3 of pregnancies following a female sterilization procedure will be ectopic
- Infection
- Surgical risks

Abstinence

CONTINUOUS ABSTINENCE

Abstaining from vaginal intercourse at any time. It is the only 100% effective way to prevent pregnancy.

FERTILITY AWARENESS-BASED (FAB) METHODS

Also known as "natural family planning (NFP)," this form of birth control is based on the timing of intercourse during a patient's menstrual cycle. It can be an effective, low-cost, and safe way to prevent an unwanted pregnancy. The success or failure of this methods will depend on the patient's ability to recognize the signs that ovulation is about to occur and abstain from having intercourse or use another form of contraception such as a barrier method during the fertile period.

Methods of FAB:
1. Basal body temperature (BBT) method
2. Ovulation/cervical mucus method
3. Symptothermal method
4. Standard days method

Basal Body Temperature

The BBT is the body's temperature fully at rest. A patient must take and record a temperature every morning after waking up, before any activity, getting out of bed, or having anything to eat or drink. The body's normal temperature should ↑ by 0.5–1°F during ovulation and remains high until the end of the menstrual cycle. The most fertile days are the 2–3 days before this increase in temperature when she has a progesterone surge, indicating that she is ovulating. The couple can abstain if they do not desire pregnancy or have intercourse if they are trying to conceive. BBT alone is not a good way to prevent pregnancy, since it only shows when ovulation has already occurred.

Ovulation/Cervical Mucus Method

This method involves a patient recognizing changes in cervical mucus to determine the fertile window. Most patients will secrete noticeably more cervical mucus as they move closer to ovulation. At time of ovulation, cervical mucus becomes more clear, profuse, wet, stretchy, and slippery, and is referred to as the "peak day" of fertility. After the peak day, the mucus will become thick again and will decrease and become less noticeable. If couple does not desire pregnancy, they are advised to abstain from intercourse or use a barrier method at the first signs of cervical mucus until 4 days after the peak day.

Symptothermal Method

This method involves a combination of the previous two methods. In addition to taking the temperature and checking for mucus changes every day, the patient checks for other signs of ovulation: abdominal pain or cramps, spotting, and changes in the position and firmness of the cervix. This method can be more effective than either of the other two methods because it uses a variety of signs.

Standard Days Method

This method follows a "standard rule" of what days during the menstrual cycle are the most fertile. It is most appropriate for women with a cycle length between 26 days and 32 days. This method considers days 8–19 to be the most fertile days. Abstinence or barrier methods should be used on these days to prevent pregnancy.

ADVANTAGES OF NFP

- No side effects, allergies, breakthrough bleeding, bloating, or hormonal impact on libido
- Low cost

- Reversible
- Improved knowledge and understanding of fertility and normal menstrual cycle
- Improved communication and shared responsibility between the patient and partner
- No impact on breast-feeding—no risk to baby

DISADVANTAGES OF *NFP*

- Abstinence isn't always easy.
- Requires both patient and partner to be committed.
- No protection against STIs.
- Takes time to learn fertility awareness.
- Method must be used consistently and correctly.

Menstruation

Puberty

- Puberty is the transition from childhood (sexual immaturity) to the final stage of sexual maturation that allows for reproduction.
- Puberty is believed to begin with **disinhibition** of the pulsatile gonadotropin-releasing hormone (GnRH) secretion from the hypothalamus. GnRH stimulates the anterior pituitary gland to secrete follicle-stimulating hormone (FSH) and luteinizing hormone (LH).
- In girls, FSH stimulates growth of ovarian follicles, and along with LH, stimulates production of estradiol in the ovaries.
- Estradiol production causes breast development, skeletal growth, and stimulation of the endometrium. Later, FSH and LH lead to ovulation and menstruation.

SECONDARY SEX CHARACTERISTICS (PUBERTAL DEVELOPMENT)

The timing of pubertal events is impacted by genetics, gender, ethnicity, and body weight. Development of the secondary sexual characteristics proceeds in the following order:

1. **Thelarche** (breast budding): Due to increase in estradiol produced by the ovaries
2. **Pubarche** (axillary and pubic hair growth): Due to increase in androgens produced by the adrenal glands
3. **Menarche** (first menses): Due to increase in estradiol acting on the endometrial lining

TANNER STAGES

The Tanner stages of development refer to the sequence of events of breast and pubic hair development.

- **Stage 1:** Prepuberty
- **Stages 2–4:** Development stages
- **Stage 5:** Adult development

PRECOCIOUS PUBERTY

Appearance of the secondary sexual characteristics at an age that is 2 to 2.5 standard deviations (SD) earlier than population norms is referred to as precocious puberty and requires investigation into the etiology. Traditionally, this is defined as pubertal development before 8 years of age in girls. The cause may be a variant of normal development or a pathologic condition, and may be categorized as central (gonadotropin-dependent) or peripheral (gonadotropin-independent).

ETIOLOGY (NOT AN EXHAUSTIVE LIST)

Central Causes: Caused by early maturation of the hypothalamic-pituitary-ovarian (HPO) axis
- Idiopathic: Most common (80–90%)
- Neurogenic: Caused by tumors of the hypothalamic-pituitary stalk and prevents negative feedback
- Inflammation of the hypothalamus: ↑ GnRH production
- 21-hydroxylase deficiency

EXAM TIP

The first menstrual bleeding is usually caused by the effects of estradiol stimulating the endometrial lining, rather than by ovulation.

EXAM TIP

Characteristic	Average Age	Hormone
Thelarche	10	Estradiol
Pubarche	11	Adrenal hormones
Menarche	12	Estradiol

WARD TIP

A female age 13 or older without any breast development should be evaluated for delayed puberty.

Peripheral Causes: Caused by excess secretion of sex hormones either from the ovaries, adrenal glands, or from exogenous sources

- Ovarian cysts (such as functioning follicular cyst): Most common peripheral cause
- Estrogen-secreting tumors ovarian tumors (such as Granulosa cell tumors)
- Excess exogenous estrogen
- Primary hypothyroidism: Proposed mechanism is cross-reactivity and stimulation of FSH receptor by high levels of thyroid-stimulating hormone (TSH), since they share a common alpha subunit
- McCune–Albright syndrome (triad of precocious puberty, café au lait spots, fibrous bone dysplasia)

Menstrual Cycle

The menstrual cycle is the cyclical changes that occur in the female reproductive system (see Figure 14-1 and Table 14-1). The HPO axis and uterus interact to allow ovulation approximately once per month [average 28 days (+/– 7 days)]. The following description is based on a 28-day menstrual cycle.

- Many follicles are stimulated by FSH, but *the follicle that secretes more estrogen than androgen will be released.* This dominant follicle releases the most estradiol so that its positive feedback causes an LH surge.

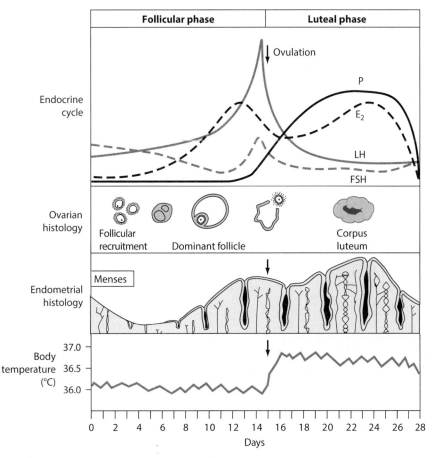

FIGURE 14-1. The menstrual cycle. (Modified, with permission, from Fauci AS, Braunwald E, Isselbacher KJ, et al. *Harrison's Principles of Internal Medicine.* 14th ed. New York: McGraw-Hill; 1998:2101.)

TABLE 14-1.   Summary of Menstrual Cycle

Menstruation: Withdrawal of progesterone causes endometrial sloughing.
Follicular phase: ▪ FSH causes follicle maturation and estrogen secretion. ▪ Estrogen causes endometrial proliferation.
Ovulation: LH surge causes oocyte to be released.
Luteal phase: Corpus luteum secretes progesterone, which causes: ▪ Endometrial maturation. ▪ ↓ FSH, ↓ LH.

FSH, follicle-stimulating hormone; LH, luteinizing hormone.

WARD TIP

Prostaglandins released from the endometrium cause dysmenorrhea.

▪ Average duration of menses = 5 days.
▪ Normal menstrual cycle length = 21–35 days.
▪ Blood loss in menstruation averages 30–50 mL and should not form clots; >80 mL is considered heavy menstrual bleeding; however, heavy menstrual bleeding should be based on patient perception.

DAYS 1–14: FOLLICULAR PHASE

▪ The follicular phase begins on the first day of menses. All hormone levels are low. Without any negative feedback, **GnRH** from the hypothalamus causes **FSH** release from the pituitary.
▪ **FSH** stimulates maturation of granulosa cells in the ovary. The granulosa cells secrete **estradiol** in response.
▪ **Estradiol** inhibits **LH** and **FSH** due to negative feedback. In the meantime, the **estradiol** secretion also causes the endometrium to proliferate.
▪ **LH** acts on the theca cells to ↑ secretion of **androgens** (which are converted to estradiol), prepare the cells for progesterone secretion, and cause further granulosa maturation.

WARD TIP

Ovulation takes place 24–36 hours after LH surge and 12 hours after LH peak.

WARD TIP

The length of the follicular phase is highly variable. The luteal phase is usually about 14 days due to the length of time the corpus luteum is able to secrete progesterone. Individuals who have changes in their cycle length typically experience changes in the follicular phase.

DAY 14: OVULATION

▪ A critical level of estradiol triggers an LH surge.
▪ The **LH surge** causes the oocyte to be released from the follicle. The ruptured follicle then becomes the corpus luteum, which secretes progesterone.

DAYS 14–28: LUTEAL PHASE

▪ The corpus luteum secretes progesterone for only about 14 days in the absence of human chorionic gonadotropin (hCG).
▪ **Progesterone** causes the endometrium to mature in preparation for possible implantation. It becomes highly vascularized and ↑ glandular secretions (see Table 14-2).
▪ **Progesterone** also inhibits the release of **FSH** and **LH**.
▪ If fertilization does not occur, the corpus luteum involutes, **progesterone** and **estradiol** levels fall, with subsequent endometrial sloughing (menses). The HPO axis is released from inhibition, and the cycle begins again.

EXAM TIP

The corpus luteum is maintained after fertilization by hCG, which is released by the embryo.

TABLE 14-2. **Ovarian Hormone Effect on Uterus**

	OVARIAN PHASE	DOMINANT HORMONE	UTERINE PHASE
Before ovulation	Follicular	Estrogen	Proliferative
After ovulation	Luteal	Progesterone	Secretory

NOTES

CHAPTER 15

Premenstrual Syndrome/Premenstrual Dysphoric Disorder

Premenstrual syndrome (PMS) and premenstrual dysphoric disorder (PMDD) have many symptoms that overlap with anxiety and depression. A differentiation should be made because each has a different treatment. PMS and PMDD both have similar symptoms, but PMDD has markedly severe symptoms. The symptoms of PMS **do not impair** daily activities; however, the symptoms of PMDD **do affect** the activities of daily living. The symptoms occur in the luteal phase for both conditions.

Definition

- Characterized by the presence of both behavioral and physical symptoms.
- Occurs during the luteal phase of the menstrual cycle and resolves shortly after menses begins.
- May interfere with work and personal relationships.
- Symptoms are followed by a symptom-free period.
- Monitor for 3 months because symptoms can be variable month to month, and the diagnosis relies on symptoms for 3 consecutive months.

Premenstrual Syndrome (PMS) Diagnostic Criteria

A 26-year-old G2P2 patient reports feeling sad and irritable before her menses. She experiences headaches and breast pain. She feels better when she is alone, but she is able to work and take care of her two children. Once she begins menses, she no longer has these symptoms. What is the most likely diagnosis? What is the best way to make the diagnosis?

Answer: PMS. This patient has behavioral and physical symptoms that resolve with menses. She is able to continue her daily activities despite the symptoms. The best diagnostic method is keeping a prospective symptom diary for 3 months.

- Prospective monitoring of menstrual and symptom history is necessary to confirm the relationship between symptoms and menstrual cycle phase. There are several validated symptom inventory tools available.
- The diagnosis of PMS can be made by documenting the presence of at least one behavioral or physical symptom during the luteal phase that leads to impaired functioning, and resolves at the onset of menses or shortly thereafter, resulting in a symptom-free interval:
  - Behavioral symptoms:
    - Mood swings (most common).
    - Sad or depressed mood.
    - Irritability.
    - Anxiety.
    - Increased appetite or food cravings.
    - Social withdrawal.
  - Physical symptoms:
    - Breast tenderness.
    - Abdominal bloating.
    - Headache.
    - Fatigue.
- Symptoms occur in three prospectively monitored menstrual cycles.
- Exclude other diagnoses—depression and anxiety may present all throughout the cycle.

Premenstrual Dysphoric Disorder (PMDD) Diagnostic Criteria (Diagnosis Made Using DSM-V Criteria)

 A 17-year-old G0 patient reports feeling sad 4 days right before she starts menstruating. She reports low energy, fatigue, hopelessness, anxiety, mood swings, bloating, breast tenderness, headache, and sleep disturbances during these days. These symptoms disappear 2 days after the start of menses. They occur on a monthly basis. She reports that she misses school on a monthly basis because she cannot get out of bed for 3 days. What is the most likely diagnosis? What is the best objective test to confirm the diagnosis?

Answer: PMDD. This patient has symptoms consistent with PMS, but with markedly severe symptoms that affect daily activities. She should monitor her symptoms in relation to her menses and record them prospectively.

DSM-V DIAGNOSTIC CRITERIA

- Physical and behavioral symptoms documented with prospectively monitored cycles for most of the preceding year.
- Symptoms must cause significant stress or interference with normal daily activities.
- One or more of the following symptoms must be present:
  - Depressed mood, hopelessness, or having self-deprecating thoughts.
  - Anxiety, tension, feeling on edge.
  - Mood lability, increased sensitivity to rejection.
  - Persistent irritability, anger, ↑ interpersonal conflicts.
- In addition, one or more of the following symptoms must be present to reach a total of five symptoms overall:
  - Problems concentrating.
  - Changes in appetite or food cravings.
  - Anhedonia.
  - Decreased energy, fatigue.
  - Feeling overwhelmed.
  - Physical symptoms, i.e., breast tenderness, bloating.
  - Sleep disturbances.

 EXAM TIP

Diagnosis of PMS should be made from recording symptoms on a prospective calendar. Irritability is the most common symptom.

Tests

- Prospective calendar of symptoms in relation to menses
- Validated prospective self-administered questionnaire: Daily Record of Severity of Problems (DRSP) form

Treatment

A clear diagnosis of PMS or PMDD should be documented before starting treatment. Other conditions with similar symptoms should be excluded, such as anxiety disorders, depression, substance abuse, and thyroid disorders. Treatment can be recommended based on severity of symptoms. Patients with mild symptoms that do not cause distress or impairment can be treated initially with supportive measures and lifestyle modifications. Women with more severe PMS or PMDD which cause distress or impairment may be treated with pharmacotherapy or behavioral therapies.

- **Supportive therapy and lifestyle modification:**
  - Reassurance and information counseling.
  - Relaxation therapy for severe symptoms has been shown to help.
  - Stress reduction techniques.
  - Regular aerobic exercise reduces both physical and behavioral symptoms.
  - Dietary supplementation: Vitamin E ↓ mastalgia.
- **Selective serotonin reuptake inhibitors (SSRIs): Increases central serotonin transmission**
  - Fluoxetine, sertraline, citalopram, and escitalopram have been well studied and shown to help. Other SSRIs and serotonin-norepinephrine reuptake inhibitors (SNRIs) may have similar efficacy.
  - Typically more effective for behavioral rather than physical symptoms.
  - Can be administered in three different regimens with effective outcomes:
  - Continuously throughout the menstrual cycle.
  - Luteal phase therapy, usually starting on day 14 of the cycle and discontinued at the onset of menses or a few days after.
  - Symptom onset therapy: Used occasionally beginning at symptoms onset and continued through the start of menses or a few days after.
- **Oral contraceptives: Suppresses the hypothalamic-pituitary-ovarian (HPO) axis to limit cyclic changes in gonadal steroids**
  - Cyclic combined oral contraceptives (COCs) with 4- rather than 7-day placebo may be more effective.
  - If symptoms do not improve with cyclic COCs, consider continuous COCs.
  - Monophasic COCs are best.
- **Other therapies:**
  - Nonsteroidal anti-inflammatory drugs (NSAIDs).
  - Gonadotropin-releasing hormone (GnRH) agonists: Severe symptoms that do not respond to or cannot tolerate SSRIs or COCs.
  - Bilateral salpingo-oophorectomy (+/− hysterectomy): Reserved as a last resort for severe, disabling cases of PMDD. Patients must have improvement with GnRH agonists and have completed childbearing.
  - Cognitive behavioral therapy: May be a beneficial addition to treatment for women with moderate to severe symptoms who have had a suboptimal response to pharmacologic therapy.

Infertility

Infertility is a common condition that is unique in that it involves two patients rather than one. The probability of achieving a pregnancy in one menstrual cycle, or fecundability, is 20% in normal fertile couples. Infertility ↑ with increasing age of the female partner and increasing amount of time spent trying to achieve pregnancy. Approximately 85% of couples will conceive within 12 months.

- Female factors account for 50–60% of infertile couples.
- Male factors account for 26% of infertile couples.
- About 28% of cases of infertility are unexplained.
- In 40% of infertile couples, there are multiple causes.

Definition: Infertility

- The inability of a couple to conceive **after 12 months** of regular unprotected intercourse in a woman under age 35, and after **6 months** of regular intercourse in a woman over age 35.
- Affects 15% of couples.

Types

- **Primary infertility:** Infertility in the absence of previous pregnancy
- **Secondary infertility:** Infertility after previous pregnancy

Female Factors Affecting Infertility

- Multifactorial: 40%
- Unexplained: 28%
- Ovulatory dysfunction: 25%
- Tubal blockage or other abnormality: 22%
- Endometriosis: 15%
- Pelvic adhesions: 12%

Male Factors Affecting Infertility

- Abnormal sperm function or concentration: 80%
- Abnormal sperm production: 75%
- Sperm transport disorders: 2–5%
- Endocrine and systemic disorders: 5–15%
- Unexplained (normal semen analysis): 15%
- Multifactorial: 50%

Infertility Workup

The workup should include a complete history and physical examination. Both partners should be evaluated concurrently.

See Table 16-1.

TABLE 16-1. **Evaluation of Infertile Couple**

Male factor: Semen analysis
Ovulation factor: Serum progesterone, day 3 FSH, prolactin
Uterine factor: Ultrasonography, saline infused sonogram, hysterosalpingogram (HSG), and possible hysteroscopy
Tubal factor: HSG, laparoscopy
Endometriosis: Laparoscopy

MALE FACTOR

Semen Analysis

Performed after at least 48 hours of ejaculatory abstinence. Ideally the sample should be collected by masturbation at the doctor's office; otherwise, it may be collected at home and delivered within one hour. Two properly performed semen analyses should be obtained at least 1–2 weeks apart. The analysis reflects sperm production that occurred 3 months ago.

CHARACTERISTICS [REFERENCE LIMITS ARE PUBLISHED BY THE WORLD HEALTH ORGANIZATION (WHO)]

- Volume: Normal >1.5 mL
- Sperm concentration: Normal >15 million spermatozoa/mL
- Total sperm number: Normal >38 million spermatozoa per ejaculate
- Total motility (progressive and nonprogressive): Normal >40%
- Morphology: Normal >4%

TREATMENT FOR ABNORMAL SEMEN ANALYSIS

- Depends on the cause.
- Refer to urologist.
- Smoking and alcohol cessation.
- Avoid lubricants with intercourse.
- Clomiphene citrate or aromatase inhibitors (for the male partner) to block negative feedback of estrogens and increase luteinizing hormone (LH), follicle-stimulating hormone (FSH), and testosterone production.
- Assisted Reproductive Technologies (ARTs) (with partner or donor sperm):
  - Intrauterine insemination (IUI): Sperm injected through cervix.
  - Intracytoplasmic sperm injection (ICSI).
  - In vitro fertilization.
- If semen analysis is normal, continue workup of other factors.

OVARIAN FACTOR

 A 28-year-old G0 patient has been unable to conceive with her husband over 1 year of regular, unprotected intercourse. Her periods are irregular. She has a BMI of 30, displays coarse facial hair, and a dark velvety pigmentation on the back of her neck. What is the likely diagnosis in this patient? What is the most likely reason she is unable to conceive?

Answer: Polycystic ovarian syndrome (PCOS) affects approximately 5% of all women, and is a leading cause of infertility. Her exam shows evidence of hyperandrogenism and insulin resistance. She is anovulatory and will likely need an ovulation induction agent to conceive.

EXAM TIP

Androgen ("steroid") use is associated with azoospermia and infertility in males.

WARD TIP

Most male infertility is idiopathic.

WARD TIP

Initial workup for infertility:
- Assess ovulatory function and ovarian reserve
- Semen analysis
- Hysterosalpingogram

METHODS OF ASSESSING OVULATION

- **History of regular monthly menses** is a strong indicator of normal ovulation, especially if accompanied by molimina symptoms of breast tenderness, bloating, etc.
- **Day 21 (mid-luteal) serum progesterone:** If >3 ng/mL, the patient is likely to be ovulatory.
- **Urinary ovulation predictor kit:** Available over the counter and tests for LH surge, which is highly predictive of ovulation.

POSSIBLE CAUSES AND TREATMENTS OF ANOVULATION

- **Hypogonadotropic hypogonadism:** hypothalamic amenorrhea from stress or starvation. Treat with lifestyle modification +/− ovulation induction.
- **Hyperprolactinemia:** Administer bromocriptine, a dopamine agonist, which suppresses prolactin. May also require ovulation induction.
- **Normogonadotropic normoestrogenic:** PCOS. Treat with ovulation induction agent +/− metformin, weight loss. Ovulation induction agents include clomiphene citrate, gonadotropins, and aromatase inhibitors.
- **Hypergonadotropic hypoestrogenic:** Primary ovarian insufficiency. Treat with In vitro fertilization (IVF) with donor eggs.

METHODS OF ASSESSING OVARIAN RESERVE

- **Day 3 FSH:** Early low levels of FSH indicate adequate production of ovarian hormones.
- **Clomiphene Citrate Challenge Test (CCCT):** 100 mg clomiphene citrate on days 5–9 with measurement of FSH on days 3 and 10, and estradiol on day 3.
- **Antral Follicle Count (AFC):** Transvaginal ultrasound (TVUS) in early follicular phase to count antral follicles; a low count indicates poor reserve.
- **Anti-Müllerian Hormone (AMH):** Biochemical marker of ovarian function; serum levels decline as the primordial follicle pool declines with age.

UTERINE FACTORS

A 30-year-old G0 patient is undergoing an evaluation of her uterus as part of the workup for infertility. What procedure in evaluating the uterus would potentially be both diagnostic and therapeutic?

Answer: Hysteroscopy allows diagnosis and treatment of certain uterine anomalies (i.e., uterine septum) at the same time.

In addition to ovulation analysis and semen analysis, an analysis of the internal architecture of the uterus and fallopian tubes is also performed to determine if there is an anatomic etiology impacting infertility. In most cases, an internal architecture study is part of the initial workup.

- **Hysterosalpingogram (HSG):**
  - First-line test for evaluation of tubal patency and also allows visualization of the uterine cavity.
  - Radiopaque dye is injected into the cervix and uterus. Dye passes through the fallopian tubes to the peritoneal cavity. It should outline the inner uterine contour and both fallopian tubes when imaged with fluoroscopy.
  - Performed during follicular phase (avoid possibility of pregnancy).
  - Subfertile women who undergo HSG have higher pregnancy rates than subfertile women who do not undergo HSG. Appears to be both diagnostic and therapeutic.

- **Hysteroscopy:**
    - A hysteroscope is a telescope that is introduced into the uterus through the cervix and allows visualization of the uterine cavity.
    - It is the definitive method to evaluate abnormalities of the uterine cavity. This is usually only performed if there is concern for abnormality seen on ultrasound, HSG or sonohysterogram (i.e., not a first-line test).
    - It can be both diagnostic and therapeutic when performed in the operating room because it offers the opportunity for treatment at the time of diagnosis (i.e., resection of a uterine septum).
    - Operative hysteroscopy is useful in:
        - Asherman syndrome (lyse intrauterine adhesions).
        - Endometrial polyps (polypectomy).
        - Congenital uterine malformations (i.e., resect uterine septum).
        - Submucosal fibroids (resect).
- **Sonohysterogram:**
    - Fluid is instilled in the endometrial cavity concurrently with a pelvic ultrasound.
    - Outlines intrauterine pathology (i.e., polyps, submucosal fibroids).
    - Can be done with an ultrasound in an office setting.
- **Ultrasound (transvaginal or abdominal):**
    - In-office study. Can allow diagnosis of fibroids and certain uterine anomalies.
- **Laparoscopy:**
    - A telescope is placed through the skin of the abdominal wall into the peritoneal cavity.
    - The timing and role of laparoscopy is controversial, but it may be important to consider in women suspected of having endometriosis, pelvic adhesions, or tubal disease based on history, physical exam, or HSG.
    - Can be used to evaluate for endometriosis, to visualize outside of the uterus to assist in diagnosis of some müllerian malformations, and to perform chromotubation to assess tubal patency. Often performed in conjunction with hysteroscopy in the OR.

CAUSES AND TREATMENTS FOR UTERINE FACTOR INFERTILITY

- Submucosal fibroid: Resection, myomectomy
- Intrauterine septum: Hysteroscopic resection of septum
- Uterine didelphys: Metroplasty—a procedure to unify the two endometrial cavities (rarely performed)
- Asherman syndrome: Hysteroscopic lysis of intrauterine adhesions

TUBAL FACTOR

 A 30-year-old G0 patient has been having unprotected intercourse for 18 months without getting pregnant. She reports regular menstrual cycles. She had two episodes of pelvic inflammatory disease (PID) in the past. What is the best diagnostic modality to evaluate this patient? What will be the best treatment for her infertility?

Answer: HSG will help determine if there is tubal blockage due to PID. If tubal blockage is present, the patient will need in vitro fertilization.

EXAM TIP

Damage from tubal surgery can result in ectopic pregnancy. Most reproductive endocrinologists recommend in vitro fertilization if tubal factor is present.

EVALUATION

- HSG
- Laparoscopy

CAUSES AND TREATMENTS FOR TUBAL FACTOR INFERTILITY

- Adhesions:
  - Lysis of adhesions via laparoscopy.
  - Microsurgical tuboplasty.
  - Neosalpingostomy (blocked tubes are opened).
  - IVF, preferred in most cases.
- If the evaluation up to this point is within normal limits, then a diagnostic laparoscopy may be performed to assess for peritoneal factors.

PERITONEAL FACTORS

Laparoscopy is diagnostic and therapeutic.

CAUSES AND TREATMENTS FOR PERITONEAL FACTOR INFERTILITY

- **Adhesions:** Lysis of adhesions via laparoscopy
- **Endometriosis:** Excision or ablation of implants

Assisted Reproductive Technologies (ARTs)

The ARTs include clinical and laboratory techniques that are used to achieve pregnancy in infertile couples. A thorough infertility evaluation should be performed on both partners first. ARTs are employed when correction of the underlying cause of infertility is not feasible. ARTs can utilize patient or donor egg and/or sperm. The American College of Obstetricians and Gynecologists (ACOG) supports unrestricted access to family-building resources and fertility services for individuals who identify as lesbian, gay, bisexual, transgender, queer, intersex, and asexual (LGBTQIA), and gender nonconforming. Thus, ARTs may be used in a variety of combinations, both with and without donor egg and sperm, to support these communities.

Types of Assisted Reproductive Technologies (ARTs)

ARTIFICIAL INSEMINATION (AI)

- AI refers to the introduction of semen into the vagina, uterus, or fallopian tube by a method other than sexual intercourse. The semen may be from a patient's partner or from a sperm donor (in which case it is referred to as therapeutic donor insemination).
- IUI is a type of AI whereby washed and concentrated motile sperm are directly injected into the uterine cavity.
- Requires an ovulatory cycle and at least one patent fallopian tube for fertilization to take place.

IN VITRO FERTILIZATION (IVF) AND EMBRYO TRANSFER

- Egg cells are fertilized by sperm outside the uterus.
- Consists of ovarian stimulation with fertility medication, oocyte retrieval, fertilization in the laboratory ("in vitro"), embryo selection, and embryo transfer into uterus.

WARD TIP

IVF ↑ the chances of multiple gestation if multiple embryos are transferred.

- These steps occur over approximately two weeks and are referred to as an "IVF cycle."
- Pregnancy rate: 20% per cycle.
- Expensive with limited coverage by insurance companies in most locations.
- In some situations, may also be used in the setting of preimplantation genetic diagnosis (PGD), prevention of mitochondrial disorders, and genetic parenthood for same-sex couples.

INTRACYTOPLASMIC SPERM INJECTION (ICSI)

- Used in conjunction with IVF for couples whose infertility is primarily male factor: Severe oligospermia (low number), azoospermia (absence of live sperm), asthenospermia (low motility), teratospermia (abnormal morphology).
- Consists of direct injection of a single spermatozoon into the cytoplasm of an oocyte.
- Pregnancy rate: 20% per cycle.
- Success rates are not influenced by the cause of abnormal sperm.
- Can use spermatozoa from testicular aspiration/biopsy or from ejaculate.

WARD TIP

Individuals who will undergo systemic chemotherapy should be referred for fertility preservation counseling. Cryopreservation techniques to freeze oocytes, spermatozoa, and embryos provide the highest likelihood of successfully producing offspring.

NOTES

Amenorrhea

EXAM TIP

Oligomenorrhea is fewer than nine menstrual cycles per year or cycle length of 35 days or more.

WARD TIP

When evaluating a patient with primary amenorrhea, note presence/absence of breasts and uterus. Most patients with primary amenorrhea have a uterus.

Amenorrhea, or the absence of menses, has a variety of causes. The hypothalamic-pituitary-ovarian (HPO) axis is involved in the regulation of the menstrual cycle, the uterus responds to the HPO axis, and an anatomically normal cervix and vagina allow the outflow of menstrual blood. An abnormality in any one of these components will result in amenorrhea.

- **Primary amenorrhea:** Absence of menses by age 15 with normal growth and secondary sexual characteristics, or absence of menses by age 13 with no secondary sexual characteristics. Usually caused by a genetic or anatomic abnormality.
- **Secondary amenorrhea:** Absence of menses for ≥3 months in a woman who previously had a regular menstrual cycle, or >6 months in a woman who had irregular menses. Usually caused by an underlying medical condition.

Primary Amenorrhea

The many causes of primary amenorrhea are typically the result of an anatomic or genetic abnormality. It has traditionally classified based on where the abnormality takes place along the HPO axis. It is more clinically useful to group the causes of primary amenorrhea on the basis of whether secondary sexual characteristics (breasts) and female internal genitalia (uterus) are present or absent. The external female genitalia are present for these patients, but focusing the physical exam on noting whether breast and uterus development are present can direct the rest of the evaluation and diagnostic testing.

BREASTS ABSENT, UTERUS PRESENT

When patients present without breasts and with a uterus, is due to the absence of ovarian estrogen. It is important to identify the underlying cause because it can have an impact on fertility.

- **Gonadal dysgenesis (hypergonadotropic hypogonadism):** The most common cause of primary amenorrhea, and is usually due to a chromosomal deletion or disorder. The ovaries are replaced by a band of fibrous tissue called *gonadal streak*. Due to the absence of ovarian follicles, there is no synthesis of ovarian steroids. Due to low levels of estrogen, breast development does not occur. Follicle-stimulating hormone (FSH) and luteinizing hormone (LH) levels are markedly elevated because the ↓ levels of estrogen do not provide negative feedback. Estrogen is not necessary for Müllerian duct development or Wolffian duct regression, so the internal and external genitalia are phenotypically female.
- **Turner syndrome (45,X):** In addition to primary amenorrhea and absent breasts, these patients have other phenotypic changes such as short stature (most prevalent), webbing of the neck, short fourth metacarpal, and cubitus valgus. Also may have structural cardiac abnormalities (coarctation of the aorta), structural renal abnormalities, and hypothyroidism. At puberty, the patient is given estrogen and progesterone to allow secondary sexual characteristics to develop. These patients also receive growth hormone.
- **Structurally abnormal X chromosome:** May have the same abnormalities as Turner syndrome patients.
- **17α-hydroxylase deficiency:** Can occur in 46,XX or 46,XY. Patients have ↓ cortisol and adrenal/gonadal sex steroid secretion. They may present with hypertension, hypernatremia, and hypokalemia due to excess mineralocorticoid. These patients need replacement with sex steroids and cortisol. Despite low levels of sex steroids, pregnancies have been

achieved with in vitro fertilization (IVF). Those with karyotype 46,XY and 17α-hydroxylase deficiency will have no breasts or female internal genitalia.

- **Hypothalamic-pituitary disorders:** Low levels of estrogen are due to low gonadotropin release.
    - **Anatomic lesions:** Anatomic lesions of the hypothalamus or pituitary can result in low gonadotropin production.
        - Congenital: Stenosis of aqueduct, absence of sellar floor.
        - Acquired: Prolactinoma, chromophobe adenoma, craniopharyngiomas.
    - **Inadequate gonadotropin-releasing hormone (GnRH) release (hypogonadotropic hypogonadism):** Patients will have normal levels of gonadotropins if stimulated with GnRH. These patients should receive estrogen-progesterone supplementation to induce breast development and allow for epiphyseal closure. Human menopausal gonadotropins or pulsatile GnRH is administered for fertility. Clomiphene does not work due to low levels of endogenous estrogen.
        - **Kallmann syndrome:** Idiopathic hypogonadotropic hypogonadism associated with anosmia, caused by a genetic mutation.
    - **Isolated gonadotropin deficiency (pituitary disorder):** Associated with:
        - Prepubertal hypothyroidism.
        - Kernicterus.
        - Mumps encephalitis.
        - Thalassemia major: Iron deposits in the pituitary.
        - Retinitis pigmentosa.

BREASTS PRESENT, UTERUS ABSENT

 An 18-year-old G0 patient presents with primary amenorrhea. Her sister experienced menarche at age 12. She reports no use of drugs, heavy exercise, or significant weight loss. She is 5'5" and 130 lb. Her blood pressure is 110/60. Physical exam demonstrates Tanner stage IV breasts, no axillary or pubic hair, and a blind vaginal pouch. What is the most likely diagnosis?

Answer: Androgen insensitivity. Breasts are present; uterus and axillary/pubic hair is absent in androgen insensitivity.

- **Complete androgen insensitivity:** This condition results from the absence of androgen receptors or lack of responsiveness to androgen stimulus. These patients have a 46,XY karyotype and normally functioning male gonads that produce normal male levels of testosterone and dihydrotestosterone. The Müllerian ducts regress due to the presence of anti-Müllerian hormone, and the Wolffian ducts do not develop because they are not stimulated by testosterone. Patients with this condition have no male or female internal genitalia, have normal female external genitalia, and have either a short or absent vagina. These patients have normal breast development and scant or absent axillary and pubic hair. Testes may be located intra-abdominally or in the inguinal canal, and have an ↑ risk of developing a malignancy (gonadoblastoma or dysgerminoma), usually after age 20. The gonads are removed after puberty and estrogen is given to allow for breast development and adequate bone growth.
- **Müllerian agenesis (Mayer-Rokitansky-Kuster-Hauser syndrome):** In this condition, the patients have no uterus and have a shortened vagina, but have normally ovulating ovaries, normal breast development, and normal axillary and pubic hair. These patients may also have associated renal

EXAM TIP

Primary amenorrhea + elevated serum FSH = Gonadal dysgenesis. Most common cause of primary amenorrhea ~40–45%.

EXAM TIP

17α hydroxylase deficiency:
46,XX: Breast absent, uterus present
46,XY: Breast absent, uterus absent

EXAM TIP

Androgen insensitivity: Patients look female externally. No pubic hair. Remove gonads after puberty to avoid risk of malignancy (gonadoblastoma or dysgerminoma).

and skeletal abnormalities and should be screened with an ultrasound or magnetic resonance imaging (MRI). They have normal endocrine function and do not need supplemental hormones. They may undergo surgical reconstruction of the vagina or use vaginal dilators to make the vagina functional (see Table 17-1).

BREASTS ABSENT, UTERUS ABSENT

17α-hydroxylase deficiency: These patients may be 46,XX or 46,XY. Patients with 46,XY karyotype have testes, but lack the enzyme needed to synthesize sex steroids. They have female external genitalia. Anti-Müllerian hormone causes the regression of the Müllerian ducts. Low testosterone levels do not allow the development of internal male genitalia. There is insufficient estrogen to allow breast development. Those with karyotype 46,XX, will have no breasts, but a uterus will be present.

BREASTS PRESENT, UTERUS PRESENT

- This is the second largest category of individuals with primary amenorrhea (chromosomal/gonadal dysgenesis #1).
- **Imperforate hymen and transverse vaginal septum**: These patients present with cyclic pelvic pain due to menstrual blood not having an egress. A hematocolpos (accumulation of menstrual blood in the vagina from an imperforate hymen) may be palpated as a perirectal mass on physical exam. A transverse vaginal septum may occur at any level between the hymenal ring and cervix. The treatment is to excise the obstruction.

Evaluation of Primary Amenorrhea

HISTORY

- Other stages of puberty reached? Lack of any pubertal development suggests ovarian/pituitary cause.
- Family history of delayed puberty.
- Height compared to other family members.
- Neonatal/childhood health problems.
- Symptoms of excess androgens.

TABLE 17-1. Comparison of Androgen Insensitivity and Müllerian Agenesis

	ANDROGEN INSENSITIVITY	MÜLLERIAN AGENESIS
Karyotype	XY	XX
Breast	Present	Present
Uterus	Absent	Absent
Pubic/axillary hair	Absent	Normal
Testosterone	Normal male levels	Female levels
Further evaluation	Need gonadectomy	Renal/skeletal abnormalities

- Recent stress, weight change, exercise.
- Drugs: Heroin/methadone can affect hypothalamus.
- Galactorrhea: Antipsychotics, metoclopramide can cause hyperprolactinemia.
- Headaches, vision problems, fatigue, polyuria, polydipsia: Hypothalamic/pituitary disorders.

PHYSICAL EXAM

- Height, weight, growth chart, arm span
- Blood pressure:
  - Turner syndrome with coarctation of aorta
  - Adrenal disorders
- Breast development (Tanner staging): Marker of ovary function and estrogen action
- Genital exam:
  - Clitoral size
  - Tanner staging of pubic hair
  - Hymen
  - Vaginal depth
  - Vaginal or rectal exam to evaluate internal organs
- Skin: Hirsutism, acne, striae, acanthosis nigricans, vitiligo
- Turner stigmata: Low hairline, web neck, shield chest, widely spaced nipples

WARD TIP

Check FSH to distinguish between gonadal failure and hypogonadotropic hypogonadism. FSH is high with gonadal failure and low with hypogonadotropic hypogonadism.

STUDIES

- Confirm presence of uterus: Ultrasound, rarely MRI.
- Uterus absent: Karyotype, serum testosterone: Müllerian anomalies have 46,XX with normal female levels of testosterone. Androgen insensitivity has 46,XY with male levels of testosterone.
- Uterus present. No other anatomic findings:
  - β-human chorionic gonadotropin (β-hCG) to rule out pregnancy.
  - FSH
    - High: Indicative of primary ovarian insufficiency. Karyotype: Turner syndrome (46,X); 17α-hydroxylase deficiency—(46, XX) electrolytes, ↑ progesterone, ↑ deoxycorticosterone, ↓ 17α-hydroxyprogesterone. Remove testes if Y chromosome present.
    - Low/normal: Functional hypothalamic amenorrhea, GnRH deficiency, hypothalamic/pituitary disorders. Head computed tomography (CT) or MRI to evaluate for infiltrative disease or adenoma. Prolactin, thyroid-stimulating hormone (TSH). Testosterone and dehydroepiandrosterone sulfate (DHEA-S) if signs of hyperandrogenism.
    - Normal: With normal breast and uterus. Focus workup on secondary amenorrhea.

EXAM TIP

Ovarian insufficiency may be due to hypothalamus not producing GnRH or ovaries not responding to FSH.

Secondary Amenorrhea

A 30-year-old G2P2002 patient, with last menstrual period (LMP) 8 weeks ago, presents with no menses for 2 months. She usually has menses every 28 days lasting for 5 days. She reports no medical or surgical history. She has had two vaginal deliveries at term. She uses combination oral contraceptive pills (OCPs), and has not missed any pills recently. What is the next step in management of this patient?

Answer: The most common cause of amenorrhea in a reproductive-age woman is pregnancy, so a urine or serum β-hCG should be checked. Contraception use does not prevent pregnancy 100% of the time.

EXAM TIP

The most common cause of secondary amenorrhea is pregnancy. Always check a pregnancy test in a reproductive-age woman.

CAUSES

- Pregnancy
- Hypothalamus (35%)
- Pituitary (19%)
- Ovary (40%)
- Uterus (5%)
- Other (1%): Cervical, endocrine

Hypothalamic amenorrhea

Characterized by low levels of gonadotropins, estrogen, absent withdrawal bleed with progesterone.
- **Lesions:** Hypothalamic tumors or infiltrative disorders such as craniopharyngiomas, granulomatous disease, lymphomas, encephalitis sequelae.
- **Drugs:** Combined OCPs act at the level of the hypothalamus and pituitary. Post-pill amenorrhea can occur up to 6 months after stopping the pill. (Other combined contraceptive options may also have amenorrhea after stopping, as can Depo-provera.)
- **Systemic disease:** Celiac disease, type 1 diabetes, chronic kidney disease
- **Functional hypothalamic amenorrhea:**
    - Many factors may contribute, such as excessive exercise, emotional stress, eating disorders or excessive weight loss (e.g., anorexia nervosa), and nutritional deficiencies.
    - In rare cases, no underlying precipitating factor is identified.

Pituitary (Hypoestrogenic Amenorrhea)

- **Neoplasms:** Chromophobe adenomas are the most common non-prolactin-secreting pituitary tumors. Prolactinomas will be discussed in a later section. Treatment may involve suppression with medication (prolactinomas) or excision.
- **Lesions:** The pituitary gland can be damaged from anoxia, thrombosis, or hemorrhage. May be associated with ↓ secretion of other pituitary hormones like adrenocorticotropic hormone (ACTH), TSH, LH, and FSH. The patients may have hypothyroidism and adrenal insufficiency.
    - **Sheehan syndrome:** Pituitary cell infarction occurs due to severe postpartum hemorrhage resulting in hypotension and often requiring blood transfusion. Treatment includes replacement of pituitary hormones.

Ovarian (Hypergonadotropic Hypogonadism)

 A 35-year-old G3P3003 patient presents with absence of menses for 8 months. She reports menarche at age 12 with menses every 40–50 days until recently. She reports a 20-lb weight gain over the last year. She used letrozole to become pregnant with her last two pregnancies. Vitals show height 5'4", weight 220 lb, BP 120/80. She has hair on her upper lip and chin, acne, and oily skin on her face. What is the most likely diagnosis? If left untreated, what is this patient at ↑ risk for?

Answer: Polycystic ovarian syndrome (PCOS). Diagnosis of PCOS is established with two out of three of the following: a history of oligomenorrhea/amenorrhea, features of hyperandrogenism (acne, hirsutism), and multiple ovarian cysts seen on ultrasound. This patient is at ↑ risk for endometrial hyperplasia or cancer if left untreated.

 A 35-year-old G2P2002 patient with LMP 1 year ago presents with hot flashes and vaginal dryness. Her serum FSH is very high. What is the most likely diagnosis?

Answer: Primary ovarian insufficiency. Symptoms are similar to those in menopause and diagnosis is confirmed with elevated FSH.

- **Primary ovarian insufficiency (POI):** Primary hypogonadism with depletion of oocytes, resulting in amenorrhea before the age of 40. The cause is unknown in 75–90% of cases, but could be due to:
  - Ovarian toxins such as radiation or systemic chemotherapy.
  - Autoimmune conditions such as polyglandular autoimmune failure.
  - Genetic causes such as Turner syndrome and fragile X premutation carriers.
  - Treatment includes hormone replacement to reduce the risk of cardiovascular disease, osteoporosis, and urogenital atrophy.
- **Surgical:** Bilateral salpingo-oophorectomy.
- **PCOS:**
  - **Diagnosis:** Established if two out of three of the following are present (Rotterdam criteria):
    - Polycystic ovaries on ultrasound.
    - Clinical or biochemical evidence of androgen excess (hirsutism, acne).
    - Oligomenorrhea/amenorrhea.
  - **Signs:**
    - Hirsutism.
    - Acne.
    - Oligomenorrhea/amenorrhea.
    - Obesity.
    - Acanthosis nigricans (gray, brown velvety skin discoloration present most commonly on neck and axilla).
    - Premature pubarche and/or precocious puberty.
  - **Treatment:**
    - Manage hirsutism, i.e., cosmetic methods, spironolactone.
    - Treat infertility (ovulation induction).
    - Protect the endometrium from endometrial hyperplasia or cancer: start cyclic or continuous OCPs/hormone therapy.
    - Evaluate and treat metabolic issues, i.e., insulin resistance, impaired glucose tolerance, obesity, dyslipidemia.

Uterine

- **Asherman syndrome:** Intrauterine adhesions can obliterate the endometrial cavity and cause amenorrhea.
  - Most frequent cause is endometrial curettage associated with pregnancy.
  - Adhesions may form after myomectomy, metroplasty, or cesarean delivery.
  - Confirm the diagnosis with hysterosalpingogram (HSG) or hysteroscopy.
  - Treat via hysteroscopic resection of adhesions. Estrogens may be administered to stimulate regrowth of endometrium.
- **Endometrial ablation:** Surgical procedure performed to treat heavy menstrual bleeding.
- **Infection:** Endometritis or tuberculosis.

Cervical

Stenosis, most commonly due to loop electrosurgical excision procedure (LEEP) or cold-knife cone. Treat with cervical dilation.

Endocrine

Can cause secondary amenorrhea.
- Hyper/hypothyroidism
- Diabetes mellitus
- Hyperandrogenism (neoplasm, exogenous androgens)

WARD TIP

Progestin challenge test: Give oral progestin for 10 days. If the endometrium has been primed with estrogen from ovaries or peripheral fat, the withdrawal of progestin after 10 days will cause endometrial sloughing with resultant withdrawal bleed. No withdrawal bleeding indicates absence of ovaries, estrogen deficiency, or outflow obstruction.

EXAM TIP

Asherman syndrome is intrauterine adhesions secondary to uterine curettage associated with pregnancy (including after SAB, for retained placenta, or PPH) or shortly thereafter with resultant scarring.

EXAM TIP

The most common symptoms associated with Asherman syndrome include amenorrhea or light periods, infertility, cyclic pelvic pain, recurrent pregnancy loss.

EVALUATION

HISTORY

- Recent stress, weight change, new diet or exercise habits, illness
- Acne, hirsutism, deepening of voice
- Symptoms of hypothalamic-pituitary disease:
  - Headaches
  - Galactorrhea
  - Visual field defects
  - Fatigue
  - Polyuria, polydipsia
- Symptoms of estrogen deficiency:
  - Hot flashes
  - Vaginal dryness
  - Poor sleep
  - ↓ libido
- Obstetric emergency with hemorrhage (Sheehan syndrome)
- Medications:
  - Initiation or discontinuation of OCPs
  - Androgenic drugs
  - High-dose progestins
  - Metoclopramide, antipsychotics: Cause ↑ prolactin leading to amenorrhea

PHYSICAL EXAM

- Body mass index (BMI): >30 kg/m² in women with PCOS
- Signs of systemic illness/cachexia, anorexia
- Genital tissue with signs of estrogen deficiency: POI
- Breast exam for galactorrhea
- Neurologic exam for visual fields: Pituitary adenoma
- Skin:
  - Hirsutism, acne, acanthosis nigricans: PCOS
  - Thin/dry skin, thickened skin: Thyroid disorders

STUDIES

- Serum hCG, prolactin, TSH, FSH. FSH is high in POF. Consider karyotype.
- Total testosterone if signs of hyperandrogenism.
- Assessment of estrogen status:
  - Serum estradiol.
  - Progestin withdrawal test with oral medroxyprogesterone 10 mg for 10 days. If bleeding occurs, then adequate estrogen is present in the body.

TREATMENT

Treatment is individualized based on the etiology of amenorrhea.

Hyperandrogenism

Definitions

- **Hirsutism:** Presence of hair in locations where it is not normally found in a woman, specifically in the midline of the body (upper lip, chin, back, intermammary region). Also known as male-pattern hair growth.
- **Virilization:** Signs of masculinization in a woman (temporal balding, deepening voice, clitoromegaly, ↑ muscle mass).
- **Hypertrichosis:** Generalized ↑ in the amount of androgen-independent vellus body hair in its normal location.
- **Vellus (lanugo) hairs:** Fine, soft, unpigmented short hairs found on most parts of the body.
- **Terminal hairs:** Coarse, darker hairs found, for example, in the axilla and pubic region. Androgens facilitate the conversion of vellus to terminal hairs.

Sources of Androgens

EXAM TIP

Ovary makes testosterone. Adrenal gland makes DHEA-S.

Androgens are produced in the ovary and the adrenal gland. The ovary primarily makes testosterone. It also secretes androstenedione and dehydroepiandrosterone (DHEA) to a smaller degree, and these are converted to testosterone in peripheral tissue. The adrenal gland makes DHEA and dehydroepiandrosterone sulfate (DHEA-S). To produce a biologic effect, the enzyme 5α-reductase in the peripheral tissue converts testosterone to more potent 5α-dihydrotestosterone (DHT).

ADRENAL PRODUCTION OF ANDROGENS

- The **zona fasciculata** and the **zona reticularis** of the adrenal cortex produce androgens, as well as cortisol. Adrenocorticotropic hormone (ACTH) regulates production.
- A third layer of the adrenal cortex, the **zona glomerulosa**, produces aldosterone and is regulated by the renin-angiotensin system.
- All three hormones—cortisol, androgens, and aldosterone—are derived from cholesterol. Androgen products from the adrenal are found mostly in the form of DHEA and DHEA-S. Elevation in these products represents ↑ adrenal androgen production.

OVARIAN PRODUCTION OF ANDROGENS

Luteinizing hormone (LH) stimulates the ovarian theca cells to produce androgens (androstenedione and testosterone). Next, follicle-stimulating hormone (FSH) stimulates ovarian granulosa cells to convert these androgens to estrone and estradiol. When LH levels become disproportionately greater than FSH levels, androgens become elevated.

Idiopathic Hirsutism (Peripheral Disorder of Androgen Metabolism)

 A 35-year-old G3P3003 patient reports increasing facial hair that began 2 years ago. Her menses occur every 30 days and lasts for 4 days. The patient reports her sister has similar symptoms. On physical examination, the patient is normotensive, has normal

(continued)

external female genitalia, and demonstrates moderately dark hair on the upper lip and chin. Serum levels of testosterone and DHEA-S are normal. What is the most likely diagnosis?

Answer: Idiopathic hirsutism. Gradual onset of hirsutism with normal menses, testosterone, and DHEA-S indicates idiopathic hirsutism.

hirsutism. This disorder is due to ↑ activity of 5α-reductase activity in the periphery. Antiandrogens that block the peripheral activity of testosterone or inhibit the enzyme 5α-reductase can be used to treat the hirsutism.

Adrenal Etiologies

CUSHING'S SYNDROME AND CUSHING DISEASE

- **Cushing's syndrome:** An adrenal tumor produces ↑ levels of cortisol with clinical findings—hirsutism, menstrual irregularity, central obesity, moon face, buffalo hump, abdominal striae, weakness, and muscle wasting. Exogenous or endogenous cortisol can be the cause. Confirm diagnosis with dexamethasone suppression test.
- **Cushing disease** (pituitary disease) is a subset of Cushing's syndrome. A benign pituitary adenoma causes an ↑ in the secretion of ACTH which results in ↑ cortisol levels. It accounts for 70% of Cushing's syndromes. Virilization and hirsutism are associated with this condition because the ACTH stimulates androgen production as well.
- **Paraneoplastic syndromes,** in which tumors (usually small cell lung cancer) produce ectopic ACTH, also cause ↑ cortisol. These account for 15% of Cushing's syndromes.
- **Adrenal tumors** (adenoma or carcinoma) account for the remaining 15% of Cushing's syndromes. In general, adenomas produce only cortisol, so no hirsutism or virilization is present. Carcinomas, by contrast, often produce androgens as well as cortisol, so they may present with signs of hirsutism and virilization. DHEA-S is markedly elevated, and hirsutism and virilization have a rapid onset. Computed tomography (CT) or magnetic resonance imaging (MRI) can confirm the diagnosis.

EXAM TIP

Rapid onset of hirsutism or virilization = Tumor (ovarian or adrenal)

 ZEBRA ALERT

A baby with ambiguous genitalia, severe hypotension, and elevated 17-hydroxyprogesterone. *Think: 21-Hydroxylase deficiency.*

CONGENITAL ADRENAL HYPERPLASIA (CAH)

- Caused by a congenital defect in an enzyme that produces cortisol.
  - **21-hydroxylase deficiency:** The most common form of CAH. The condition has various levels of severity. Affected individuals lack an enzyme crucial to cortisol and mineralocorticoid production. Therefore, the ↑ precursors of cortisol are shunted to androgen production. Elevated serum 17-hydroxyprogesterone is used as a marker for establishing the diagnosis of 21-hydroxylase deficiency. In the severe form, affected females have ambiguous genitalia at birth, along with severe salt wasting and cortisol insufficiency. Late-onset 21-hydroxylase deficiency presents with varying degrees of virilization and hirsutism in females after puberty.
  - **11β-hydroxylase deficiency:** Associated with ↓ cortisol, but ↑ mineralcorticoids and androgens. A typical patient with this enzyme deficiency has severe hypertension with virilization/hirsutism (which results in ambiguous genitalia of female newborns). The levels of 11-deoxycortisol are high in 11β-hydroxylase deficiency (see Table 18-1).

WARD TIP

Most common cause of ambiguous genitalia in a newborn: CAH due to 21-hydroxylase deficiency

TABLE 18-1. Clinical Findings in Congenital Adrenal Hyperplasia

	21-HYDROXYLASE DEFICIENCY	11B-HYDROXYLASE DEFICIENCY
Androgens	High	High
Cortisol	Low	Low
Mineralacorticoids	Low → hypotension	High → hypertension
Marker	↑ 17-hydroxyprogesterone	↑ 11-deoxycortisol

Ovarian Etiologies

POLYCYSTIC OVARIAN SYNDROME (PCOS)

- PCOS is a common condition (affecting 5–10% of reproductive-age women) and is diagnosed by the presence of two out of three clinical findings (Rotterdam criteria): Hyperandrogenism (i.e., acne, hirsutism), oligomenorrhea/amenorrhea, and multiple ovarian cysts on ultrasound.
- An abnormal release of gonadotropin-releasing hormone (GnRH) causes a persistently elevated LH. The LH:FSH ratio is often >3:1. There are ↑ levels of androgens produced from the adrenal gland and the ovary. Serum testosterone is elevated. These women also have higher levels of estradiol that is not bound to sex hormone-binding globulin (SHBG), although the total estradiol level is not elevated. There is ↑ estrone due to adipose conversion of androgens.
- These patients may also may have acanthosis nigricans, obesity, insulin resistance, dyslipidemia, and infertility. In the future, they are at ↑ risk for metabolic syndrome with diabetes mellitus, hypertension, cardiovascular disease, and endometrial cancer. The risk of endometrial cancer is reduced with the use of oral contraceptive pills (OCPs).

OVARIAN STROMAL HYPERTHECOSIS

- LH stimulates theca cells in the ovary resulting in stromal hyperplasia. Theca cells produce large amounts of testosterone, resulting in severe hyperandrogenism and insulin resistance.
- Presents primarily in postmenopausal women with gradual onset of acne, hirsutism, and virilization.
- The increase in ovarian testosterone secretion results in an increase in peripheral estrogen conversion, which increases the risk of endometrial hyperplasia and malignancy.

THECA LUTEIN CYSTS

- These cysts are the result of stimulation by high levels of human chorionic gonadotropin (hCG) or by extreme sensitivity to hCG.
- Theca cells produce androgens, and granulosa cells transform the androgens to estrogens.
- Theca lutein cysts produce abnormally high levels of androgens, in excess of the amount that can be converted to estrogens.
- Diagnosis is made by ovarian biopsy.

WARD TIP

The most common cause of hirsutism and irregular menses is PCOS.

WARD TIP

A 24-year-old obese woman with facial hair presents with amenorrhea. Serum testosterone is elevated. *Think: PCOS.*

ZEBRA ALERT

A baby with ambiguous genitalia is born to a mother who reports ↑ facial hair growth over last few months. *Think: Luteoma of pregnancy.*

LUTEOMA OF PREGNANCY

- A benign solid tumor that grows in response to hCG.
- Virilization may occur in both the mother and the female fetus.
- The tumor usually disappears postpartum, as do maternal clinical features.

ANDROGEN-SECRETING OVARIAN NEOPLASMS

A 25-year-old G0 patient reports a 2-month history of increasing dark hair on her upper lip and chin, thinning hair on her head, and deepening of her voice. On exam, she is normotensive, has hair growth as stated above, and has temporal balding. Her pelvic exam demonstrates clitoromegaly. What is the most likely diagnosis? What is the next step in management?

Answer: Due to the rapid presentation of virilization, this is most likely an adrenal or ovarian tumor. Drawing serum total testosterone and DHEA-S will help differentiate the source. Pelvic ultrasound will confirm the presence of an ovarian mass. A CT or MRI will confirm the presence of an adrenal mass.

- **Sertoli-Leydig cell tumors** and **hilar (Leydig) cell tumors** are rare conditions in which the neoplasms secrete androgens.
- Sertoli-Leydig cell tumors are distinguished from hilar cell tumors in that Sertoli-Leydig tumors usually present in young women with palpable masses and hilar cell tumors are found in postmenopausal women with nonpalpable masses.
- Neoplasms present with rapid signs of virilization.

History

- Pregnancy: Theca lutein cysts, luteoma of pregnancy
- Timing of hirsutism, virilization: Rapid onset suggestive of ovarian or adrenal tumors and gradual onset suggestive of idiopathic etiology

Physical Exam

- Note distribution of terminal hair
- Note signs of virilization
- Bimanual exam: Pelvic mass
- Hirsutism, menstrual irregularity, central obesity, moon face, buffalo hump, abdominal striae, weakness, and muscle wasting: Cushing's syndrome

Studies

- Serum total testosterone (ovarian), DHEA-S (adrenal): Distinguish ovarian versus adrenal source.
- Ultrasound: Confirm ovarian mass.
- CT/MRI: Confirm adrenal mass.
- Dexamethasone suppression test: Distinguish the etiology of the ACTH stimulation.
- Serum 17-hydroxyprogesterone: Elevated in 21-hydroxylase deficiency.
- Serum 11-deoxycortisol: Elevated in 11β-hydroxylase deficiency.

WARD TIP

If cortisol levels are low after an overnight dexamethasone suppression test, Cushing's syndrome is excluded from the differential.

Treatment

- Ovarian and adrenal tumors:
  - Sertoli-Leydig cell tumors: Unilateral salpingo-oophorectomy if not completed childbearing.
  - Hilar cell tumors: Usually in postmenopausal women. Hysterectomy with bilateral salpingo-oophorectomy (BSO).
  - Adrenal adenoma or carcinoma: Surgical removal.
  - Stromal hyperthecosis: Hysterectomy with BSO.
- Late-onset 21-hydroxylase deficiency:
  - Androgen excess and menstrual irregularities can be treated as PCOS.
  - Infertility: Supplement with glucocorticoids to suppress androgens and allow ovulation.
- PCOS:
  - Weight loss.
  - OCPs for acne and menstrual irregularity. Estrogen component in the OCP ↑ SHBG; SHBG binds androgens; free androgen levels are then ↓. Progestin in the OCP inhibits 5α-reductase activity in the skin.
  - Cyclic progesterone for menstrual irregularity.
  - Infertility: Ovulation induction with letrozole.
- Skin disorders:
  - Peripheral antiandrogens: Spironolactone, finasteride, cyproterone acetate.
  - Androgenic acne responds quickly to treatment. Hirsutism moderately responsive; alopecia least responsive to treatment.
- Idiopathic hirsutism:
  - Peripheral androgen activity inhibitor. May take 3 months to work (length of hair life cycle).
  - Electrolysis, laser, or intense pulsed light therapy.
  - OCPs, medroxyprogesterone acetate.
  - Eflornithine hydrochloride cream: Topical treatment for unwanted facial hair.
  - Spironolactone: Blocks androgen receptors, ↓ ovarian testosterone production, inhibits 5α-reductase.
  - Finasteride (5α-reductase inhibitor), flutamide (nonsteroidal antiandrogen): Similar effectiveness to spironolactone.

EXAM TIP

Treatment of choice for idiopathic hirsutism: Spironolactone

CHAPTER 19

Hyperprolactinemia and Galactorrhea

Definitions

- **Hyperprolactinemia:** Elevated levels of the hormone prolactin (PRL)
- **Galactorrhea:** Physiologic watery or milky nipple discharge that is non-pathologic and is unrelated to pregnancy
- **Prolactinoma:** Prolactin-secreting pituitary tumor

Etiology

 A 35-year-old G2P2002 patient presents with a 6-month history of milky-appearing nipple discharge and amenorrhea. She used to have menses every 28 days, lasting for 4 days. She does not take any medications. No masses are palpated on the breast exam, but a milky-appearing nipple discharge is expressed from both breasts. Her serum β-human chorionic gonadotropin (β-hCG) is negative. What is the most likely diagnosis? What studies should be ordered next?

Answer: This patient has galactorrhea and amenorrhea, most likely due to hyperprolactinemia. The next steps in the evaluation are to order serum PRL and thyroid-stimulating hormone (TSH).

- PRL is a peptide hormone produced by the anterior pituitary gland and is important for lactation. The main function of PRL is to stimulate growth of mammary tissue as well as produce and secrete milk into the alveoli. ↑ secretion of PRL, hyperprolactinemia, may lead to galactorrhea. PRL secretion is stimulated by thyrotropin-releasing hormone (TRH) and serotonin; it is inhibited by dopamine.
- Hyperprolactinemia inhibits the pulsatile release of gonadotropin-releasing hormone (GnRH), resulting in amenorrhea/oligomenorrhea, anovulation, inappropriate lactation, and galactorrhea.
- **Causes** of hyperprolactinemia:
  - Drugs: Antipsychotics (most common), antidepressants [both tricyclic antidepressants (TCAs) and selective serotonin reuptake inhibitors (SSRIs)], antihypertensives (verapamil, methyldopa), opioid analgesics, antiemetics (metoclopramide), oral contraceptive pills (OCPs).
  - Hypothyroidism: ↓ negative feedback of thyroxine (T4) on the hypothalamic-pituitary axis causing an increase in TRH. TRH stimulates PRL secretion.
  - Hypothalamic: Any disease in or near the hypothalamus, such as craniopharyngioma, sarcoidosis, histiocytosis, metastatic breast carcinoma, or leukemia, may interfere with portal circulation of dopamine.
  - Pituitary: Prolactinoma. Microadenoma (<1 cm) and macroadenoma (>1 cm). See the following section on prolactinoma.
  - Hyperplasia of lactotrophs (lactotroph adenoma): Present very similarly to microadenomas.
  - Empty sella syndrome: Intrasellar extension of subarachnoid space which causes compression of the pituitary gland and an enlarged sella turcica.
  - Acromegaly: Pituitary gland secretes growth hormone as well as PRL.
  - Acute/chronic renal disease: ↓ metabolic clearance of PRL.
  - Chest surgery or trauma: Breast implants, herpes zoster at breast dermatome.

Prolactinoma

- One-tenth of people in the general population have an incidental prolactinoma.
- Fifty percent of women with hyperprolactinemia have prolactinoma.
- Most prolactinomas are microadenomas.
- Majority of microadenomas do not enlarge.
- Hyperprolactinemia with or without a microadenoma is benign and treatment is not necessary unless estrogen levels are low or pregnancy is desired.
- Microadenoma growth is **not** stimulated by:
  - Pregnancy.
  - OCPs.
  - Hormone replacement.

HISTORY

- Amenorrhea/oligomenorrhea
- Galactorrhea
- Headaches
- Bitemporal visual field deficit

PHYSICAL EXAM

- Visual field testing if macroadenoma is present. Macroadenomas can exert pressure on the optic chiasm.
- Breast exam.

STUDIES

- PRL level.
- TSH, triiodothyronine (T_3), T_4: Evaluate for hypothyroidism if PRL is elevated.
- Magnetic resonance imaging (MRI): Most sensitive for diagnosis of pituitary masses and empty sella syndrome due to greater soft tissue contrast.

TREATMENT

- **Drugs:** Stop the suspected drug, and repeat PRL after 1 month. If medication cannot be stopped and PRL level above 100 ng/mL, image the sella turcica to determine the presence of macroadenoma.
- Patient with galactorrhea and normal menses: **No further therapy** if normal PRL, normal TSH.
- **Cabergoline:** Long-acting ergot dopamine receptor agonist, first-line treatment.
  - For patients with macroadenoma: Can reduce tumor mass.
  - For those that desire to conceive, are anovulatory, with hyperprolactinemia: Discontinued after conception as it crosses the placenta. Not known to be teratogenic.
  - For those with galactorrhea only: Inhibits secretion of PRL.
  - Favorable side effect profile.
  - Administered once or twice a week.
- **Bromocriptine:** Dopamine receptor agonist, second-line therapy.
  - Causes more severe side effects of nausea and orthostatic hypotension.
  - Administered twice daily.
- **Transsphenoidal microsurgical resection:**
  - Recommended only if medical therapy has failed and bothersome signs or symptoms persist.
  - Risk of diabetes insipidus, iatrogenic hypopituitarism.

WARD TIP

Most macroadenomas enlarge with time. Most microadenomas do not.

EXAM TIP

The most common symptoms of hyperprolactinemia are galactorrhea and amenorrhea.

WARD TIP

Sixty percent of women with galactorrhea have hyperprolactinemia. Ninety percent of women with galactorrhea, amenorrhea, and low estrogen have hyperprolactinemia.

EXAM TIP

MRI: Modality of choice to diagnose pituitary adenomas or empty sella syndrome

EXAM TIP

Cabergoline is the drug of choice for women with PRL-secreting microadenoma who want to conceive.

ZEBRA ALERT

Cabergoline at high doses (such as those used to treat Parkinson disease) has been shown to increase valvular heart disease, but does not appear to cause this at lower doses used to treat hyperprolactinemia.

EXAM TIP

Pregnancy ↑ the likelihood that PRL levels will ↓ or become normal overtime.

EXAM TIP

Bromocriptine or cabergoline induction of pregnancy is not associated with ↑ congenital abnormalities, spontaneous abortion, or multiple gestation.

WARD TIP

Cabergoline is more effective and better tolerated than bromocriptine.

- Fifty percent cure for microadenomas, 25% cure for macroadenoma: The entire adenoma is not able to be resected in many patients (especially macroadenomas), and the adenoma and hyperprolactinemia may recur.
- **Radiation:** Adjunctive treatment following incomplete removal of large tumors.
- **Osteoporosis treatment/prophylaxis:** Low levels of estrogen resulting from hyperprolactinemia can result in bone loss.

CHAPTER 20

Abnormal Uterine Bleeding

Definitions

Abnormal uterine bleeding (AUB) refers to uterine bleeding in reproductive-aged patients that is of abnormal volume, duration, regularity, or frequency.

The PALM-COEIN system was developed in 2011 by the International Federation of Gynecology and Obstetrics (FIGO) and adopted by the American College of Obstetricians and Gynecologists (ACOG) in order to standardize the terminology used to describe AUB. This system provides terminology to describe uterine bleeding by bleeding pattern and etiology. The term "AUB" is paired with descriptive terms heavy menstrual bleeding (HMB) instead of menorrhagia, and intermenstrual bleeding (IMB) instead of metrorrhagia. AUB is further classified by one of the following letters that describes the etiology:

PALM: Refers to *structural* causes of AUB.
P—Polyp (AUB-P)
A—Adenomyosis (AUB-A)
L—Leiomyoma (AUB-L)
M—Malignancy and hyperplasia (AUB-M)

COEIN: Refers to *nonstructural* causes of AUB.
C—Coagulopathy (AUB-C)
O—Ovulatory dysfunction (AUB-O)
E—Endometrial (AUB-E)
I—Iatrogenic (AUB-I)
N—Not yet classified (AUB-N)

Abnormal Uterine Bleeding (AUB): Reproductive Age

A 24-year-old G0P0 patient presents with irregular menses occurring every 3–4 months. Her periods are heavy and last 7–9 days. She reports severe acne since puberty, and she was recently diagnosed with type 2 diabetes. Her body mass index (BMI) is 40, and her exam is otherwise normal. What initial lab tests should be ordered in the evaluation of this patient?

Answer: β-human chorionic gonadotropin (β-hCG), follicle-stimulating hormone (FSH), thyroid-stimulating hormone (TSH), prolactin (PRL). These tests cover the top differential diagnosis of pregnancy, primary ovarian insufficiency (POI), thyroid dysfunction, and hyperprolactinemia as the cause of AUB.

A normal menstrual cycle occurs every 21–35 days (28 ± 7 days) with menstruation for 2–7 days. The normal blood loss is <80 mL total, which represents eight or fewer soaked pads per day with usually no more than 2 heavy days. AUB is any disturbance of the above.

Most cases of reproductive-age bleeding are related to pregnancy, structural uterine pathology, anovulation, coagulopathy, or neoplasia. Less common causes include trauma and infection.

ETIOLOGY

- Organic:
  - Reproductive tract disease.
  - Pregnancy complications: Threatened, incomplete, missed abortion; ectopic pregnancy; trophoblastic disease.

- Malignancy: Most commonly endometrial and cervical cancers. Estrogen-producing ovarian tumors (i.e., granulosa-theca cell tumors) may present with excessive uterine bleeding.
- Infection: Endometritis presents with episodic intermenstrual bleeding. Cervicitis, sexually transmitted infections (STIs), and severe vaginal infections can present with bleeding.
- Structural causes (fibroids, polyps, adenomyosis).
- Foreign bodies: Tampons retained in the vagina or intrauterine devices for contraception can cause bleeding.
- Traumatic vaginal lesions.
- **Systemic:**
  - von Willebrand disease.
  - Prothrombin deficiency.
  - Leukemia.
  - Sepsis.
  - Idiopathic thrombocytopenic purpura.
  - Hypersplenism.
  - Thyroid dysfunction: Both hypothyroidism (more common) and hyperthyroidism may be associated with AUB.
  - Cirrhosis: Excessive bleeding secondary to the reduced capacity of the liver to metabolize estrogens.
- **Iatrogenic:**
  - Anticoagulation medications.
  - Oral or injectable steroids used for contraception.
  - Menopausal hormone therapy (MHT).
  - Psychotropic drugs: Interfere with neurotransmitters responsible for inhibition and release of hypothalamic hormones, leading to anovulation and AUB.
  - **Ovulatory:** Occurs during reproductive years due to abnormal endometrial hemostasis (due to many causes). Usually presents as heavy and/or intermenstrual bleeding.
  - **Anovulatory:** There is continuous estradiol production without corpus luteum formation or progesterone production. This steady state of estrogen stimulation results in constant endometrial proliferation without progesterone-mediated maturation and shedding. Fragments of overgrown endometrium shed sporadically. Anovulation can be seen in:
    - Polycystic ovarian syndrome (PCOS).
    - Obesity.
    - Adolescents (peri-menarchal).
    - Perimenopause.

HISTORY

Assess menstrual history, bleeding pattern, pertinent history with the following questions:
- Last menstrual period (LMP) and any bleeding pattern changes over last several periods?
- Bleeding history: Frequency, interval, duration?
- Intermenstrual bleeding or postcoital bleeding?
- AUB since menarche or new?
- How many days of heavy bleeding versus light bleeding/spotting?
- Assess heaviness of bleeding: How often change pad/tampon, how many pads/tampons used per day, need to change protection at night, passage of clots/size of clots, bleeding onto clothes or bedding? (This is very subjective, but provides an indication of the inconvenience the bleeding causes.)
- Associated symptoms such as pelvic pain, dysmenorrhea, or dyspareunia?
- Family history of bleeding?

The classic patient who presents with AUB due to adenomyosis is in her 40s, parous, with a "globular" (diffusely enlarged), "boggy" (soft) uterus on examination.

Ovarian tumors (benign and malignant) may present with AUB—most commonly granulosa cell tumors.

Anovulation → ↑ estradiol → endometrial proliferation → disorganized shedding

Signs of PCOS
- Oligomenorrhea
- Hyperandrogenism (i.e., hirsutism, acne)
- Obesity
- Cystic ovaries on ultrasound (US)

- History of epistaxis, gum bleeding, postpartum bleeding, surgical bleeding?
- Precipitating factors such as intercourse, trauma, procedure?

PHYSICAL EXAM

- Bimanual may reveal bulky uterus/discrete fibroids.
- Obesity, hirsutism/acne (PCOS), acanthosis nigricans (insulin resistance).
- Exophthalmos, goiter/thyroid nodule, delayed DTRs, dry skin/hair (thyroid disorder).
- Visual field deficits, galactorrhea (hyperprolactinemia).
- Petechiae/ecchymoses (coagulopathy).

DIAGNOSTIC TESTS

- Pap test
- Pregnancy test
- CBC
- TSH
- *Chlamydia trachomatis*
- FSH
- Prolactin
- Coagulation panel (targeted screening for bleeding disorders): von Willebrand factor for adolescents
- Endometrial biopsy (EMB) for women ≥45 years of age as a first line test, or in women <45 years of age with history of unopposed estrogen exposure (i.e., morbid obesity, PCOS), failed medical management, persistent AUB
- Pelvic US
- Sonohysterogram (pelvic US combined with intrauterine saline infusion to outline the uterine cavity)
- Hysteroscopy

TREATMENT

A 28-year-old G2P2002 patient presents to the Emergency Department reporting a 1-week history of heavy vaginal bleeding that has worsened over the past 24 hours. She also reports shortness of breath and dizziness. On physical exam, she appears pale and diaphoretic; vitals show HR 110, BP 85/60. Speculum exam demonstrates active bright-red bleeding and a normal-appearing cervix. What is the best next step in the management of this patient?

Answer: Dilation and curettage (D&C) is the treatment of choice for a patient with heavy bleeding and hemodynamic instability because its effect is immediate.

- Address organic, systemic, iatrogenic causes as indicated.
- Medical management: First-line treatment. Used for patients who desire future fertility or those who will reach menopause within a short period of time.
    - Nonsteroidal anti-inflammatory drugs (NSAIDs).
    - Tranexamic acid (anti-fibrinolytic agent used only during days of heavy bleeding).
    - Hormones: Estrogen/progesterone (E/P) oral contraceptive pill (OCP) is often first-line management of AUB, but other combination E/P methods such as the transdermal contraceptive patch or the vaginal contraceptive ring may also be used. Levonorgestrel intrauterine device (IUD) is also FDA approved for the treatment of AUB. Progesterone-only methods such as oral progesterone or depot medroxyprogesterone acetate (DMPA) may be used, especially if there is a contraindication to estrogen. OCPs or estrogens are used in the management of acute bleeding.

- D&C: Indicated mainly for patients with heavy bleeding leading to hemo-dynamic instability. Once the acute episode of bleeding is controlled, the patient can be started on medical management.
- Uterine artery embolization: A minimally invasive option for patients with uterine fibroids; reserved for patients who have completed childbearing.
- Endometrial ablation: A minimally invasive alternative to hysterectomy when medical management fails, or when there are contraindications to their use. It should **not** be used in patients who wish to become pregnant, and contraception is still required after this procedure.
- Myomectomy: Can be hysteroscopic for submuscosal fibroids, abdominal/laparoscopic/robotic approach for large intramural fibroids, reserved mostly for patients with uterine fibroids who desire fertility.
- Hysterectomy: Definitive treatment for patients with AUB in whom medical and/or minimally invasive options have failed or are contraindicated and who are have completed child-bearing

Postmenopausal Bleeding (PMB)

> A 55-year-old G3P3003 patient with LMP 5 years ago presents with vaginal spotting. She also reports painful intercourse but the spotting is not related to sexual activity. She has no medical problems, and does not take any medications. Pelvic exam reveals pale, dry vaginal mucosa with ↓ rugae and no blood in the vagina. What is the most likely diagnosis?
>
> **Answer:** Bleeding due to endometrial atrophy is the most common cause of postmenopausal bleeding (PMB).

PMB is defined as bleeding that occurs after 12 months of menopausal amen-orrhea. All vaginal bleeding in postmenopausal patients must be evaluated. PMB can be due to benign or malignant causes.

Etiology

- Endometrial or vulvovaginal atrophy (most common): Hypoestrogenism causes atrophy (thinning of the tissue) of the endometrium and vagina. In the uterus, the collapsed, atrophic endometrial surfaces contain little or no fluid to prevent intracavitary friction, resulting in microerosions of the surface epithelium which present as light bleeding or spotting. The terms "vaginal atrophy" and "atrophic vaginitis" are being replaced by the more comprehensive term "genitourinary syndrome of menopause" (GSM). It may present with bleeding from the walls of the vagina after intercourse due to trauma/friction.
- MHT: Many postmenopausal patients who take MHT develop vaginal bleeding.
- Endometrial hyperplasia: Postmenopausal patients should have low levels of estrogens and thus should not have stimulation of the endometrium resulting in bleeding.
    - Possible sources of estrogen include endogenous estrogen production from ovarian or adrenal tumors or exogenous estrogen therapy.
    - Obesity may also lead to high levels of endogenous estrogen due to the peripheral conversion in adipose tissue of androstenedione to estrone and the aromatization of androgens to estradiol.
- Medications: A good medication history is key!
    - Anticoagulants: Iatrogenic effect.
    - Tamoxifen: Predisposes patients to endometrial polyps, hyperplasia, and malignancy.

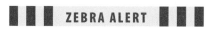

ZEBRA ALERT

Uterine fibroids and adenomyosis are conditions that **should not** cause PMB, unless the patient is using MHT. Leiomyosarcoma should be considered in postmenopausal patients with rapidly enlarging fibroids and bleeding, although the incidence of this is quite small.

- - - - - - - - - - - - - -

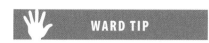

WARD TIP

MHT for menopausal patients with a uterus must contain progestin with estrogen to prevent endometrial hyperplasia/carcinoma.

WARD TIP

PMB = Endometrial cancer until proven otherwise by tissue biopsy, as 5–20% of women who present with PMB will have endometrial cancer.

WARD TIP

A thorough history is required to exclude genitourinary or gastrointestinal causes of bleeding. Some patients who present with PMB actually have a source in another organ system.

WARD TIP

Differential diagnosis for thickened endometrial stripe in a postmenopausal woman:
- Endometrial cancer
- Endometrial hyperplasia
- Leiomyoma
- Polyp

WARD TIP

Endometrial stripe >4–5 mm in a patient with PMB should prompt an evaluation for malignancy.

- Supplements: Soy and other phytoestrogens taken in large doses may cause endometrial stimulation.
- Endometrial polyps: Endometrial growths that may be stimulated by estrogen or tamoxifen. Usually benign, but may be premalignant or malignant.
- Infection: Endometritis or STIs.
- Cancer:
  - Endometrial cancer. Risk increases with increasing age.
  - Cervical cancer. Vaginal bleeding occurs because the cancer outgrows its blood supply. The necrotic and denuded tissue bleeds easily and may cause a malodorous discharge.
  - Estrogen-secreting ovarian tumor.
  - Leiomyosarcoma (**uterine sarcoma**) should be considered in postmenopausal women with rapidly growing fibroids and bleeding.

History

- Onset, frequency, duration, and amount of bleeding
- Associated signs/symptoms, i.e., weight loss, changes in bowel/bladder function, fever
- History of trauma or bleeding in relation to sexual activity or use of a pessary
- Medication—hormones, anticoagulants, tamoxifen, over the counter herbal supplements
- Past medical and surgical history
- Family history of bleeding, colon cancer, gynecologic cancer, breast cancer

Physical Exam

- The goal is to determine the source of bleeding.
- Note any suspicious lesions/ulcerations, lacerations, discharge, or foreign bodies.
- Classic signs of atrophy include pale, dry vaginal epithelium that has lost its rugae.
- Assess the size, contour, mobility, and tenderness of the uterus and assess for adnexal masses.

Studies

- Endometrial biopsy to evaluate for endometrial hyperplasia or cancer (most common initial diagnostic test).
- Testing for STIs and wet mount microscopy.
- Pap test for cervical cancer screening (biopsy any visible cervical lesions).
- Transvaginal ultrasound (TVUS) to assess endometrial stripe thickness. If endometrial stripe is <4 mm, endometrial sampling may be deferred unless the patient has persistent bleeding. Rationale is thin lining due to endometrial atrophy.
- Hysteroscopy with D&C may be both diagnostic and therapeutic.

Treatment

A 65-year-old G1P1001 patient presents with postmenopausal vaginal bleeding. Her final menstrual period (FMP) was 15 years ago. She reports 3 days of dark-red spotting that has now resolved. An office endometrial biopsy demonstrates endometrial hyperplasia with atypia. What is the next best step in management?

Answer: The next step is hysteroscopy with D&C. Approximately 30% of women with this diagnosis on biopsy will have a concurrent endometrial cancer. Once cancer is diagnosed or excluded, the patient should undergo hysterectomy with possible surgical staging.

Treatment of PMB is dependent on the cause:

- Topical vaginal estrogen (cream, ring, tablet) is used to treat GSM.
- Hysteroscopy with D&C +/− polypectomy can be offered if the TVUS suggests an intracavitary lesion or polyp, if the endometrial stripe is very thickened and/or cystic and requires further evaluation, if the patient is at increased risk of endometrial cancer, if the patient has an insufficient or nondiagnostic office endometrial biopsy, or if the patient has persistent unexplained PMB with a benign office endometrial biopsy.
- Endometrial hyperplasia without atypia can be managed with progestin (oral or levonorgestrel IUD) and ongoing monitoring.
- Endometrial hyperplasia with atypia should be treated as if there is underlying cancer. Approximately 30% will have underlying cancer. Hysteroscopy D&C can rule this out prior to performing hysterectomy as the treatment of choice.
- If endometrial carcinoma is diagnosed, consult gynecologic oncology to direct surgical evaluation and staging. Chemotherapy and/or radiation may also be required. Endometrial carcinoma associated with endometrial hyperplasia with atypia is usually low grade, and can be managed with hysterectomy alone.

NOTES

Pelvic Pain

WARD TIP

Causes of CPP unrelated to the female reproductive system include irritable bowel syndrome (IBS), interstitial cystitis (IC), pelvic floor muscle tenderness, and depression.

     ZEBRA ALERT

Mittelschmerz is pelvic pain associated with ovulation. It occurs at the time an egg is released from the ovary.

WARD TIP

CPP etiologies—Think of "**LEAP²ING**" pain
Leiomyoma
Endometriosis/Endometritis
Adhesions/Adenomyosis
Psychological/Psychiatric (i.e., abuse history, depression)
Pelvic floor myalgia, myofascial pain
Infections [i.e., urinary tract infection (UTI), sexually transmitted infections (STIs), pelvic inflammatory disease (PID)]
Neoplasia
Gastrointestinal (GI) tract [i.e., inflammatory bowel disease (IBD), diverticulosis, or irritable bowel syndrome (IBS)]

Chronic Pelvic Pain (CPP)

A 35-year-old G2P2 patient, with a history of uterine fibroids, presents with a 1-year history of pelvic pain lasting 20 minutes, 3–4 times a week. The pain is not relieved by acetominophen. Pelvic exam reveals a 16-week size uterus with tenderness directly over the fundus. Her cervix and adnexa are nontender. Her pregnancy test is negative. What is the most likely diagnosis? What diagnostic test should be ordered? What is the next best step in management?

Answer: The most likely diagnosis is a fibroid uterus with degeneration. It can be diagnosed with a pelvic ultrasound. Medical therapy is instituted first, typically with nonsteroidal anti-inflammatory drugs (NSAIDs). If the pain persists despite conservative therapy, a surgical intervention may be considered.

CPP is usually defined as noncyclic pain that may be constant or episodic, is located in the pelvis, has been present for at least 6 months, and is not related to pregnancy. It is a symptom that may be attributed to an identifiable pathophysiological process (i.e., endometriosis) or to various functional somatic pain syndromes without any identifiable cause. CPP often has a multifactorial etiology. There is increasing recognition among experts, including the American College of Obstetricians and Gynecologists (ACOG), that CPP is often associated with negative cognitive, behavioral, sexual, and emotional consequences, and patients with CPP are more likely to be stigmatized by society and the health care system. In addition, recent evidence supports the role of "central sensitization" in CPP, whereby peripheral pain provokes an exaggerated response by the interneurons, which amplifies pain perception, and ultimately increases psychologic distress.

Workup

- **Detailed history** (focusing on above etiologies): It can be very helpful to use a standardized questionnaire (such as the International Pelvic Pain Society's Pelvic Pain Assessment Form) to elicit and document history, symptoms, prior evaluations and treatments, and physical exam findings.
  - Temporal pattern: Timing and duration of symptoms.
  - Pain characteristics: Pain may be constant, intermittent, or cyclic (occurs with monthly menses).
  - Associated symptoms/relieving factors: Pain may be associated with positional changes, fever, or nausea/vomiting.
  - Prior surgeries: Adhesions (fibrous tissue that forms between two internal organs) may form after surgery and may be a source of pain.
  - Last menstrual period (LMP) and menstrual history.
  - GI symptoms such as nausea, vomiting, diarrhea, dyschezia, or constipation associated with the pain.
  - Sexual history: Presence of dyspareunia (deep versus insertional), history of PID (may also cause pelvic adhesions).
  - Social history (marital discord, depression, stress, history of physical or sexual abuse): Pelvic pain may be associated with psychiatric factors and childhood sexual abuse.
- **Physical exam:**
  - Abdominal exam: Evaluate for mass, hernia, scars.
  - Bimanual exam: Evaluate uterine size, mobility, uterine or ovarian tenderness or masses, cervical motion tenderness.
  - Pelvic floor exam: Evaluate for both tone and tenderness of the pelvic floor muscles with a single digit exam.

- External genitalia: Evaluate for vulvar tenderness or lesions.
- Rectovaginal exam: Uterosacral nodularity or a fixed, tender, retro-verted uterus may suggest endometriosis.
- Bladder exam (palpate anterior vagina): Tenderness may suggest IC.
- Speculum exam: Evaluate for lesions, erythema, discharge.
- **Labs: Performed to exclude other causes of CPP**
    - Complete blood count (CBC): An elevated white blood cell count (WBC) may indicate an infection.
    - Pregnancy test.
    - Testing for gonorrhea and chlamydia.
    - Urinalysis (UA) and urine culture.
    - Fecal occult blood.
- **Imaging studies: Performed to identify structural causes of CPP**
    - Pelvic ultrasound: Best to evaluate for ovarian cysts/masses/endometrio-mas or uterine fibroids. May be suggestive of adenomyosis.
    - Computed tomography (CT)/magnetic resonance imaging (MRI)—best to evaluate for abdominopelvic masses or suspected malignancies. May also better define masses seen on ultrasound. MRI can help diag-nose adenomyosis or deep infiltrating endometriosis.
- **Referrals**
    - Gastroenterology referral for colonoscopy to evaluate for diverticulosis, IBS, or IBD.
    - Urology referral for cystoscopy to evaluate for IC.
    - Psychiatry referral to evaluate psychosomatic pain and depression.

Acute Pelvic Pain

A 22-year-old G0 patient presents with a 2-day history of severe, sharp right lower quadrant pain. Her LMP was 13 days ago, and she has no significant medical or surgical history. Her pain is not relieved with ibuprofen. Her vitals show T = 98.2, P = 100, BP 85/60. A pregnancy test is negative. Her hematocrit dropped from 38 to 30%. On exam, her abdomen is soft and tender with rebound and guarding. An ultrasound reveals a normal left ovary and a 4-cm right ovary, with a moderate amount of fluid in the cul-de-sac (pouch of Douglas). What is the most likely diagnosis? What is the best next step in management?

Answer: The most likely diagnosis is a ruptured corpus luteal cyst. She recently ovulated, since her period was 2 weeks ago. She has vitals and an exam consistent with an acute abdomen. Given her drop in hematocrit, the fluid in the cul-de-sac is likely blood from the ruptured cyst. She needs surgical treatment with a diagnostic laparoscopy to diagnose and treat.

Acute pelvic pain is any lower abdominal or pelvic pain that has been present <3 months. Acute pelvic pain differs from CPP in that it usually arises from an inflammatory, infectious, or anoxic event or traumatic injury that resolves over time with treatment and/or repair.

ETIOLOGIES

- Gynecologic: May require surgery if pain is severe:
    - Ruptured ovarian cyst
    - Adnexal torsion
    - Tubo-ovarian abscess, PID
    - Endometriosis
    - Uterine fibroid (degenerating or not)

WARD TIP

The pain history can be characterized by using the mnemonic "PQRST": (provoking/palliating, quality, radiation, associated symptoms/setting, and timing).

WARD TIP

Laparoscopy is the final, conclusive step in diagnosing and/or treating CPP, and shared decision making between the patient and physician should be used to determine the best time to proceed with surgery.

WARD TIP

Differential for acute pelvic pain—
A ROPE
Appendicitis/**A**bscess/**A**bortion
Ruptured ovarian cyst
Ovarian torsion
PID (or tubo-ovarian abscess)
Ectopic pregnancy

WARD TIP

An elevated WBC may be due to infection (PID or appendicitis), inflammation/necrosis related to adnexal torsion, or a degenerating leiomyoma.

- Obstetric:
  - Ectopic pregnancy
  - Abortion
- GI/genitourinary (GU):
  - Diverticulitis
  - Appendicitis
  - IBD or IBS.
  - UTI or pyelonephritis
  - Nephrolithiasis

WORKUP

- The initial goal in the work up is to exclude life-threatening conditions.
- **History:** Include temporal characteristics (cyclic, intermittent, or noncyclic), timing of onset, location, and severity of pain.
- **Physical exam:** Evaluate for localized/point tenderness, cervical motion tenderness, adnexal tenderness, pelvic or adnexal masses, abdominal tenderness, guarding or rebound tenderness.
- **Labs:**
  - Pregnancy test.
  - CBC.
  - UA and culture.
  - Tests for chlamydia and gonorrhea.
- Pelvic ultrasound: Look for ovarian cysts/neoplasm, ovarian torsion (check Dopplers), an intrauterine/ectopic pregnancy, uterine fibroids, or a tubo-ovarian abscess.

TREATMENT

- Depends on the etiology of the pain.
- Start with conservative management, i.e., NSAIDs or other pain management.
- Surgical therapy: Consider if signs of an acute abdomen, if the diagnosis is unclear, or if the differential diagnosis includes potentially life-threatening or organ-threatening conditions, such as appendicitis, or ovarian torsion.
- Surgery: May consist of a diagnostic laparoscopy (if hemodynamically stable) or an exploratory laparotomy (if hemodynamically unstable).

CHAPTER 22

Endometriosis and Adenomyosis

Endometriosis

👤 A 32-year-old G0P0 patient presents with a 3-year history of infertility. She experienced menarche at age 13, and has regular menses every 28 days. She reports severe pain 2–3 days before her period, pain during her period, and pain with intercourse. She reports no history of sexually transmitted infections (STIs). Her husband has one child from a previous marriage. On exam, she has uterosacral nodularity and a fixed, retroflexed uterus. How should the suspected diagnosis be confirmed? What findings would be present on a tissue biopsy?

Answer: The patient has classic symptoms of endometriosis: dysmenorrhea and dyspareunia. Endometriosis is often associated with infertility. Although history and exam may suggest endometriosis, diagnostic laparoscopy is required to make a definitive diagnosis. The tissue biopsy would show endometrial glands, stroma, and hemosiderin-laden macrophages. The most common sites of involvement are the ovaries and pouch of Douglas.

EXAM TIP

Endometriosis is the most likely cause of infertility in a menstruating woman over the age of 30, without a history of pelvic inflammatory disease.

ZEBRA ALERT

A 37-year-old patient reports hemoptysis during her period.
Think: Endometriosis of the nasopharynx or lung.

Definition

Endometrial glands and stroma growing outside of the uterus, often causing pain and/or infertility. Symptoms can range from minimal/none to severely debilitating and do not correlate with the extent of disease. Lesions may be categorized as superficial peritoneal, ovarian, or deeply infiltrating.

Incidence

- 10–15% of reproductive-aged women.
- Occurs primarily in women in their 20s and 30s.
- Accounts for 20% of chronic pelvic pain.
- One-third to one-half of women with infertility has endometriosis.

Pathophysiology

- The ectopic endometrial tissue is physiologically functional and responds to ovarian hormones (especially estrogen).
- The result of this ectopic tissue is "ectopic menses," which cause bleeding, peritoneal inflammation, fibrosis, and adhesions.

Sites of Endometriosis

Common
- Ovary (bilateral): 60%
- Peritoneum over uterus
- Anterior and posterior cul-de-sacs
- Broad ligaments/fallopian tubes/round ligaments
- Uterosacral ligaments
- Bowel
- Appendix

Less Common
- Rectosigmoid: 10–15%
- Diaphragm
- Cervix
- Vagina
- Bladder

Rare
- Nasopharynx
- Lungs/pleural cavity

- Central nervous system (CNS)
- Abdominal wall
- Abdominal surgical scars or episiotomy scar

THEORIES OF ETIOLOGY

The pathogenesis of endometriosis is likely multifactorial. There are five theories commonly cited. It is likely that multiple theories may explain the diverse nature of this disorder:

- **Retrograde menstruation:** Endometrial tissue is transported in a retrograde fashion through the fallopian tubes, and implants in the pelvis with a predilection for the ovaries and pelvic peritoneum. It is estimated that up to 90% of women experience retrograde menstruation, yet not all of them develop endometriosis, suggesting that additional factors contribute.
- **Coelomic (peritoneal) metaplasia:** Under certain conditions, peritoneal tissue develops into functional endometrial tissue, thus responding to hormones.
- **Vascular/lymphatic transport:** Endometrial tissue is transported via blood vessels and lymphatics. This can explain endometriosis in locations outside of the pelvis (i.e., lymph nodes, pleural cavity, kidneys).
- **Altered immunity:** There may be deficient or inadequate natural killer (NK) or cell-mediated response. This can explain why some women develop endometriosis, whereas others with similar characteristics do not.
- **Iatrogenic dissemination:** Endometrial glands and stroma can be implanted during a procedure (i.e., cesarean delivery), and result in endometriosis in surgical scars.

GENETIC PREDISPOSITION

- A patient with a first-degree relative with endometriosis has a 7% chance of being similarly affected, as compared with 1% in unrelated persons.
- Patients with a positive family history may develop endometriosis at an earlier age.

CLINICAL PRESENTATION

- Pelvic pain (may be dysmenorrhea or chronic pelvic pain):
  - Secondary dysmenorrhea (pain usually begins 2–3 days before menses, lasts throughout menses, and may persist several days after menses).
  - Dyspareunia (typically with deep penetration rather than insertion) results due to endometriotic implants in the pouch of Douglas and rectovaginal septum.
  - Dyschezia (pain with defecation): Also due to deep implants in the pouch of Douglas and rectovaginal septum.
- Infertility.
- Ovarian mass.
- Cyclic bowel or bladder symptoms (i.e., hematuria).
- Up to one-third of women may be asymptomatic.

SIGNS

- Fixed, tender, retroflexed uterus, with scarring posterior to uterus.
- "Nodular" uterosacral ligaments or thickening and induration of uterosacral ligaments.
- Ovarian endometriomas: Tender, palpable, and freely mobile adnexal masses that arise from implanted endometrial tissue within the ovary. This creates a small blood-filled cavity in the ovary, classically known as a "chocolate cyst."
- Blue/brown vaginal implants (rare).

WARD TIP

Severity of symptoms does not necessarily correlate with quantity of ectopic endometrial tissue, but may correlate with the depth of penetration of the ectopic tissue.

WARD TIP

Long-term complications of endometriosis:

- Prolonged bleeding of ectopic tissue causes scarring (adhesions).
- Adhesions may contribute to infertility, small bowel obstruction, pelvic pain, and difficult surgeries.

ZEBRA ALERT

Congenital anomalies that promote retrograde menstruation may be found in adolescents with endometriosis.

WARD TIP

Chronic pelvic pain may result from endometriosis with associated adhesive disease.

EXAM TIP

Classic symptoms of endometriosis: Dysmenorrhea, dyspareunia, and dyschezia.

DIAGNOSIS

- **Laparoscopy or laparotomy:** The gold standard for definitive diagnosis is laparoscopy with biopsy, but visual inspection is considered satisfactory for diagnosis. If surgery is planned for diagnostic purposes, consent should be obtained to treat the endometriosis at the same time with ablation or excision.
- **Clinical diagnosis:** A presumptive diagnosis based on symptoms, exam findings, and imaging can be sufficient to initiate therapy.
- The colors of endometrial implants vary widely:
    - Red or red-blue implants.
    - Yellow-brown implants.
    - White or opaque implants.
    - Translucent "blebs."
    - Blue/brown implants—"powder burn lesions."
    - Peritoneal surfaces may also be scarred, puckered, or have defects.
    - The cardinal features of a tissue biopsy include endometrial glands, stroma, and hemosiderin-laden macrophages.

CLINICAL COURSE

- Thirty-five percent are asymptomatic (i.e., diagnosis is made incidentally at the time of surgery for another indication).
- Symptomatic patients may have increasing pelvic pain and possible bowel and bladder pain.
- There is often improvement during pregnancy secondary to temporary cessation of menses and decidualization of lesions due to the changing hormonal environment.
- Can be associated with infertility, which may be due to anatomic distortion from adhesions, and/or production of cytokines and other substances that inhibit normal ovarian function, fertilization, and implantation.

TREATMENT

Medical

The primary goal is to induce amenorrhea and cause regression of the endometriotic implants. Many of these options suppress estrogen. Medical treatment does not improve fertility.

- First-line treatments are nonsteroidal anti-inflammatory drugs (NSAIDs) and oral contraceptive pills (OCPs), as these treatments are inexpensive and well tolerated.
    - Combined estrogen-progestin OCPs: May use cyclic or continuous regimen.
    - NSAIDs: Treats dysmenorrhea.
    - Gonadotropin-releasing hormone (GnRH) agonists (i.e., leuprolide): Suppresses follicle-stimulating hormone (FSH) and induces a pseudomenopause. (May provide add-back progestin therapy to reduce hypoestrogenic side effects.)
    - Progestins: Depot medroxyprogesterone acetate, oral progestins, etonogestrel implant, levonorgestrel intrauterine device (IUD).
    - Danazol: An androgen derivative that suppresses FSH/LH (luteinizing hormone), causing pseudomenopause. Not often used due to androgenic side effects.
    - Aromatase inhibitors (i.e., letrozole): Used off-label, best for severe, refractory pain, often used in combination with progestin.

Surgical

- Conservative (retain reproductive potential): Laparoscopic lysis, ablation, and/or excision of adhesions and endometriotic implants.
- Definitive: Hysterectomy +/− bilateral salpingo-oophorectomy. Reserved for refractory cases when childbearing is complete.

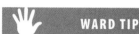

WARD TIP

Acupuncture has been shown to reduce endometriosis-related dysmenorrhea.

EXAM TIP

The pulsatile release of endogenous GnRH stimulates FSH secretion. GnRH agonists cause down regulation of pituitary receptors and suppress FSH secretion. This creates a pseudomenopause state.

WARD TIP

The only way to definitively diagnose adenomyosis is with microscopic examination of the uterus after hysterectomy.

Adenomyosis

 A 39-year-old G4P4 patient presents with worsening heavy menstrual bleeding (HMB) and dysmenorrhea. On physical exam, the uterus is 14 weeks' size, globular, boggy, slightly tender, and mobile. What is the next best step in management?

Answer: There is no proven medical therapy for adenomyosis, and hysterectomy is the only guaranteed treatment. However, conservative management with hormonal therapy is a reasonable next step. NSAIDs and OCPs can improve dysmenorrhea and regulate the heavy menses.

DEFINITION

Ectopic endometrial glands and stroma are found *within the myometrium*, resulting in a symmetrically enlarged and globular uterus due to hypertrophy of the surrounding myometrium.

INCIDENCE

- Occurs in 30% of women.
- Usually presents in parous women in their 40s to 50s. Rare in nulliparous women.
- May coexists with other processes that cause heavy menses and dysmenorrhea, such as uterine fibroids, endometrial polyps, and endometriosis.

SIGNS AND SYMPTOMS

Common:
- Chronic pelvic pain
- Symmetrical uterine enlargement
- Dysmenorrhea (25%)
- HMB (60%)

DIAGNOSIS

Transvaginal ultrasound is the first-line study to evaluate an enlarged uterus, pelvic pain, and/or HMB. Magnetic resonance imaging (MRI) can be used to differentiate between adenomyosis and uterine fibroids and may be used to help with conservative surgical planning.

TREATMENT

- **Medical therapy is directed at managing symptoms.**
- GnRH agonist, NSAIDs, aromatase inhibitors, oral progestins, levonorgestrel IUD, and OCPs may be used to treat pain and bleeding.
- Hysterectomy: Definitive therapy if childbearing is complete. The diagnosis is usually confirmed after histologic examination of the hysterectomy specimen.
- Endometrial ablation and uterine artery embolization have both been shown to be helpful for some women who have completed childbearing.

Adenomyosis Versus Endometriosis

- **Adenomyosis:**
  - Typically found in older, multiparous women.
  - Tissue is not as responsive to hormonal stimulation.
  - Noncyclic pain.
- **Endometriosis:**
  - Typically found in young, nulliparous women.
  - Tissue is responsive to hormonal stimulation.
  - Cyclic pain.

WARD TIP

When an enlarged uterus is found on exam, ultrasound can help differentiate between adenomyosis and uterine fibroids.

WARD TIP

The diagnosis of adenomyosis is suggested by characteristic clinical findings (i.e., heavy menses, dysmenorrhea, enlarged uterus) after endometriosis and leiomyomas have been ruled out.

EXAM TIP

Adenomyosis is classically described as an enlarged, globular, "boggy" uterus on physical exam.

NOTES

Differential Diagnoses of Pelvic Masses

Pelvic masses may be cystic or solid, benign or malignant, and can occur at any age. They can originate from the cervix, uterus, or adnexa, or from other organ systems.

DIFFERENTIAL DIAGNOSES

- Physiologic/functional cyst (follicular, corpus luteal, or theca lutein)
- Pregnancy (ectopic pregnancy)
- Infection/inflammation [tubo-ovarian abscess (TOA), diverticular abscess, appendicitis]
- Benign: Fibroid, ovarian neoplasms (most common—cystic teratoma), endometriomas
- Malignant: Ovaries, fallopian tubes, colon, cervix, metastatic

Diagnostic Tests for Various Causes of Pelvic Masses

The primary diagnostic tests are physical exam, pelvic ultrasound (US), and a pregnancy test.
- **Pregnancy:** Pregnancy test
- **Functional/Physiologic ovarian cysts:** Physical exam + US to confirm
- **Leiomyoma:** Physical exam + US to confirm
- **Malignant ovarian neoplasm:** US, computed tomography (CT) scan to look for metastatic disease, cancer antigen-125 (CA-125), surgical exploration if malignancy suspected due to imaging studies, age, family history
- **Benign ovarian neoplasm:** Physical exam, US, CA-125
- **TOA:** Physical exam, US or CT, history of pelvic inflammatory disease (PID) with a palpable adnexal mass on exam (see Figure 23-1)

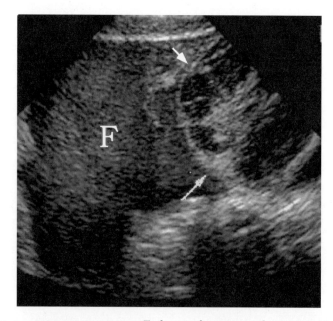

FIGURE 23-1. Tubo-ovarian abscess. Endovaginal sonogram of a patient with pelvic pain, vaginal discharge, and fever. The sonogram demonstrates echogenic fluid (F) in the cul-de-sac and a large cystic mass with internal echoes (arrows) in the left adnexa. This patient was known to have pelvic inflammatory disease and was successfully treated with antibiotics. (Reproduced, with permission, from Callen PW. *Ultrasonography in Obstetrics and Gynecology*. 5th ed. Philadelphia, PA: Saunders; 2007.)

Functional Ovarian Cysts

 A 24-year-old G0 patient with a LMP 1 week ago presents with sudden severe right-sided pelvic pain. She also reports dizziness and feeling "weak." A urine pregnancy test is negative. What is the best next step in management?

Answer: US. This patient presents with symptoms common for a ruptured ovarian cyst, which may require surgical intervention.

Functional ovarian cysts include follicular cysts and corpus luteum cysts.

FOLLICULAR CYSTS

Follicular cysts are the most common functional ovarian cysts.

PHYSIOLOGY

Failure of rupture or incomplete resorption of the ovarian follicle results in a cyst. Just like the original follicle, the ovarian cyst is lined with granulosa cells and contains a clear to yellow estrogen-rich fluid.

SIGNS AND SYMPTOMS

- Usually asymptomatic when small (<5 cm). The larger the size, the more pain they cause and the higher the risk of ovarian torsion.
- Abnormal uterine bleeding.
- Unilateral abdominal and pelvic pain.
- Acute pelvic pain with findings of rebound and guarding on exam often signify rupture of the ovarian cyst.

DIAGNOSIS

- Physical exam: Pelvic and abdominal exams.
- US confirms the diagnosis and is also helpful to see whether the cyst is ruptured. May show a simple (fluid-filled) ovarian cyst or fluid in the cul-de-sac, which is consistent with a ruptured cyst.

TREATMENT

- No treatment is necessary for most cysts, since they usually resolve spontaneously within 2 months. US may be repeated in 4–6 weeks to confirm resolution of the cyst.
- Oral contraceptive pills (OCPs) may help prevent formation of future cysts, especially in patients with recurrent cysts.
- If the cyst is unresolved after 2 months, it is more likely to be a neoplasm rather than follicular cyst, and laparoscopy with ovarian cystectomy or oophorectomy may be indicated to diagnose and treat the cyst.
- Laparoscopic cystectomy or oophorectomy can also be considered for symptomatic or asymptomatic cysts >5 cm, which are at an increased risk for ovarian torsion.

LUTEIN CYSTS

There are two types of lutein cysts: **corpus luteum cysts** and **theca lutein cysts**.

Corpus Luteum Cyst

- The corpus luteum fails to involute and continues to enlarge. It can produce progesterone for weeks longer than normal, and may delay menses.
- **Corpus hemorrhagicum** is formed when there is hemorrhage into a corpus luteum cyst.
- If this ruptures, the patient can present with acute lower-quadrant pain and vaginal bleeding, and may develop signs of shock and hemoperitoneum.
- These cysts rarely grow >5 cm.

SIGNS AND SYMPTOMS

- Unilateral adnexal tenderness and pain
- Abnormal uterine bleeding

DIAGNOSIS

History and pelvic exam, US

TREATMENT

- Observe for 2 months. Can start OCPs.
- If symptomatic: Nonsteroidal anti-inflammatory drugs (NSAIDs), OCPs, laparotomy/laparoscopy if exam shows an acute abdomen and torsion or rupture is suspected.

Theca Lutein Cyst

↑ levels of human chorionic gonadotropin (hCG) can cause **follicular overstimulation** and lead to theca lutein cysts, which are often multiple and bilateral.

Tubo-Ovarian Abscess (TOA)

An abscess involving the ovary and fallopian tube that most often arises as a consequence of PID.

PHYSIOLOGY

- Primary TOA may arise as a complication of an ascending infection of the reproductive tract.
- Secondary TOA may develop as a result of bowel perforation (appendicitis, diverticulitis) from intraperitoneal spread of infection.
- TOA can also develop in association with pelvic surgery or malignancy.

SIGNS AND SYMPTOMS

- Pelvic and/or abdominal pain
- Leukocytosis
- Fever
- Vaginal discharge
- Palpable mass

DIAGNOSIS

- Physical exam: Pelvic and abdominal.
- US or CT confirms the diagnosis and allows the opportunity to assess for other abscesses.

TREATMENT

- Antimicrobial therapy
- Laparoscopic or US-guided drainage if no response to antibiotics

Endometriomas

Endometriomas arise as a result of ectopic endometrial tissue in the ovary. They are commonly referred to as "chocolate cysts" due to the thick, brown, tarlike fluid that they contain (see Figure 23-2).

PHYSIOLOGY

Endometriomas arise in women who have endometriosis. Endometriosis is a condition in which endometrial glands and stroma occur outside the uterine cavity.

SIGNS AND SYMPTOMS

- Pelvic pain
- Dysmenorrhea
- Dyspareunia

DIAGNOSIS

- Clinical diagnosis can be made in women with a history of endometriosis, pelvic pain, and an ovarian cyst. As many as 50% of women with endometriosis will develop an endometrioma.
- Definitive diagnosis is made by laparoscopy and a biopsy containing hemosiderin-laden macrophages. However, it can be strongly suspected based on history, physical exam, and US.

TREATMENT

- **Only surgical; medical therapy is not effective treatment for an endometrioma**.
- Conservative surgery (ovarian cystectomy): Entire cyst (endometrioma) can be excised by laparoscopy of laparotomy. Aspiration has proven to be ineffective.
- Definitive surgery (oophorectomy): Alternative to cystectomy. Endometriomas are less likely to recur after oophorectomy, and it is a good option for women who have completed childbearing.

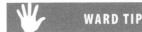

WARD TIP

An ovarian endometrioma = Chocolate cyst

Benign Cystic Teratomas

A 25-year-old G1P1 patient presents for an annual exam. She reports a 3-month history of left-sided intermittent dull pelvic pain. She is afebrile and a urine pregnancy test is negative. Pelvic exam demonstrates left adnexal enlargement and tenderness. The right adnexa is nontender without palpable masses. An US reveals a 5-cm, left hypoechoic unilocular cyst containing calcifications and internal debris. What is the most likely diagnosis? What is the best treatment for this patient?

Answer: Diagnosis: benign cystic teratoma. Treatment: laparoscopy with an ovarian cystectomy.

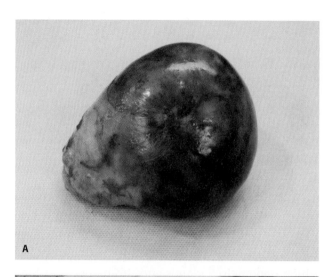

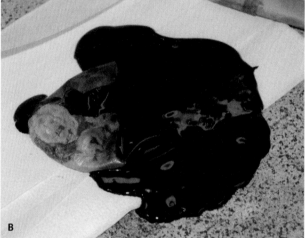

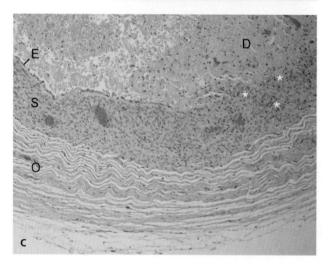

FIGURE 23-2. **Endometrioma.** A. Surgical specimen of an ovary containing an endometrioma. B. Dark, chocolate-like fluid had filled this cyst. (Photographs contributed by Dr. Roxanne Pero, with permission.) C. In ovarian endometriomas, endometrial-type epithelium (E) and subjacent stroma (S) line the cyst and are bordered peripherally by ovarian stroma (O). The golden brown pigment in the cyst wall (asterisk) is hemosiderin, indicating remote hemorrhage. Debris composed of necrotic and degenerating cells and remote hemorrhage occupies the interior of the cyst (D). It is the remote hemorrhage that confers the chocolate-like color to cyst fluid. (Reproduced, with permission, from Hoffman BL, Schorge JO, Halvorson LM, et al. *Williams Gynecology.* 4th ed. McGraw Hill; 2020.)

- Benign mature cystic teratomas (dermoid cysts) are the most common ovarian germ cell tumor.
- Germ cell tumors arise primarily in young women age 12–30 and account for 70% of tumors in this age group.

PHYSIOLOGY

- Teratomas contain tissue of ectodermal, mesodermal, and endodermal origin. The tissue is mature (benign) and may include skin, bone, teeth, and hair.
- The diverse tissue found within a teratoma is believed to develop from the genetic material in a single oocyte.
- Oocytes that are able to develop into teratomas undergo an arrest in development after meiosis I.
- Almost all mature cystic teratomas have a 46,XX karyotype.
- Malignant transformation develops in only 1–3% of cases.

DIAGNOSIS

US is the primary imaging tool used for diagnosis. Teratomas have a characteristic appearance, which usually includes cystic and solid components along with calcifications.

TREATMENT

- Excision of the teratoma by laparotomy or laparoscopy.
- An ovarian cystectomy is preferred in women who have not completed childbearing.
- If there is no viable ovarian tissue, if the patient is >40, or if the patient has completed childbearing, then an oophorectomy is preferred.
- Evaluate other ovary carefully—teratomas are bilateral in 15% of cases.

EXAM TIP

A young woman with a dermoid cyst can be treated with an ovarian cystectomy rather than an oophorectomy—the ovary can be preserved.

Malignancies

Malignant ovarian tumors are the leading cause of death from reproductive tract cancer. The lifetime risk of developing ovarian cancer is 1.6%. This risk is ↑ to 5% with one affected first-degree relative.

PATHOLOGY

Origins of the three main types of ovarian tumors:
- Epithelial: Repeated stimulation (i.e., ovulation) of the ovarian surface epithelium is hypothesized to result in malignant transformation. These tumors include serous, mucinous, endometrioid, clear cell, and transitional cell. Ninety-five percent of ovarian cancers are epithelial.
- Sex-cord stromal: These include granulosa cell, Sertoli cell, Sertoli-Leydig, and fibromas/fibrothecomas.
- Germ cell: These include teratoma, dysgerminoma, yolk sac, and embryonal choriocarcinoma.

RISK FACTORS

- Family history in first-degree relative
- Age (>50)
- Nulliparity
- History of breast cancer

SIGNS AND SYMPTOMS

- GI symptoms: Abdominal pressure, fullness, swelling, or bloating.
- Urinary urgency.

TABLE 23-1. Pelvic Sonographic Findings Suggestive of Malignancy

Solid component of mass, not hyperechoic, presence of nodularity
Multiloculated (fluid trapped in different compartments)
Thick septations (thick walls between compartments)
Presence of ascites
Peritoneal masses, **matted bowels, enlarged nodes**

- Pelvic discomfort or pain.
- Often ovarian neoplasms are **asymptomatic**.

DIAGNOSIS

- An elevated serum CA-125 (>35 units) indicates an ↑ likelihood that an ovarian tumor is malignant. Note that CA-125 is typically only elevated in epithelial ovarian cancers.
- Ultrasound is helpful in distinguishing between masses that are likely to be malignant and benign (see Table 23-1).
- Definitive diagnosis is tissue biopsy (which typically occurs at time of surgical resection or staging).

TREATMENT

- Complete surgical staging must be conducted for all women with ovarian cancer.
- In a woman with early-stage ovarian cancer, a hysterectomy with bilateral salpingo-oophorectomy, omentectomy, lymphadenectomy, appendectomy, and peritoneal washings should be performed.
- With more advanced disease, aggressive removal of all visible disease improves survival ("optimal cytoreduction" is residual disease <1 cm in diameter).
- Ovarian cancer is one of the few cancers in which "surgical debulking" even in the presence of distant metastasis is helpful.
- Postoperative chemotherapy with a platinum and a taxane agent is indicated for women with advanced epithelial ovarian cancer.

PROGNOSIS

- Seventy-five percent of women are diagnosed with advanced disease after regional or distant metastases have occurred.
  - Overall 5-year survival.
  - 17% with distant metastases.
  - 36% with local spread.
  - 89% with early disease.

Leiomyomas (Fibroids)

EXAM TIP

Ovarian cancers usually present with vague GI symptoms (fullness, early satiety, bloating) at a more advanced cancer stage.

WARD TIP

CA-125 is elevated in 80% of women with epithelial ovarian cancer overall but in only 50% of women with early disease.

WARD TIP

The most common fibroid symptom is heavy/prolonged menses.

 A 40-year-old G1P1 patient presents with heavy, painful menses. She also reports occasional bleeding in between her periods, along with pelvic pain and pressure. On exam, the uterus is 16 weeks in size and irregular. The adnexae are not palpable. What is the next step in management?

Answer: This patient likely has uterine fibroids. Imaging with US should be done next to confirm the diagnosis.

Leiomyomas are localized, benign, **smooth muscle tumors** of the uterus, which are hormonally responsive.

EPIDEMIOLOGY

- Clinically found in 25–33% of reproductive-age women and in up to 50% of Black women.
- They are almost always multiple.
- The most common indication for hysterectomy.

SEQUELAE

Changes in uterine fibroids over time include:
- Hyaline degeneration
- Calcification
- Red degeneration (painful interstitial hemorrhage, often with pregnancy)
- Cystic degeneration—may rupture into adjacent cavities

UTERINE LOCATIONS OF LEIOMYOMAS: BASED ON THE INTERNATIONAL FEDERATION OF GYNECOLOGY AND OBSTETRICS (FIGO) CLASSIFICATION SYSTEM

- **Submucous:** Just below endometrium, protruding into the uterine cavity; more likely to cause abnormal bleeding. The extent of protrusion into the uterine cavity is further classified by FIGO:
  - Type 0: Completely within the endometrial cavity.
  - Type 1: Extends <50% into myometrium.
  - Type 2: Extends ≥50% into the myometrium.
- **Intramural:** Within the uterine wall. May enlarge enough to distort the uterine cavity or serosal surface. *Transmural* fibroids extend from the serosal to the mucosal surface of the uterus.
- **Subserosal:** Just below the serosa. May have a broad or pedunculated stalk.
- **Cervical:** Located in the cervix rather than uterine corpus.
- **Other descriptors:**
  - **Parasitic:** The fibroid obtains blood supply from another organ (i.e., omentum).
  - **Interligamentous:** The fibroid grows laterally into the broad ligament (likely started out subserosal).

SYMPTOMS

- **Asymptomatic** in >50% of cases. Symptoms are related to the number, size, and location of the fibroids.
- **Bleeding +/−** anemia: One-third of cases present with heavy or prolonged menstrual bleeding.
- **Pain:** Secondary dysmenorrhea, dyspareunia.
- **Bulk symptoms:** Pelvic pressure, urinary symptoms (i.e., frequency, difficulty emptying bladder), or bowel symptoms (i.e., constipation, painful defecation).
- **Infertility:** May distort uterine cavity and lead to difficulty conceiving (i.e., tubal obstruction) or increased risk of miscarriage.

DIAGNOSIS

- **Physical exam** (bimanual pelvic and abdominal exams): Fibroids are usually midline, enlarged, irregularly shaped, and mobile.
- **Ultrasound:** May also be visualized by X-ray, magnetic resonance imaging (MRI), CT, hysterosalpingogram (HSG), hysteroscopy.
- Depending on patient characteristics, abnormal bleeding may be evaluated with Pap test, endocervical curettage (ECC), endometrial biopsy, hysteroscopy with dilation and curettage (D&C).

EXAM TIP

Leiomyomas are the most common pelvic tumor found in females.

ZEBRA ALERT

Rapidly enlarging fibroid = (Think) Leiomyosarcoma

WARD TIP

Submucosal and intramural types of fibroids usually present with heavy menses. Subserosal fibroids may become pedunculated and present with acute pain and torsion.

EXAM TIP

Pregnancy with fibroids carries ↑ risk of:
- Placental abruption
- Fetal growth restriction
- Dysfunctional labor
- Malpresentation
- Cesarean delivery
- Preterm labor and birth

WARD TIP

The most common location for a uterine fibroid = Subserosal

EXAM TIP

About one-third of fibroids recur following myomectomy.

WARD TIP

The treatment for *asymptomatic* fibroids is observation.

WARD TIP

Definitive treatment for fibroids = Hysterectomy

TREATMENT

- **No treatment** is indicated for asymptomatic women, as this hormonally sensitive tumor will likely shrink with menopause.
- Pregnancy is usually **uncomplicated**. Some fibroids may grow in size during pregnancy. Bed rest and analgesics are recommended for pain due to fibroid degeneration.
- Treatment is usually initiated when:
    - Bleeding is not able to be managed with medications.
    - Hematocrit falls.
    - Fibroids compress adjacent structures (i.e., bladder or bowel symptoms, hydronephrosis).
    - Symptoms interfere with quality of life.
- Medical management:
    - OCPs or progestins (implants, injections, pills) may be used to manage bleeding, but are inconsistently effective.
    - Levonorgestrel-containing IUD may be used to manage bleeding if the uterus is not significantly enlarged and if the uterine cavity is not distorted.
    - Gonadotropin-releasing hormone (GnRH) agonists can be given for up to 6 months to shrink tumors (i.e., before surgery) and control bleeding (i.e., allow improvement of anemia).
- Surgical management:
    - **Endometrial ablation:** Women who have completed childbearing and have small fibroids (<4 cm) may be candidates.
    - **Uterine artery embolization:** Minimally invasive option for women who want to preserve their uterus but not their fertility; contraindicated for pedunculated fibroids.
    - **Myomectomy:** Surgical removal of the fibroid by hysteroscopy, laparoscopy, or laparotomy. A myomectomy is reserved for women who desire to retain their uterus for childbearing.
    - **Hysterectomy:** Indicated for symptomatic women who have failed conservative management and completed childbearing.

Cervical Dysplasia

Cervical Dysplasia

Cervical dysplasia describes abnormal cells of the cervix that can be precursors to cancer. Papanicolaou (Pap) tests are performed as a method for screening cervical cancer and assessing cervical dysplasia. Further workup and treatments include colposcopy, cone biopsy, loop electrosurgical excision procedure (LEEP), cryotherapy, and laser therapy. Approximately 80% of cervical dysplasia is related to oncogenic or high risk strains of human papillomavirus (HPV or hrHPV) infection. A vaccine against hrHPV can be offered to individuals as a primary approach to prevent cervical dysplasia.

Cervical dysplasia and cervical cancer lie on a continuum of conditions. Cervical dysplasia can take one of three paths:
1. Progress to cancer
2. Remain the same and not progress
3. Regress to normal

WARD TIP

Vaccines against high-risk strains of HPV are currently FDA approved for females and males between the ages of 9 and 45 years.

Risk Factors for Cervical Dysplasia and Cervical Cancer

- HPV infection:
  - Eighty percent of cases
  - Risk highest if infected >6 months
  - Types 16, 18, 31, 33, 45, 52, 58—high oncogenic potential or hrHPV strains
- ↑ sexual activity (↑ risk of viral/bacterial infections):
  - Multiple sexual partners
  - Intercourse at early age (<18 years)
- Low socioeconomic status (likely due to limited access to health care and screening)
- Genetic predisposition
- Cigarette smoking (increases risk for squamous cell cancers but not adenocarcinomas)
- Oral contraceptive pills (OCPs), particularly with use >5 years (condoms ↓ risk in these women)
- Immunosuppression

EXAM TIP

HPV typical associations:
- Types 6 and 11: Associated with low-grade lesions and 90% of anogenital warts
- Types 16 and 18: Associated with >50% of high-grade lesions and 70% of cervical cancer

Human Papillomavirus (HPV)

- HPV is a double-stranded DNA virus that is sexually transmitted. Infection can occur through sexual contact—infected intact skin, mucous membranes, or bodily fluids from an infected partner.
- Abstinence, condoms, and decreasing the number of sexual partners can lower the risk of acquiring HPV.
- There is a high prevalence of HPV in sexually active women, but most infections are subclinical (asymptomatic).
- Most young women will clear the virus within 24 months.
- There are more than 200 genotypes of HPV.

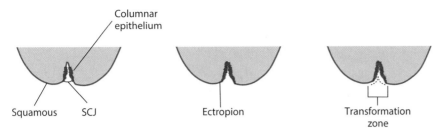

FIGURE 24-1. **Sites of cervical cancers.**

Squamocolumnar Junction (SCJ)

■ The terms "squamocolumnar junction" (SCJ) and "transformation zone" (TZ) and are often used interchangeably; however, they are two distinct entities.
■ The SCJ is located on the cervix and is the border where the squamous epithelium of the ectocervix meets the columnar epithelium of the endocervix.
■ The cervical TZ is the area of metaplasia that changes throughout a patient's life and is histologically the area where the glandular epithelium has been replaced by squamous epithelium (see Figure 24-1).
■ The SCJ is part of the TZ, but the TZ comprises a larger area than just the SCJ.
■ Most cervical cancers arise at the SCJ.
■ In nulliparous women, it is usually located at the external cervical os.
■ In pregnancy, it migrates out and is visible to the naked eye.

WARD TIP

The ectocervix is comprised of squamous epithelium, and the endocervix (including cervical canal) is comprised of glandular epithelium.

Pap Test

 A 21-year-old G2P2 patient desires contraception. She has been sexually active for 4 years, with three lifetime partners. Her menses are irregular. Before prescribing combined OCPs, what tests need to be performed?
Answer: A pregnancy test, Pap test, and STI screening.

A Pap test is a cytologic **screening test** for cervical dysplasia.

EXAM TIP

The methods available for cervical cancer screening are the Pap test (i.e., cytology), HPV testing, and co-testing with both cytology and HPV.

TECHNIQUE

■ A speculum is placed in the vagina to expose the uterine cervix.
■ Cells are circumferentially scraped from the ectocervix with a spatula and from the endocervix using an endocervical brush.
■ A conventional Pap test involves spreading the cells from the spatula and rolling the cytobrush on a glass slide, spraying with fixative, and sending to cytopathology for evaluation.
■ Liquid-based thin layer cytology has largely replaced the conventional Pap test technique. The spatula and cytobrush are placed into a liquid fixative solution and swirled vigorously to collect the cells. This specimen is processed by the cytology laboratory, where loose cells are trapped onto a filter and then plated in a monolayer on a glass slide to be evaluated.
■ If liquid-based cytology is used, the sample may also be tested for presence of gonorrhea, chlamydia, and/or HPV.

SUCCESS RATE

↓ incidence of invasive cervical cancer in the United States by 50% in the last 30 years due to widespread screening.

SCREENING GUIDELINES

According to the American College of Obstetricians and Gynecologists (ACOG) recommendations as of 2021 are:

■ Individuals aged 21–29 should be screened with cervical cytology (Pap test) alone every 3 years.
■ There are now three recommended options for cervical cancer screening in individuals aged 30–65 years:
  ■ Cytology alone every 3 years.
  ■ FDA-approved primary hrHPV testing alone every 5 years.
  ■ Co-testing with cytology and hrHPV testing every 5 years.
■ Frequency of Pap test screening should be individualized, and may need to occur earlier/more often in women who have HIV, are immune compromised, were exposed to diethylstilbestrol (DES) in utero, or have been previously treated for CIN2, CIN3, or cancer.
■ Women under age 21 should not be screened, because the incidence of cervical cancer is very low, and they have an effective immune response that will usually clear the HPV infection in 8–24 months.
■ Pap tests may be discontinued after age 65 in healthy women with adequate negative prior screening test (Pap test) results and no history of CIN2 or higher.
■ A Pap test may be discontinued after hysterectomy (with removal of the cervix) for benign disease.

CLASSIFICATION OF ABNORMALITIES

■ The Bethesda System is used to describe both cytologic (on Pap test) and histologic (on biopsy) findings.
  1. Cytologic (Pap test) abnormalities are described using the term "squamous intraepithelial lesion" (SIL) (see below).
     ■ Each cytology report consists of: (1) a description of specimen adequacy, (2) a general categorization (i.e., negative, epithelial cell abnormality), and (3) ancillary testing (i.e., HPV test).
     ■ Management of abnormal Pap tests in women ages 21–24 differs from those age ≥25 because of the low incidence of cervical cancer in this age group.
  2. Histologic (biopsy) abnormalities are described using the term "cervical intraepithelial neoplasia" (CIN). In 2012, the Lower Anogenital Squamous Terminology (LAST) project of the College of American Pathology (CAP) and the American Society for Colposcopy and Cervical Pathology (ASCCP) published changes in the terminology used to describe HPV-associated squamous lesions of the anogenital tract, whereby histologic cervical findings are described using the same terminology as cytologic findings.
     ■ CIN1 is a low-grade lesion with mild atypical changes in the lower one-third of the epithelium. It is referred to as low-grade SIL (LSIL) in the LAST system.
     ■ CIN2 is considered a high-grade lesion, with atypical changes confined to the lower two-thirds of the epithelium. The diagnosis of CIN2 has poor reproducibility and can be difficult to differentiate from CIN3. Thus, CIN2 is stratified according to p16 immunostaining to identify precancerous lesions. Specimens that are p16-negative are referred to as LSIL and those that are p16-positive are referred to as high-grade SIL (HSIL).

WARD TIP

Two things to remember about a Pap test:
1. It is a screening test.
2. It provides cytologic information, not histologic.

- CIN3 is a high-grade lesion, where atypical cells encompass >2/3 of the epithelium, and is referred to as HSIL in the LAST system. CIN2 and CIN3 are often treated the same.
- The recommendations for management of CIN differs for women ages 21–24 from those age ≥25 because the risk of cervical cancer is very low in this population.

PAP TEST RESULTS, WORKUP, AND FOLLOW-UP

- **Negative for intraepithelial lesion or malignancy:** Repeat Pap test per age-based protocol described above.
- **Atypical squamous cells of undetermined significance (ASCUS):**
  1. Reflex HPV testing if under age 30, concurrent HPV testing if age 30 and above.
  2. If HPV negative—continue routine screening per protocol.
  3. If HPV positive—colposcopy if age ≥25, repeat cytology (Pap test) in 1 year if age 21–24.
- **Atypical squamous cells, cannot exclude HSIL (ASC-H):** Colposcopy with indicated biopsies.
- **Atypical glandular cells (AGC):** Colposcopy with indicated biopsies, endocervical curettage (ECC), and endometrial biopsy.
- **LSIL:** Colposcopy with indicated biopsies if age ≥25, repeat cytology (Pap test) in 1 year if age 21–24.
- **HSIL:** Colposcopy with ECC and indicated biopsies.
- The algorithms are very complex and vary based on age and history. Protocols are available online at www.asccp.org. (This organization also has an handy app that keeps this information at your fingertips.)

Colposcopy with Cervical Biopsy

A 45-year-old G4P4 patient presents for a routine annual exam. Her Pap test returns with a report of ASCUS. Her Pap tests have always been normal in the past. What is the next best step to evaluate her cancer risk?

Answer: High-risk HPV DNA testing. If high-risk HPV DNA testing is "positive," indicating the presence of a hrHPV strain, then a colposcopy and indicated biopsies should be performed. If the HPV testing is negative, she can be managed as per her age-based protocol.

DEFINITION

- A procedure that utilizes staining and a low-magnification microscope, mounted on a stand, for the viewing of the cervix, vagina, and vulva.
- Provides illuminated, magnified view, which aids in identifying lesions and biopsying suspicious areas to *obtain histologic diagnosis.*

INDICATIONS FOR A COLPOSCOPY

- Performed to evaluate abnormal Pap tests, as per the guidelines described above
  - ASCUS with high-risk HPV subtypes (age ≥25)
  - ASC-H
  - AGC
  - LSIL (age ≥25)
  - HSIL

WARD TIP

An abnormal *screening* test (Pap test) needs a *diagnostic* test for confirmation (colposcopy with biopsies).

EXAM TIP

Pap test screening should not begin until age 21, regardless of sexual activity.

WARD TIP

Colposcopy and directed biopsies are needed to make a histologic diagnosis.

WARD TIP

On biopsy, 5–17% of cases of ASCUS and 24–94% of ASC-H demonstrate CIN2–CIN3 (HSIL).

PROCEDURE

1. Speculum is inserted to expose the cervix.
2. **Acetic acid is applied**. After 30 seconds, the acetic acid dehydrates cells and causes precipitation of nucleic proteins in the superficial layers. The neoplastic cells appear whiter because of a higher nucleus/cytoplasm ratio ("acetowhite epithelium").
3. **Colposcopy:** Next, a low-power microscope (colposcope) is used to look for dysplasia. Signs of dysplasia include acetowhite epithelium and abnormal vessels (punctations, mosaicism). The transformation zone must be visualized in its entirety. If the TZ or the entire extent of the lesion is not entirely visualized, then the colposcopy is considered inadequate.
4. **Cervical biopsy:** Neoplastic and dysplastic areas are then biopsied under colposcopic guidance. Contraindications include acute pelvic inflammatory disease (PID) and cervicitis. Pregnancy is **not** a contraindication.
5. **ECC:** A curette is used to scrape the cervical canal to obtain endocervical cells for cytologic examination. An ECC should **not** be performed during pregnancy.

INFORMATION PROVIDED BY COLPOSCOPY AND ECC

If biopsy results or ECC is positive for CIN2 or CIN3 (HSIL), then a cone biopsy or a LEEP should be performed as both a diagnostic and therapeutic procedure.

WARD TIP

Ninety percent of women with abnormal cytologic findings can be adequately evaluated with colposcopy.

WARD TIP

What must be completely visualized for adequate colposcopic evaluation?
1. TZ
2. Extent of lesion in its entirety

Cone Biopsy and Loop Electrosurgical Excision Procedure (LEEP)

These are both excisional procedures which involve excising a cone-shaped portion of the cervix, including the endocervical canal and TZ. They are intended to be both diagnostic and therapeutic.

- **Cold knife cone biopsy:** Performed in the operating room using a scalpel to excise a cone-shaped portion of the cervix. Requires use of anesthesia.
- **LEEP:** Usually performed in an office setting (may be performed in an operating room). A small wire loop with an electric current is used to excise the TZ and the endocervix. Local anesthesia/analgesia is required (i.e., paracervical block with 1% lidocaine with epinephrine).

INDICATIONS FOR CONE BIOPSY/LEEP

- Inadequate view of TZ on colposcopy
- Positive ECC
- Treatment for CIN2–CIN3 (HSIL)
- Treatment for adenocarcinoma in situ
- When cancer cannot be excluded after colposcopy, biopsy, and ECC

COMPLICATIONS AND SIDE EFFECTS OF CONE BIOPSY/LEEP

- Intraoperative bleeding (rare).
- Postoperative (delayed) bleeding.
- Infection (rare enough that routine use of perioperative antibiotics is not recommended).
- Reproductive effects:
  - Cervical stenosis: Risk <10% and related to amount of tissue removed. It may block menstrual flow, prevent passage of instruments through endocervical canal, possibly impede cervical dilation during labor.

- Increased risk of preterm birth, risk varies according to amount of tissue removed.
- Second trimester pregnancy loss: Twofold increased risk in pregnancy loss between 16 and 22 weeks, typically due to cervical insufficiency.
- Does not appear to impact pregnancy rates or first trimester loss risk.

WARD TIP

Evaluation of biopsy margins may be challenging with LEEP, because of thermal artifact.

ABLATIVE TECHNIQUES

Cryotherapy and laser ablation may be used in certain circumstances to ablate the cervical tissue. The depth of ablation for all techniques should be at least 4.8 mm.

INDICATIONS

Treatment of low-grade lesions only if it is a lesion completely visualized on colposcopic exam and invasive cancer has been excluded. Ablative techniques do not provide a pathologic specimen, so they are considered to be therapeutic but not diagnostic.

Cryotherapy ("Cryo")

- An outpatient procedure that uses a metal probe cooled with either carbon dioxide or nitrous oxide to ablate lesions.
- The tissue must be cooled to $-20°C$ to cause destruction of the lesion.

Laser Therapy

- Light amplification by stimulated emission of radiation (LASER): A high-energy photon beam generates heat at impact and vaporizes tissue. A CO_2 laser is most commonly used.
- Performed with colposcopic guidance. Causes less tissue destruction of the TZ compared to other methods.
- Expensive and requires special training and protective eyewear.

COMPLICATIONS AND SIDE EFFECTS

- Profuse, watery, vaginal discharge (cryo > laser).
- Bleeding (laser > cryo).
- Long-term complications include cervical stenosis and a small ↑ in preterm labor.

Prevention of Cervical Dysplasia

Three different vaccines have been developed to protect against acquiring HPV and developing HPV-related diseases; currently, only the 9-valent vaccine is available in the United States. The optimal timing for HPV vaccination is prior to an individual's sexual debut. These vaccines are intended to be prophylactic, and have not been shown to treat or improve existing HPV-related diseases; however, therapeutic vaccines for this purpose are currently being studied.

QUADRIVALENT VACCINE (GARDASIL)

- Licensed in 2006 by the FDA as the first quadrivalent HPV vaccine.
- Administered as three doses: 0.5 mL intramuscularly given at intervals of 0, 2, and 6 months.
- Contains virus-like particles from four HPV genotypes: 6, 11, 16, and 18.

9-VALENT VACCINE (GARDASIL-9)

- Contains high-risk HPV genotypes 6, 11, 16, 18, as well as types 31, 33, 45, 52, and 58.
- The administration intervals are the same.

CERVARIX

- Licensed in 2010 by the FDA as the first bivalent HPV vaccine.
- Administered in three doses: 0.5 mL intramuscularly given at intervals of 0, 1, and 6 months.
- Contains virus-like particles from two HPV genotypes: 16 and 18.

SUCCESS RATE

Gardasil: Protects against 70% of cervical cancers and 90% of genital warts

Cervarix: Protects against 75% of cervical cancers caused by types 16 and 18

INDICATIONS

- In the United States, HPV vaccination is FDA approved for females and males between the ages of 9 and 45 years.
- In the United States, the Advisory Committee on Immunization Practices (ACIP) recommends the following:
  1. Routine vaccination at age 11–12, but can be given as early as age 9.
  2. For adolescents and adults aged 13–26 years who have not been previously vaccinated or have not completed the series, catch-up vaccination is recommended.
  3. For adults 27 years and older, catch-up vaccination is not routinely recommended, and should be made on an individual basis. This is because the likelihood of prior exposure to HPV increases with age.
- Pregnancy Class B; not recommended for pregnant women.
- Can be given to breast-feeding women.
- Recommended even for previously exposed patients, especially if they are determined to have a future risk of HPV exposure via anticipated new sexual partners.

SIDE EFFECTS

- Pain
- Redness
- Allergic reaction

FOLLOW-UP

- Routine cervical cancer screening still necessary.
- The need for booster dose has not been established.

EXAM TIP

What HPV genotypes are contained in the Gardasil quadrivalent vaccine?
Answer: Types 6, 11, 16, and 18.

Cervical Cancer

Cervical cancer is the third most frequent malignancy of the female genital tract. Eighty percent of cervical cancers are squamous cell carcinomas. They are related to human papillomavirus (HPV) infection while adenocarcinomas comprise 20% and can be related to maternal diethylstilbestrol (DES) exposure as well as certain strains of HPV (Table 25-1). The lifetime risk in the United States of developing cervical cancer is <1%. Cervical cancer is staged clinically, not surgically. Treatment depends on the stage of disease (Table 25-2). Patients diagnosed while pregnant face unique considerations, but overall have similar survival rates as nonpregnant patients.

Epidemiology

AGE AFFECTED

- Peak incidence between ages 45 and 55.
- The incidence in the United States in patients age ≤20 is 0.1/100,000.
- The incidence in the United states in patients age 35–54 is 2.2–2.3/100,000.

ANCESTRY PREVALENCE

- More prevalent in patients of African ancestry and patients of South and Central American ancestry than in those of European ancestry. However, this may be related more to social determinants of health than actual genetic predisposition.
- Mortality rate is two times greater in patients of African ancestry than in those of European ancestry. However, this may be related more to social determinants of health than actual genetic predisposition.

Symptoms

 A 50-year-old G3P3 patient presents with postcoital bleeding and some pain during intercourse. What is the next step?
Answer: Speculum exam with a Pap test or biopsy if a lesion is visible.

TABLE 25-1. Risk Factors for Cervical Cancer

HPV-RELATED RISK FACTORS	NON-HPV RELATED RISK FACTORS
Early onset of sexual debut	Non-European ancestry*
Multiple sexual partners	Lower socioeconomic status
History of other sexually transmitted infections	Oral contraceptive use
Immunosuppression	Cigarette smoking

* However, this may be related more to social determinants of health than actual genetic predisposition.

TABLE 25-2. Presenting Symptoms for Cervical Cancer Based on Stage*

LOCALIZED DISEASE (STAGE 1A2 OR LESS)	REGIONAL DISEASE (STAGE 2B OR LESS)	ADVANCED DISEASE (STAGE 3 OR GREATER)
None	Watery or bloody, maloderous discharge	Weight loss/loss of appetite
Postcoital bleeding	Hematuria	Severe back pain (related to hydronephrosis)
Irregular vaginal bleeding	Irregular vaginal bleeding	Leg swelling (related to lymphatic blockage)

*Suggested stages are for average cases, there is some variation in patient presentation.

Types of Cervical Cancer

SQUAMOUS CELL CANCER

- Accounts for 80% of cervical cancer
- Associated with HPV infection: Types 16 and 18 are responsible for 80% of cases

ADENOCARCINOMA

- Accounts for 20% of all invasive cervical cancers.
- Arises from columnar cells lining the endocervical canal and glands.
- **Early diagnosis is difficult; the false-negative rate with Pap test is 80%.**
- May be associated with maternal DES exposure and certain strains of high risk HPV, i.e., 16 and 18. (Fifty percent of cervical adenocarcinoma is related to Type 18.)

WARD TIP

Metastasis of cervical cancer to:
RIB Eye steak
Rectal
Intra-abdominal
Bladder
Endometrial

Clinical Staging of Invasive Cervical Cancer

A 55-year-old G1P1 patient presents to clinic for evaluation of postcoital bleeding. The Pap test and colposcopy with biopsy confirm a diagnosis of squamous-cell cervical carcinoma. Physical exam demonstrates a visible lesion that is 3 cm in size and does not involve the vagina or parametrial tissue. What stage is this patient?
Answer: Based on clinical staging, she is stage IB1.

Clinical staging of cervical cancer is important for prognosis and treatment (see Tables 25-3 and 25-4).

EXAM TIP

Cervical cancer is staged clinically.

TABLE 25-3. FIGO Staging (Revised 2019)

STAGE 0—CARCINOMA IN SITU (CIN3)

STAGE I—CANCER CONFINED TO THE CERVIX ONLY

IA—Invasive cancer identified only microscopically. Gross lesions are stage IB.
  IA1—Invasion of stroma no greater than 3 mm in depth
  IA2—Invasion of stroma greater than 3 mm and less than or equal to 5 mm in depth

IB—Clinically visible lesion confined to the cervix or lesions > IA.
  IB1—Lesion confined to cervix ≤2 cm.
  IB2—Lesion confined to cervix >2 cm but ≤4 cm
  IB3—Lesion confined to cervix >4 cm

STAGE II—CANCER EXTENDS BEYOND UTERUS, BUT NOT TO THE PELVIC SIDEWALL; INVOLVES THE UPPER VAGINA, BUT NOT THE LOWER THIRD

IIA—No parametrial involvement.
  IIA1—Clinically visible lesion ≤4 cm with involvement of less than upper 2/3 of vagina.
  IIA2—Clinically visible lesion >4 cm with involvement of less than upper 2/3 of vagina.

IIB—Parametrial involvement.

STAGE III—CANCER EXTENDED TO THE PELVIC SIDEWALL; TUMOR INVOLVES THE LOWER THIRD OF THE VAGINA; HYDRONEPHROSIS OR A NONFUNCTIONING KIDNEY
IIIA—No extension to the pelvic sidewall, but involves the lower third of the vagina.

IIIB—Extension to the pelvic sidewall; hydronephrosis or a nonfunctioning kidney.
IIIC—Involvement of the pelvic and/or para-aortic lymph nodes
  IIIC1—Pelvic lymph nodes only
  IIIC2—Para-aortic lymph nodes

STAGE IV—CANCER THAT HAS EXTENDED BEYOND THE TRUE PELVIS; INVOLVES EITHER THE MUCOSA OF THE BLADDER OR RECTUM OR BOTH
Stage IVA—Spread of cancer to adjacent pelvic organs (bladder/rectum).
Stage IVB—Spread of cancer to distant organs (outside of pelvis).

CLINICAL STAGING

- Physical exam (often under anesthesia): Bimanual, speculum, and rectovaginal exams to palpate tumor. Palpation of groin and supraclavicular lymph nodes.
- Colposcopy, ECC, cervical biopsy, cervical conization.
- Endoscopic exams: Hysteroscopy to evaluate the uterine lining, proctoscopy to evaluate rectal involvement, cystoscopy to evaluate bladder involvement.
- Imaging studies: Chest X-ray, intravenous pyelogram (IVP) to evaluate for urinary tract obstruction. (CT (computed tomography) is used in some centers.)

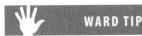

WARD TIP

Radical hysterectomy requires removal of:
- Uterus
- Cervix
- Parametrial tissue
- Upper vagina

TABLE 25-4.   Grading of Cervical Carcinoma

GRADE	INVASIVE SQUAMOUS TUMOR	ADENOCARCINOMA
X	Cannot be assessed	
1	Well differentiated	▪ Small component of solid growth and nuclear atypia ▪ Mild to moderate
2	Moderately differentiated	Intermediate-grade differentiation
3	Poorly differentiated	▪ Solid pattern ▪ Severe nuclear atypia predominate
4	Undifferentiated	

TABLE 25-5.   Nonsurgical Treatment for High Stage Cervical Cancer

CHEMOTHERAPY	RADIATION THERAPY
Response rates are higher with combination therapy.	High-dose delivery to the cervix and vagina, and minimal dosing to the bladder and rectum via:
Most combinations include platinum	– External-beam whole pelvic radiation OR – Transvaginal intracavitary cesium: Transvaginal applicators allow significantly larger doses of radiation to surface of cervix
Response rates: 50–70% for 4–6 months of life	

TREATMENT

General principles of treatment:
- Patients may undergo definitive treatment only if disease is confined to pelvis.
- Patients with local recurrence after radical hysterectomy are treated with **radiation**.
- Patients previously treated with radiotherapy are treated only by **radical pelvic surgery**.

Treatment of cervical cancer by stage:
- **0–1:** If microinvasive disease (1A1): Cold-knife cone biopsy (ectocervix); extrafascial (simple) hysterectomy.
- **1B–2A:** Radical hysterectomy or radiation, pelvic lymphadenectomy, para-aortic lymphadenectomy.
- **2B or higher:** Chemotherapy (cisplatin) and radiation (Table 25-5).

SURVIVAL

Disease stage at diagnosis is the most important predictor of survival in cervical cancer, though lymph node status and tumor volume also are important. Five-year survival after treatment for stage 1A2 disease is 95%, compared to

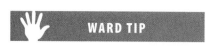

WARD TIP

How does cervical cancer spread? Direct extension and lymphatic spread. Lymph nodes involved are external, internal, common iliac, and para-aortic nodes.

75% in patients with stage 1B2 and 65% among those with stage 2B disease. Five-year survival drops markedly to about 40% for those with stage 3 disease.

Surveillance of Cervical Carcinoma

- Patients are examined every 3 months for the first 2 years, then every 6 months in years 3–5, and yearly thereafter.
- An exam consists of a history, physical, and Pap.

Recurrent Cervical Carcinoma

- Thirty percent of patients treated for cervical cancer will have a recurrence.
- Recurrence of cancer can occur anywhere, but usually occurs locally (vagina, cervix, or lateral pelvic wall) (see Table 25-6).

Cervical Cancer in Pregnancy

Three percent of all invasive cervical cancers occur during pregnancy.

SYMPTOMS

- One-third of pregnant patients with cervical cancer are asymptomatic.
- Symptoms in pregnancy include vaginal bleeding and discharge.

SCREENING

- Cervical cytology should be performed at the initial obstetric visit (if >21 years old and is needed based on timing of last Pap test).
- Colposcopy and cervical biopsies may be performed during pregnancy, but endocervical curettage (ECC) is contraindicated due to the risk of trauma to the pregnancy, and the risk of heavy bleeding.
- *Therapeutic* conization is contraindicated during pregnancy. *Diagnostic* conization is reserved for patients in whom an invasive lesion is suspected

TABLE 25-6.   Common Symptoms of Recurrence

Vaginal bleeding
Hematuria/dysuria
Constipation/melena
Pelvic and leg pain
Fistulas (in bladder or bowel)
Sacral backache or pain in sciatic distribution
Costovertebral angle and flank pain

WARD TIP

Leg pain following the distribution of the sciatic nerve or unilateral leg swelling is often an indication of pelvic recurrence.

KEY POINT

Uremia is the major cause of death in cervical cancer (found in 50% of patients).

WARD TIP

Causes of death in cervical cancer patients include uremia.

WARD TIP

What is the basic treatment for *invasive* cervical cancer?
- If confined to cervix: Radical hysterectomy, pelvic lymphadenectomy, para-aortic lymphadenectomy.
- If beyond cervix: Chemo and radiation.

but cannot be confirmed by biopsy *and* the results will alter the timing or mode of delivery. Otherwise, conization is performed postpartum. Cone biopsy, if necessary, should be performed in the second trimester. Complications may include hemorrhage and preterm labor.
- Clinical staging unchanged.

TREATMENT

- Definitive treatment is incompatible with pregnancy continuation.
- Therapy should be influenced by **gestational age, tumor stage, metastatic evaluation, and patient desires**. If the patient chooses to continue the pregnancy, therapy can be postponed until after delivery. Alternatively, a pregnancy can be terminated in order to begin treatment (subject to local laws). Chemotherapy may be used during pregnancy, but radiation therapy typically is not.
  - In early-stage disease a diagnostic CKC (cold-knife conization) can be done if the patient has a stage IA1 cancer. If the stage is > stage IA2, then after delivery, treatment can be instituted.
  - Second-trimester treatments can include platinum-based chemotherapies, which would allow prolongation of pregnancy for fetal maturity. A CKC during pregnancy can lead to complications such as hemorrhage and loss of pregnancy.
  - Third-trimester treatments include radical hysterectomy and pelvic lymphadenectomy after cesarean delivery.
  - Delays in treatment have not been reported to ↑ recurrence rates in stage I disease.

DELIVERY

- Consideration of possible tumor hemorrhage and size/shape influence delivery method.
- Patients with small-volume stage IA tumors may be candidates for vaginal delivery.
- Patients with > stage IA1 cancer require a cesarean delivery, followed by appropriate surgical treatment (hysterectomy).

PROGNOSIS

Limited data suggest **no difference** in prognosis of patients with cervical cancer diagnosed in pregnancy compared to nonpregnant patients.

Adenocarcinoma of Cervix

- Makes up 20% of cervical cancers.
- Mean age of diagnosis is early 50s (similar to squamous cell cancers).
- Carcinomas mainly arise from the endocervix.
- Cervical conization with negative margins is required to define microinvasive disease, because noncontiguous or "skip" lesions are common with adenocarcinomas (as opposed to squamous tumors).
- Treatment is largely the same as for squamous cell carcinomas.

SCREENING OF DES-EXPOSED PATIENTS

- Annual Pap test
- Careful palpation of vaginal walls to rule out adenosis or masses

TREATMENT

- Similar to treatment of squamous-cell carcinoma of cervix.
- Preferred treatment is radical hysterectomy and pelvic lymph node dissection for stage IB or IIA.
- Vaginectomy if vagina is involved.

DISEASE RECURRENCE

- Most DES-related clear-cell carcinomas recur after ≤ 3 years of initial treatment.
- Pulmonary and supraclavicular nodal metastasis common; yearly screening chest X-ray recommended.

CHAPTER 26

Endometrial Hyperplasia and Endometrial Cancer

Endometrial Hyperplasia

Hyperplasia is a proliferation of endometrial glands that may progress to or coexist with an endometrial cancer. On the histologic level, this is defined by gland-to-stroma ratio of >50%. There are 2 subtypes: **hyperplasia without atypia and atypical hyperplasia** (also known as endometrial intraepithelial neoplasm [EIN]).

Physiology pearl: Remember—estrogen stimulates endometrial proliferation and progesterone buffers and normalizes endometrium.

DIAGNOSIS OF ENDOMETRIAL HYPERPLASIA

- Endometrial **biopsy** (gold standard)
- Other procedures where endometrial hyperplasia may be found:
  - Endocervical curettage (ECC)
  - Hysteroscopy with uterine curettage
  - Hysterectomy

TREATMENT

- Hyperplasia without atypia may be treated with progestin therapy.
  - Options include oral progestins (cyclic or daily), depo medroxyprogesterone acetate (DMPA, or depo provera), or a levonorgestrel containing IUD (Mirena®).
  - The regression rate is high, and the endometrium should be reassessed in 3–6 months to ensure regression.
  - Weight loss also recommended in this population
- Atypical hyperplasia/EIN is treated with hysterectomy if childbearing is complete.
  - Consider referral to gynecologic oncology given high risk of concurrent malignancy.
  - If fertility is desired, may be treated with high-dose progestin therapy and re-biopsied in 3 months. Megestrol acetate is a very potent progesterone that is often used in this setting.

Epidemiology of Endometrial Cancer

- Endometrial carcinoma is a malignancy arising from the lining of the uterus.
- It is the most common gynecologic malignancy in the United States and is diagnosed in over 35,000 patients annually. It is 1.3 times more common than ovarian cancer and twice as common as cervical cancer.
- Because endometrial cancer usually presents with obvious symptoms, it is often diagnosed at an early stage.
- Lifetime risk is 3%.
- The average age at diagnosis is 61 years.
- Two types:
  - **Type I (most common):** An estrogen-dependent neoplasm that begins as proliferation of normal tissue. Over time, chronic proliferation becomes hyperplasia (abnormal tissue) and, eventually, neoplasia. These comprise 80% of endometrial cancers, and histologic types include endometrioid.
  - **Type II:** Unrelated to estrogen or hyperplasia. Tends to present with higher-grade or more aggressive tumors. These comprise 10–20% of endometrial cancers, and histologic types include clear cell, serous, mucinous, undifferentiated. These have a much poorer prognosis.

TABLE 26-1.   **Risk Factors of Endometrial Cancer**

ESTROGEN RELATED	NON-ESTROGEN RELATED
Estrogen-producing tumors (i.e., granulosa cell tumors)	HTN
Unopposed estrogen stimulation (e.g., menopausal estrogen replacement: 4–8 times ↑ risk	Lynch syndrome
Early menarche	Diabetes
Late menopause	Endometrial hyperplasia
Nulliparity (2–3 times ↑ risk)	Family history
Tamoxifen treatment for breast cancer (2–3 times ↑ risk)	BRCA mutations
Obesity (2–5 times ↑ risk, estrone made by fat cells)	

BRCA: HTN. hypertension.

Clinical Presentation

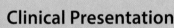 A 55-year-old G0P0 presents with a 2-month history of intermittent vaginal bleeding. The patient completed menopause 3 years ago, is obese, and has never been pregnant. What is the most likely diagnosis?
Answer: Endometrial cancer

- **Abnormal bleeding** is present in 90% of cases: (see Table 26-1)
    - Bleeding in postmenopausal patients (classic).
    - Meno/metrorrhagia (in premenopausal cases).
- Abnormal Pap test: 1–5% of cases. Pap tests are *not* diagnostic, but a finding of abnormal glandular cells (AGC) warrants further investigation.

WARD TIP

About 5–10% of patients who present with postmenopausal bleeding will have endometrial cancer.

Differential Diagnosis of Postmenopausal Bleeding

 A 59-year-old G0 postmenopausal patient comes in with a 2-month history of spotting. The patient says that the bleeding is minimal, but still requires wearing a panty liner. The patient has no pain or other symptoms. The patient weighs 300 pounds. What is the next step?
Answer: Endometrial biopsy. The most likely diagnosis is endometrial atrophy. The most lethal diagnosis is endometrial cancer.

DIFFERENTIAL DIAGNOSES OF POSTMENOPAUSAL BLEEDING

- Exogenous estrogens (i.e., hormone replacement therapy)
- Atrophic endometritis/vaginitis
- Endometrial cancer

TABLE 26-2. Comparison of Endometrial Hyperplasia Subtypes

	HYPERPLASIA WITHOUT ATYPIA	ATYPICAL HYPERPLASIA (ALSO KNOWN AS ENDOMETRIAL INTRAEPITHELIAL NEOPLASM)
General	Non-neoplastic change	Has cellular and genetic changes associated with invasive cancers
Histologic morphology	Mild crowding, cystic dilation	Crowding, cells are clonal and morphologically different from surrounding stroma
Risk of progression to cancer	~1% at 5 years, 2% at 10 years	~5% at 5 years, 9% at 10 years
Risk of co-existing cancer	Low	23–37%

- Endometrial/cervical polyps
- Coagulopathy
- Endometrial hyperplasia (see Table 26-2)

PROTECTIVE FACTORS

- Regular ovulation
- Combined oral contraceptives
- Multiparity

EVALUATION OF POSTMENOPAUSAL BLEEDING

- Endometrial biopsy.
- Hysteroscopy with D&C if endometrial biopsy is inadequate or suspicious, or if a polyp is diagnosed.
- Transvaginal ultrasound to evaluate endometrial stripe. The stripe should be thin (<5 mm) in a postmenopausal patient. A thickened stripe requires further evaluation.
- If the cause of the postmenopausal bleeding is suspected to be a polyp, office hysteroscopy or saline infusion sonohysterogram (SIS) may be used to visualize. However, tissue sampling (via endometrial biopsy) is still mandatory.

Additional Workup for Endometrial Cancer

After diagnosis of endometrial cancer is made, the following should be performed to evaluate for possible metastasis:

- Physical exam: Assess size/mobility of uterus, lymph nodes, ascites.
- Chest X-ray.
- Complete metabolic panel, complete blood count (CBC), type, and screen.
- Pelvic or abdominal imaging is NOT INDICATED if surgical staging is planned.
- Take a careful family history for other cancers to see if the patient is at risk for a hereditary cancer syndrome, i.e., Lynch syndrome.

Staging of Endometrial Cancer

Endometrial cancer is staged surgically.

- The stage of an endometrial cancer is determined by:
  1. The spread of tumor in the uterus.
  2. The degree of myometrial invasion.
  3. The presence of extrauterine tumor spread.
- This assessment is accomplished through a surgical staging operation (similar to ovarian cancer). The staging of a patient's disease directs treatment and predicts outcome (see Table 26-3 and Figure 26-1).

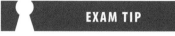

EXAM TIP

Grade is the most important prognostic indicator in endometrial cancer.

TABLE 26-3. Staging of Endometrial Cancer FIGO (Revised 2009)

STAGE	DESCRIPTION
*I: Tumor confined to the uterus	IA: Limited to endometrium or invades <½ of the myometrium IB: Tumor invades ≥½ of the myometrium
*II: Tumor invades cervical stroma, but does not extend beyond uterus**	

*III: Local and/or regional spread of the tumor	IIIA: Invasion of uterine serosa and/or adnexa
	IIIB: Invasion of vagina and/or parametrial involvement
	IIIC: Mets to pelvic/para-aortic lymph nodes
	    IIIC1: Pelvic lymph nodes
	    IIIC2: Para-aortic lymph nodes

*IV: Tumor invades bladder and/or bowel mucosa, and/or distant metastases	IVA: Invasion of bladder and/or bowel mucosa

* Endocervical gland involvement is stage I.

** Positive peritoneal cytology does not change the stage and is reported separately.

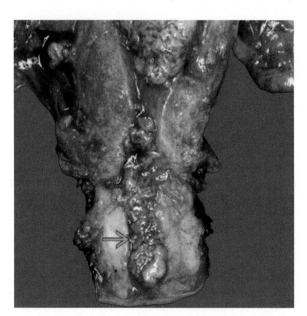

FIGURE 26-1. Pathology specimen of uterus with visible endometrial cancer in the endometrial cavity.

Grading

Grading is determined by the tumor **histology:**

G1	Well differentiated	<5% solid pattern
G2	Moderately differentiated	5–50% solid pattern
G3	Poorly differentiated	>50% solid pattern

Treatment

Basic treatment for all stages (surgical staging is always the first step):
- Hysterectomy
- Bilateral salpingo-oophorectomy (BSO)
- Pelvic and para-aortic lymphadenectomy
- Peritoneal washings for cytology ("loose or free cancer cells")

ADJUVANT THERAPY

After the above steps in treatment, adjuvant therapy is carried out. This depends on the stage of disease and histology of the tumor, which determines the risk of recurrence.

Low Risk: Grade 1, stage 1A, confined to endometrium.
- No further treatment beyond surgical staging as described above.

Intermediate Risk: Stage 1A or 1B or stage II—involves myometrium or cervical stroma.
- Radiation therapy +/− chemotherapy.

High Risk: Stage III or higher, or any patient with serous or clear-cell histology.
- Chemotherapy (carboplatin and paclitaxel) +/− radiation therapy.

Uterine Sarcoma

 A 53-year-old G1P1 postmenopausal patient presents with vaginal bleeding and pelvic pain. For the past 3 months, the patient has noticed that her abdomen has enlarged rapidly. What is the most likely diagnosis?
Answer: Leiomyosarcoma (LMS)

- Uterine sarcoma is classified separately from endometrial cancer:
  - <10% of uterine malignancies.
  - Presents as a rapidly enlarging mass with vaginal bleeding.
  - Poor prognosis.
- Risk factors are not well delineated.
- Most cases are diagnosed with exploratory surgery for what was thought to be a uterine myoma (fibroid).

TYPES

A. Homologous (mesenchymal tissue that normally forms in the uterus—most common)
B. Heterologous (foreign tissue to the uterus, i.e., cartilage, bone) (see Table 26-4)

TABLE 26-4.   Other Less Common Sarcoma Types

ENDOMETRIAL STROMAL SARCOMA (ESS)	CARCINOSARCOMA	UNDIFFERENTIATED SARCOMAS
Homologous	Heterologous	High grade
10% of uterine sarcomas	Rare, <5% of uterine sarcomas	Rare
Low grade, indolent	previously called malignant mixed Müllerian tumors	Aggressive, with poor prognosis
Peaks in fifth decade	Usually found in patients >60	
Has estrogen and progesterone receptors	Presents with postmenopausal bleeding and rapidly growing uterus	

- Leiomyosarcoma (LMS):
  - Homologous
  - One-third of uterine sarcomas
  - Presents with rapidly growing pelvic mass +/– pain or vaginal bleeding.
  - Usually large (>10 cm) and yellow/tan mass grossly

DIAGNOSIS

- >10 mitosis/10 high-powered fields with cytologic atypia
- Usually diagnosed from specimen sent after hysterectomy
- Staged just like endometrial cancer

TREATMENT

- Surgical (total hysterectomy/BSO, +/– lymphadenectomy, and peritoneal washings).
- Adjuvant therapy (chemotherapy) may decrease recurrence.
- Radiation may enhance local control after surgery. Unknown survival benefit.
- Multi-agent chemotherapy is prescribed for metastatic sarcomas. Complete responses are rare.

NOTES

Ovarian Cancer and Fallopian Tube Cancer

Ovarian cancer is the deadliest gynecologic cancer because it is difficult to detect before dissemination. It is the second most common gynecologic cancer.

Seventy percent of cases of ovarian cancer are diagnosed at stage III or IV.

Epithelial cell ovarian cancer accounts for 85% of all ovarian cancers.

Omental caking is a fixed pelvic and upper abdominal mass (metastatic tumor implanted in the omentum) associated with ascites. It is pathognomonic for ovarian cancer.

Ovarian cancer typically spreads by exfoliation of cancerous cells into the peritoneal fluid.

More than 5 years of oral contraceptive pill (OCP) use ↓ risk of ovarian cancer by 25–50%. This protection lasts 15 years after discontinuation.

The serous type of epithelial ovarian cancer is the most common type of ovarian cancer and is bilateral 65% of the time.

Ovarian cancer is a malignancy arising from the cells of the ovary. However, epithelial ovarian cancer is thought to have similar or even the same pathogenesis as fallopian tube cancer and primary peritoneal cancer. There are three categories of ovarian cancer: epithelial, germ cell, and sex cord stromal. Ovarian cancer is the most deadly gynecologic malignancy because it is most often diagnosed at an advanced stage.

Epidemiology

Second most common gynecologic malignancy.
- Seventy percent of patients are diagnosed as stage III or IV.
- Lifetime risk is 1 in 70.
- Median age at diagnosis is 63 years.

Epithelial Cell Ovarian Cancer

A 65-year-old G0P0 patient presents with a 4-month history of increasing abdominal girth and bloating. She also reports occasional shortness of breath and nausea. She doesn't understand why her pants are too small when she seems to be eating less. What is the suspected diagnosis?
Answer: Ovarian cancer. Initial steps in diagnosis: Transvaginal ultrasound and CA-125. Definitive diagnosis: Surgery.

A 61-year-old G2P2 patient is diagnosed with ovarian cancer after she presented with abdominal bloating. On pelvic ultrasound, she is found to have 6-cm bilateral ovarian masses and ascites. What would the next step be in management?
Answer: Total hysterectomy (TH) with bilateral salpingo-oophorectomy (BSO), omentectomy, pelvic and para-aortic lymph adenectomy, and then chemotherapy with carboplatinum and paclitaxel. The patient will get serial CA-125 levels on follow-up examinations.

The majority of ovarian cancers are epithelial.

HISTOLOGIC SUBTYPES

Six subtypes arising from epithelial tissue:
- Serous: 50%
- Mucinous: 25%
- Endometrioid: 10%
- Clear cell: 6%
- Brenner: 4%
- Undifferentiated: 5%

CLINICAL REMINDER

Initial stages are usually asymptomatic. Signs/symptoms are usually from metastasis to other organs.

Epithelial ovarian cancers are thought to arise from incorrect repair of the epithelial cells of the ovary after ovulation at the site of the follicular wall rupture where the repair occurs. Thus risk factors are things leading to more ovulation and protective factors are things leading to less ovulation. Figure 27-1

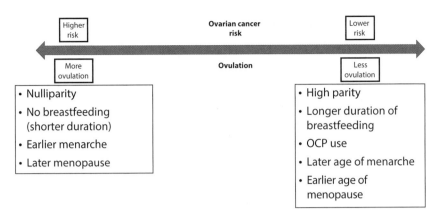

FIGURE 27-1. Risks factors and protective factors for epithelial ovarian cancers.

NON-OVULATION RELATED RISK FACTORS

- Advanced age (50–70)
- Family history of ovarian cancer
- Personal or family history of breast cancer
- European ancestry

NON-OVULATION RELATED PROTECTIVE FACTORS

- Tubal ligation or salpingectomy
- Oophorectomy
- Hysterectomy

WORKUP

- Cancer Antigen 125 (CA-125):
  - A tumor marker that is elevated in 80% of cases of **epithelial** ovarian cancers.
  - It is useful in tracking the progression of the disease and the response to treatment.
  - It may be elevated in many premenopausal medical conditions (i.e., fibroids, endometriosis) or other causes of peritoneal inflammation.
  - It is **not effective** as a screening tool.

Hereditary Ovarian Cancer Syndromes

Ten to fifteen percent of cases occur in association with genetically predisposed syndromes called **hereditary ovarian cancer (HOC) syndromes.** In these patients, ovarian cancer is diagnosed at a median age of 50 years. There are three types:
1. **Breast-ovarian cancer syndrome:** Involves cancer of the breast and ovary and is linked to the mutation of breast cancer genes, BRCA-1 and BRCA-2 genes, in 90% of HOC. BRCA is a tumor suppressor gene that is located on chromosome 17.
2. **Lynch II syndrome—hereditary nonpolyposis colon cancer (HNPCC):** Involves sites that may include breast, ovaries, uterus, and colon.
3. **Site-specific ovarian cancer:** Accounts for <1% and has an extremely strong genetic link. Usually, two or more first-degree relatives have the disease.

EXAM TIP

Ovarian cancer spread is normally through the peritoneal fluid, which carries cancer cells locally to other abdominal structures.

 ZEBRA ALERT

Ovarian cancer metastasis to the umbilicus is "Sister Mary Joseph's nodule." This is a palpable umbilical nodule.

WARD TIP

In a postmenopausal woman with a pelvic mass, CA-125 is much more specific for ovarian cancer compared to a premenopausal woman.

EXAM TIP

BRCA-1 has higher risk of ovarian cancer (40%) versus only 15% in BRCA-2.

TABLE 27-1.   **Ovarian Tumors and Their Serum Markers**

Ovarian Tumor	Serum Tumor Marker
Dysgerminoma	LDH
Endodermal sinus tumor	AFP
Embryonal and choriocarcinoma	β-hCG, AFP
Epithelial ovarian tumor	CA-125
Granulosa cell tumor	Inhibin
Sertoli-Leydig cell tumor	Testosterone

AFP, α-fetoprotein; β-hCG, β-human chorionic gonadotropin; CA; GCT, germ cell tumor; LDH, lactic dehydrogenase.

WARD TIP

Malignant conditions that cause ↑ CA-125:
- Endometrial cancer
- Lung cancer
- Breast cancer
- Pancreatic cancer

Benign conditions that cause ↑ CA-125:
- Endometriosis
- Pelvic inflammatory disease (PID)
- Leiomyoma
- Pregnancy
- Hemorrhagic ovarian cyst
- Liver disease

WARD TIP

Large ovarian tumors can cause bowel obstruction and other gastrointestinal symptoms.

Ovarian Cancer Workup

- Unfortunately, ovarian cancer is often diagnosed after the disease has spread beyond the ovary (advanced stage).
- As with any pelvic mass, the first step of evaluation is ultrasound.
- CA-125: Tumor marker for **epithelial** ovarian cancer (not very sensitive or specific).
- Surgical staging procedure if malignancy is suspected (see above). See Table 27-1.

Screening Recommendations for Genetic Cancer Syndromes

- Women with **standard risk** (<2 first-degree relatives with ovarian cancer): No routine screening recommended. A first-degree relative is considered a mother, sister, or daughter.
- Women with **high risk** (>2 first-degree relatives with ovarian cancer): Genetic testing and counseling.
- If high risk, perform:
  - Annual CA-125 (poor tool for screening).
  - Annual transvaginal ultrasound.
  - Annual pelvic exam.
  - Consider BRCA screening. Consider prophylactic oophorectomy once done with childbearing if positive.

Staging

Ovarian cancer is staged surgically (see Table 27-2). The staging surgery includes:
- Peritoneal washings (for cytology)
- TH

TABLE 27-2. **Staging of Ovarian Cancer (FIGO)**

STAGE	DESCRIPTION
I: Tumor limited to ovaries	IA: One ovary, capsule intact
	IB: Both ovaries, capsules intact
	IC: Tumor on ovary surface, capsule ruptured, ascites with malignant cells, or positive peritoneal washings
II: Pelvic spread	IIA: Involvement of uterus/tubes
	IIB: Involvement of other pelvic structures
	IIC: IIA or IIB plus tumor on ovary surface, capsule ruptures, ascites with malignant cells, or positive peritoneal washings
III: Spread to the abdominal cavity	IIIA: Positive abdominal peritoneal washings (indicates microscopic seeding)
	IIIB: <2 cm implants on abdominal peritoneal surface
	IIIC: >2 cm implants on abdominal peritoneal surface and/or positive retroperitoneal or inguinal nodes
IV: Distant metastasis	Parenchymal liver/spleen spread
	Pleural effusion, skin or supraclavicular nodes

- BSO
- Omentectomy
- Appendectomy (for mucinous only)
- Pelvic and para-aortic lymphadenectomy

TREATMENT

The purpose of surgery in patients with ovarian cancer is twofold:
1. To accurately stage the patient's disease.
2. To achieve "optimal cytoreduction" of the disease, which means removing all sites of primary or metastatic tumor >1 cm in size. This kind of debulking surgery has been shown to improve survival in patients with *any* stage ovarian cancer.

ADJUVANT THERAPY

Chemotherapy can improve survival and disease-free intervals in women with ovarian cancer.

First-line chemotherapy: Paclitaxel and cisplatin *or* paclitaxel and carboplatin. For women with stage III or IV disease—**neoadjuvant chemotherapy**—i.e., chemotherapy first and then surgery (once the tumor burden is reduced)—is associated with less perioperative morbidity and mortality, with no difference in disease-free survival. The chemotherapy agents are the same.

Chemotherapy can be given IV or intraperitoneal (IP). IP chemotherapy is best for women who are optimally debulked and not good for women with stage IV disease or who have a large residual tumor burden. Randomized controlled trials (RCTs) for IP chemotherapy are ongoing.

POOR PROGNOSTIC INDICATORS

- Short disease-free interval
- Mucinous or clear cell tumor
- Multiple disease sites
- High/rising CA-125

Before a staging surgery, a computed tomography (CT) scan of the chest/abdomen/pelvis is helpful to evaluate the extent of the disease, including retroperitoneal lymph-node enlargement and liver metastases.

Krukenberg tumors are ovarian tumors that are metastatic from another primary cancer, usually from the gastrointestinal tract.

CA-125 is elevated in 80% of cases of ovarian cancer, but only in 50% of stage I cases. It is most useful as a tool to gauge progression/regression of disease.

Surgical staging: Ovarian, endometrial, vulvar, and fallopian tube cancers
Clinical staging: Cervical and vaginal

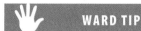
WARD TIP

While chemotherapy is traditionally administered IV, IP administration has shown promise in treating ovarian cancer.

WARD TIP

Chemotherapy can cause neutropenia. An absolute neutrophil count <500 cells/μL requires prophylactic antibiotic treatment to prevent septic complications.

WARD TIP

Approximately one-third of GCTs found in women <21 years old are malignant.

Nonepithelial Ovarian Cancer

Accounts for 15% of ovarian cancers. Histologic types include:
- **Germ cell tumors (GCTs):** 8% of all ovarian cancers and include teratomas, dysgerminomas, and choriocarcinomas
- **Sex-cord stromal tumors:** 1% of all ovarian cancers and include granulosa-theca cell tumors, and Sertoli-Leydig tumors

OVARIAN GERM CELL TUMORS (GCTS)

GCTs account for 20–25% of ovarian neoplasms, but only 5% of **malignant** ovarian neoplasms. They are the primary cause of ovarian cancer in women <30 years old. They arise from totipotential germ cells that normally are able to differentiate into three germ cell tissues. Most are benign. See Table 27-3.

CLINICAL PRESENTATION
- Abdominal pain with rapidly enlarging palpable pelvic/abdominal mass. See Table 27-4.
- Acute abdomen.
- Fever.
- Usually found in children or young women.
- Some GCTs produce hormones like hCG and AFP. These patients may present with pregnancy symptoms, abnormal uterine bleeding, or precocious puberty (due to high hCG).

Dysgerminoma

 A 7-year-old girl presents with abdominal pain, and a workup reveals an adnexal mass. She undergoes an exploratory laparotomy and an excisional biopsy. What is the most likely pathology?
Answer: Dysgerminoma

- Arises from undifferentiated totipotential germ cells.

TABLE 27-3. Malignant Germ Cell Tumors

TUMOR TYPE	PERCENT OF MALIGNANT GCT	OTHER TRAITS	TUMOR MARKER
Dysgerminoma	33%	10% bilateral Chemo/RT sensitive	LDH
Yolk sac tumor	15–20%	VERY aggressive Younger patients (median age 23) * Schiller-Duval bodies	AFP
Immature teratoma	36%	May see neural differentiation	none
Choriocarcinoma	<2%	Patients <20 years old	β-hCG
Embryonal Carcinoma	4%	Average age is 15 Presents with precocious puberty or vaginal bleeding	β-hCG and AFP
Mixed GCTs	5%	Dysgerminoma and yolk sac tumor is the most common combination	**Vary depending on components**

AFP, α-fetoprotein; β-hCG, β-human chorionic gonadotropin; GCT, germ cell tumor; LDH, lactic dehydrogenase.

TABLE 27-4. Presentation of Epithelial Ovarian Cancer*

SYMPTOMS	SIGNS
Early satiety	Fluid wave (from ascites)
Nausea/Vomiting	Pelvic mass (can be bilateral or unilateral)
Pelvic pain	Abdominal mass (from omental cake)
"Clothes don't fit anymore"—change in abdominal girth/Bloating	
Change in bowel habits	

*NB: Fallopian tube and primary peritoneal often present similarly.

Yolk Sac Tumor

- Arises from extraembryonic tissues (resembles a yolk sac).

Immature Teratoma

- Arises from tissue from ectoderm, mesoderm, and endoderm
- Haphazard tissue from the ectoderm, mesoderm, and endoderm

Choriocarcinoma

- Arises from cytotrophoblasts and syncytiotrophoblasts (extraembryonic tissues)

Embryonal Carcinoma

- Composed of primitive embryonal cells

TREATMENT OF MALIGNANT GCTs

- Surgery: **Unilateral** salpingo-oophorectomy and complete surgical staging. **Remember, because these are in young women, try to save one ovary.**
- Adjuvant chemotherapy: Recommended for all malignant GCTs except stage IA, grade I immature teratomas. Stage IA, grade 1 immature teratomas have a high cure rate with surgery alone. The BEP regimen is the standard of care:

BEP Regimen	Side Effects
Bleomycin	Pulmonary fibrosis
Etoposide	Blood dyscrasias
Cis**P**latin	Nephrotoxicity (extreme nausea and vomiting)

PROGNOSIS OF OVARIAN GCTs

Prognosis is generally good because most are discovered *early.* Five-year survival is 85% for dysgerminomas, 75% for immature teratomas, and 65% for yolk sac tumors.

WARD TIP

A benign (mature) cystic teratoma can undergo malignant degeneration, usually after menopause.

ZEBRA ALERT

Both mature and immature teratomas can produce the N-Methyl-D-aspartate (NMDA) antibodies that lead to anti-NMDA receptor encephalitis. (50% of women with NMDA receptor encephalitis have a teratoma.)

WARD TIP

Struma ovarii is a teratoma with thyroid tissue that often presents with symptoms of hyperthyroidism.

WARD TIP

Granulosa cell tumors are very chemosensitive.

EXAM TIP

The most common solid benign tumor of the ovary is a fibroma.

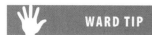

ZEBRA ALERT

Meig syndrome (hydrothorax, ascites) can occur with a fibroma of the ovary.

- - - - - - - - - - - - - -

OVARIAN SEX-CORD STROMAL TUMORS

- Arise from the sex cords and specialized stroma of the embryonic gonads (before they differentiate into ovaries or testes).
- Some of these tumors are functional tumors and secrete estrogen or testosterone.
- They behave as low-grade malignancies and usually affect older women.
- Rare—comprises only 1% of malignant ovarian neoplasms.

Granulosa Cell Tumor

- Most common type of malignant sex-cord stromal tumor. Comprise 2–5% of all ovarian malignancies.
- Secretes **estrogens**.
- Can present with **feminization, precocious puberty, menorrhagia,** or **postmenopausal bleeding.**
- Association with endometrial cancer in 5% of cases.
- Characteristic Call-Exner bodies (eosinophilic bodies surrounded by granulosa cells) (Figure 27-2).
- Inhibin is the tumor marker.

Sertoli-Leydig Cell Tumor

- Secretes **testosterone**.
- Frequently presents with **virilization, hirsutism,** and **menstrual disorders**.
- Testosterone is the tumor marker.

TREATMENT OF OVARIAN SEX-CORD STROMAL TUMORS

- Surgical:
  - TH and BSO in women who have completed childbearing.
  - **Unilateral** salpingo-oophorectomy in young women with low-stage/grade neoplasia.
- **Adjuvant therapy:** Chemotherapy and radiation are not commonly used in patients with stage I disease but is recommended for patients with stages II–IV disease and those with recurrence.

WARD TIP

Fallopian tube carcinoma, epithelial ovarian cancer, and primary peritoneal cancer likely have a common pathogenesis.

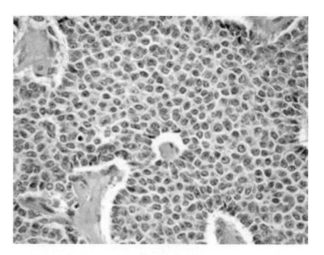

FIGURE 27-2. Call-Exner bodies granulosa cell tumor.

Fallopian Tube Carcinoma

Fallopian tube carcinomas usually are adenocarcinomas. The most common histologic subtype is **papillary serous** (90%). They spread through the peritoneal fluid in a similar fashion to ovarian cancer. As noted above, many serous epithelial ovarian carcinomas have a tubal precursor lesion.

Fallopian tube cancer behaves like and is treated like epithelial ovarian cancers and primary peritoneal cancers. Removal of fallopian tubes (at the time of hysterectomy or as method of sterilization) has been shown to decrease the lifetime risk of ovarian epithelial cancer. Even tubal ligation decreases the risk of epithelial ovarian cancer.

PRESENTATION

- Early stages often diagnosed during a laparotomy/laparoscopy for other indications.
- Later stages present like epithelial ovarian cancer and are identified on pathology.

STAGING, TREATMENT, AND PROGNOSIS

Same as ovarian cancer.

NOTES

CHAPTER 28

Vulvar Squamous Intraepithelial Lesions, Vulvar Cancer, and Vaginal Cancer

The nomenclature surrounding what was formerly referred to as Vulvar Intraepithelial Neoplasia (VIN) has changed many times throughout recent years. The most widely used and accepted classification system was proposed and published by the International Society for the Study of Vulvovaginal Disease (ISSVD) in 2015 and has also been adopted by the American College of Obstetricians and Gynecologists (ACOG). It replaces VIN with the term "Squamous Intraepithelial Lesion" (SIL) in order to be more consistent with terminology used to describe cervical SIL.

2015 ISSVD Terminology for Vulvar SIL

- **Low-grade squamous intraepithelial lesion (LSIL) of the vulva**
  - Previously referred to as VIN 1.
  - Includes vulvar LSIL, flat condyloma, or human papillomavirus (HPV) effect.
  - Not considered to be pre-cancerous lesions; often self-limited, and will resolve within 1–2 years.
- **High-grade squamous intraepithelial lesion (HSIL) of the vulva**
  - Previously referred to as vulvar SIL 2 and vulvar SIL 3.
  - These lesions are considered to be pre-cancerous and are associated with ~20% of vulvar cancers.
- **Differentiated VIN (dVIN)**
  - Previously referred to as VIN simplex type.
  - Lesions that are *not* associated with HPV.
  - <5% of vulvar SIL.
  - Highest risk of progression to vulvar cancer (~30%).
  - May be associated with lichen sclerosus and other vulvar dermatoses.

RISK FACTORS
- Vulvar HSIL and vulvar cancer are associated with HPV infection, especially high-risk subtypes 16, 18, 31, and 33.
- Vulvar LSIL and anogenital condyloma are associated with HPV subtypes 6 and 11.
- History of vulvar skin disease such as lichen sclerosus.
- Cigarette smoking.
- Vulvar SIL is more common in *premenopausal* patients, whereas dVIN is more common in *postmenopausal* patients.

PRESENTATION
- Vulvar pruritus and/or irritation (recent or longstanding).
- Pain, burning, or dysuria.
- Vulvar lesions: Wide variety of appearances—the color may be brown, red, pink, gray, or white, and the lesion may be verrucous, nodular, ulcerated, or flat.
- May be asymptomatic (~40%).

DIAGNOSIS
- **Biopsy** (most important for diagnosis)
- Colposcopy (must include vulva, vagina, cervix, and perineum)

TREATMENT
- **Vulvar LSIL:**
  - May observe if asymptomatic.
  - If symptomatic, may treat with medical or surgical options (see next page on Treatment of Vulvar HSIL).

- **Vulvar HSIL:**
    - Treatment is based on symptoms, size, location, prior treatment history, and likelihood of invasive disease.
    - Surgical excision: Especially if there is concern for invasive disease.
    - Laser ablation: Best for multifocal disease. Must rule out cancer first.
    - Topical treatment: Imiquimod, topical 5-fluorouracil.

Vulvar Cancer

A 64-year-old G1P1 patient presents with vulvar itching. On exam, she has a 1-cm white lesion on her labia that bleeds when palpated. What is the first step to make a diagnosis? What other findings in her medical and social history might put her at ↑ risk for cancer?

Answer: The first step in diagnosis is biopsy! Other findings that might put her at ↑ risk for cancer include age, itching, and bleeding on exam.

- Most often found in women age 60–70 (average age 68 years).
- HPV is associated with most squamous cell vulvar cancers.
- Vulvar cancer is the fourth most common gynecologic cancer (5% of all gynecologic cancers) and can arise as carcinoma of various types:
    - Squamous cell carcinoma (75%).
    - Melanoma (4–10%).
    - Adenocarcinoma (Bartholin's gland) (1–5%).
    - Basal cell carcinoma.
    - Metastasis.
    - Sarcoma (1–2%).
    - Paget disease (<1%).

SIGNS AND SYMPTOMS

- Pruritus (most common)
- Vulvar lesion (may be ulceration, palpable mass, or plaque)
- Bleeding
- Vulvar pain
- May be asymptomatic

RISK FACTORS

- Postmenopausal (increasing age)
- Cigarette smoking
- HIV
- HPV infection
- Vulvar HSIL
- Cervical HSIL
- Vulvar skin disease, i.e., lichen sclerosus

DIAGNOSIS

- Biopsy of the suspicious lesion.
- Lesions may be multifocal, so all vulvar and perianal tissue as well as the cervix and vagina should be evaluated.
- Cervical SIL or cancer may also be present (~20%) and should be assessed.

STAGING (SEE TABLE 28-1)

- The current staging system for vulvar cancer was introduced in 2017 and is a hybrid of clinical and surgical staging.

EXAM TIP

Condyloma acuminata: Genital warts associated with HPV, which have a pearly, and plaque-like or cauliflower appearance versus

Condyloma lata: Genital warts in secondary syphilis, which are non-painful, raised, grayish-white lesions

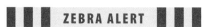

ZEBRA ALERT

Remember that a dark-pigmented vulvar lesion could be a melanoma and requires biopsy. It is the second most common vulvar cancer histology.

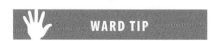

WARD TIP

Most common site of vulvar SIL and cancer is labia majora.

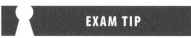

EXAM TIP

Lichen sclerosus is associated with dVIN, which may be a precursor to vulvar cancer.

TABLE 28-1. NEW (2021) FIGO STAGING FOR CARCINOMA OF THE VULVA

STAGE	DESCRIPTION
I	Tumor confined to the vulva
IA	Tumor size ≤2 cm and stromal invasion ≤1 mm[a]
IB	Tumor size >2 cm or stromal invasion >1 mm[a]
II	Tumor of any size with extension to lower one-third of the urethra, lower one-third of the vagina, lower one-third of the anus with negative nodes
III	Tumor of any size with extension to upper part of adjacent perineal structures, or with any number of nonfixed, nonulcerated lymph node
IIIA	Tumor of any size with disease extension to upper two-thirds of the urethra, upper two-thirds of the vagina, bladder mucosa, rectal mucosa, or regional lymph node metastases ≤5 mm
IIIB	Regional[b] lymph node metastases >5 mm
IIIC	Regional[b] lymph node metastases with extracapsular spread
IV	Tumor of any size fixed to bone, or fixed, ulcerated lymph node metastases, or distant metastases
IVA	Disease fixed to pelvic bone, or fixed or ulcerated regional[b] lymph node metastases
IVB	Distant metastases

[a]Depth of invasion is measured from the basement membrane of the deepest, adjacent, dysplastic, tumor-free rete ridge (or nearest dysplastic rete peg) to the deepest point of invasion.

[b]Regional refers to inguinal and femoral lymph nodes.

Used, with permission, from Olawaiye AB, Cotler J, Cuello MO, et al. FIGO staging for carcinoma of the vulva: 2021 revision. *Int J Gynecol Obstet*. 2021:155:43-47. https://doi.org/10.1002.

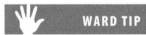

WARD TIP

Vulvar cancer and vaginal cancer both metastasize by a variety of mechanisms, including direct extension to adjacent structures, lymphatic spread, and hematogenous dissemination.

- Tumor size, depth of invasion, and extension are evaluated by physical exam and biopsy.
- Lymph nodes are evaluated by physical exam, imaging studies, and either lymphadenectomy or sentinel lymph node biopsy (SLNB).

TREATMENT

- Surgical excision based on size and extent of lesion, the histologic type, and the status of lymph nodes.
  - **Radical local excision:** T1 lesions with no extension to adjacent perineal structures (referred to as "wide local excision").
  - **Modified radical vulvectomy:** T2 lesions of any size with extension to adjacent perineal structures (i.e., urethra, vagina, anus).
  - **Chemoradiation + selective surgical excision:** T3 lesions with extension to more distant structures, i.e., bladder mucosa, upper 2/3 of urethra or vagina, rectal mucosa, fixed to pelvic bone.
  - **Inguinofemoral lymph nodes:** Assessment of lymph nodes is essential for staging purposes, and may vary from lymph node biopsy, SLNB, to full inguinofemoral lymphadenectomy, which involves the removal of the inguinal (superficial) and femoral (deep) lymph nodes. High morbidity.
  - **Adjuvant therapy:** For select patients, the risk of recurrence may be reduced with adjuvant radiation therapy or chemotherapy.

Vaginal Cancer

> A 72-year-old G1P1 patient presents reporting a 4-week history of vaginal spotting. She had a vaginal hysterectomy at age 45 for heavy menses. On exam, a 2-cm ulcerated lesion is noted on the posterior wall of the vagina. What is the next step in management?
> **Answer:** Biopsy the lesion.

- A rare primary cancer that arises in vagina (3% of gynecologic cancers).
- Many vaginal malignancies are metastatic (via direct extension or via lymphatic or hematogenous spread) from the endometrium, cervix, vulva, ovary, breast, rectum, or kidney.
- Usually presents in **postmenopausal women** (average age 60 years).
- Increased risk in premenopausal women exposed to diethylstilbestrol (DES) in utero. These patients should have more frequent screening for vaginal and cervical cancer.
- Most common type is **squamous cell carcinoma** (other types are similar to vulvar cancer types: melanoma, sarcoma, adenocarcinoma).
- HPV infection and/or history of cervical or vulvar SIL is a risk factor for development of vaginal cancer.
- Patients who have undergone hysterectomy (with removal of the cervix) for cervical HSIL or who have a history of cervical HSIL should continue to undergo cytologic screening and HPV testing for at least 25 years following diagnosis.

WARD TIP

Vaginal cancer typically presents with vaginal bleeding.

SIGNS AND SYMPTOMS

- Ulcerated lesion
- Exophytic mass
- Abnormal or malodorous vaginal discharge
- Vaginal bleeding
- Asymptomatic (~20%)
- Pelvic pain in advanced cases

DIAGNOSIS

- Complete pelvic examination and biopsy of suspicious lesion.
  - A lesion may be easily missed because the blades of a speculum can obscure visualization of the entire vagina; use of a plastic lighted speculum can assist with this evaluation. If a metal speculum is used, the vaginal walls should be inspected as the speculum is removed.
  - The posterior wall of the upper third of the vagina is the most common location of a vaginal cancer.

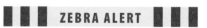

ZEBRA ALERT

Clear cell adenocarcinoma of the vagina may develop in young women as a result of in utero DES exposure.

TABLE 28-2. Staging of Vaginal Cancer (Clinical Staging System) Stage

I: Limited to vaginal mucosa
II: Beyond mucosa but not involving pelvic wall
III: Pelvic wall involvement
IV: Involvement of bladder, rectum, or distant mets

STAGING

See Table 28-2. Vaginal cancer is **clinically** staged. Clinical staging is based on physical exam, biopsies, cystoscopy, proctoscopy, and chest and skeletal X-rays. The stage of tumor is the most important predictor of prognosis.

TREATMENT

- Treatment is based on the size and extent of the lesion, clinical stage, status of lymph nodes, and histologic type of the lesion.
    - **Stage I:** Surgical resection ± radiation.
    - **Stages II–IV:** Often not candidates for surgery due to extensive disease. Chemoradiation with concurrent use of radiation with chemotherapy (usually fluorouracil or cisplatin).

CHAPTER 29

Vulvar Disorders

Inflammatory Vulvar Skin Disorders

Vulvar skin disorders associated with inflammation include contact dermatitis, lichen simplex chronicus (LSC), lichen sclerosus (LS), and lichen planus (LP). They, along with other vulvar dermatologic conditions, range from isolated local findings to systemic illnesses. They all typically present with vulvar itching and burning. A good understanding of the vulvar anatomy will help to identify these disorders. Visible lesions must be biopsied to rule out vulvar squamous intraepithelial lesions (SIL) or malignancy.

 A 60-year-old G1P1 patient reports vulvar itching. She has a history of LS that previously responded well to topical high potency steroids. On exam, she has a raised, white lesion on her vulva. What is the best next step in the management of this patient? Is this patient at ↑ risk for malignancy? What microscopic changes contribute to the white appearance?
Answer: The next step in diagnosis is a punch biopsy. An ↑ risk of vulvar carcinoma is associated with LP and LS. The white appearance is secondary to lichenification.

CONTACT DERMATITIS

- Nonscarring inflammatory reaction that may present at any age.
- Very common.
- Most common symptom is chronic itching or burning.
- May be initiated by contact with irritants such as sweat, urine, or topical products such as cleansers and fragrances.

LICHEN SIMPLEX CHRONICUS (LSC)

- Chronic, nonscarring inflammatory disorder that occurs primarily in adults.
- Most common symptom is chronic or intermittent intense itching (often at night) with vigorous scratching (classic history is "itch-scratch-itch" cycle).
- Lesions may be raised, white, and thickened, or may appear red and irritated due to scratching. Microscopic examination reveals acanthosis and hyperkeratosis.
- Commonly associated with a personal or family history of seasonal allergies, asthma, or eczema.

LICHEN SCLEROSUS (LS)

- Chronic, progressive, scarring dermatologic condition that affects both postmenopausal women and prepubertal girls.
- Affects anogenital skin and is characterized by white, atrophic papules that may coalesce into plaques and may extend to the perineum and around the anus in a classic "keyhole" pattern. It results in epidermal contracture which leads to loss of vulvar architecture such as obliteration/fusing of the labia minora, phimosis of the clitoral hood, and shrinkage of the perineum.
- Most common symptoms are pruritis, anal discomfort, dyspareunia/sexual dysfunction, and dysuria.
- Microscopic examination reveals epithelial thinning with a layer of collagen and inflammatory cells (see Figure 29-1). There is also loss of the rete ridges.

LICHEN PLANUS (LP)

- Scarring, inflammatory disorder of the skin that may also affect skin, nails, oral mucosa, and scalp.
- Uncommon condition that usually affects women 50–60 years of age.

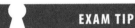

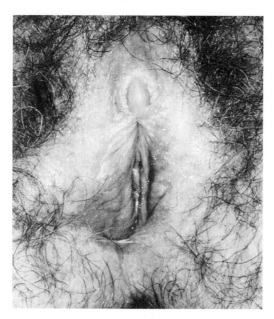

FIGURE 29-1. Vulvar lichen sclerosus. Notice the paper-thin appearance, bilateral distribution, and pale color, with a loss of architecture. In severe cases, contractures and fissures can occur in the posterior fourchette. (Reproduced, with permission, from DeCherney AH, Nathan L, Goodwin TM, et al. *Current Diagnosis & Treatment: Obstetrics & Gynecology.* 10th ed. New York: McGraw-Hill;2007:617.)

- May present with shiny, purple erosive or papular lesions on the inner vulva and/or vagina.
- Most common symptoms are vulvar pain, pruritis, burning, and dyspareunia.
- Often associated with significant architectural distortion such as obliteration of labia minora and narrowing of the introitus, as well as adhesions causing shortening of the vagina.
- May present as vulvo-vaginal-gingival syndrome.

WARD TIP

Up to 70% of patients with LP will have oral involvement.

DIAGNOSIS OF VULVAR SKIN DISORDERS

At least a 5-mm punch biopsy of most abnormal or atypical part of the lesion(s).

TREATMENT OF INFLAMMATORY/PRURITIC VULVAR SKIN DISORDERS

- Educate patients about vulvar skin care and hygiene.
- High potency steroid ointment (i.e., clobetasol propionate 0.05%) and oral steroids may be used in severe cases.
- Pruritis may be treated with oral antihistamines: Sedating options at night (i.e., diphenhydramine), and nonsedating options during daytime (i.e., cetirizine). Avoid topical antipruritic medications as they may contribute to allergic contact dermatitis.

PAGET DISEASE OF THE VULVA

A 65-year-old G2P2 patient presents with a 2-year history of an itchy genital lesion. She has been menopausal for 10 years. On exam, there is a red eczematous lesion on her vulva. A biopsy of the lesion demonstrates Paget disease. What is the next step in management?

Answer: Solitary lesions need wide local excision down to subcutaneous fat. Paget disease of the vulva may be associated with underlying invasive adenocarcinomas (4–17%). Patients with Paget disease are also more likely to have a noncontiguous cancer (20–30%) and should be evaluated for a synchronous neoplasm.

PRESENTATION

- Pruritis is the most common presenting symptom (70%).
- May present with a well-demarcated, erythematous, eczematoid lesion that is often multifocal. Can be located anywhere on the vulva, mons, perineum, perianal area, or inner thigh.
- Most commonly found in postmenopausal white females.
- May be associated with adenocarcinoma within the lesion or beneath the surface of the lesion (~25%), or with other synchronous carcinomas (~25%), i.e., adenocarcinoma of the gastrointestinal (GI) tract or breast.

DIAGNOSIS

Direct biopsy of the lesion. Microscopic examination will reveal Paget cells (large cells with clear cytoplasm (clear halo) and eccentric, hyperchromic nuclei).

TREATMENT

- If solitary lesion without synchronous malignancy: Wide local excision down to subcutaneous fat with a 2-cm margin.
- Local recurrences are common after treatment (>50%), so long-term follow-up is warranted.

FOLLOW-UP

Patients with Paget disease of the vulva will need long-term follow-up due to the risk of recurrence and of noncontiguous carcinoma. Patients should be followed annually with:

- Breast exam and appropriate breast cancer screening
- Vulvar exam with low threshold for biopsy
- Cytologic evaluation of the cervix
- Screening for GI malignancy (i.e., colorectal) and tumors at other sites (i.e., lung, ovary, pancreas)

Psoriasis

- A common dermatologic condition characterized by sharply demarcated red plaques covered by silver scales.
- Commonly occurs over the knees and/or elbows, and lesions can also be found on the vulva and gluteal cleft in up to 75% of patients.
- The most common presenting symptom is pruritus, and there may also be pain, burning, and dyspareunia.

DIAGNOSIS

- Clinical diagnosis based on examination alone is acceptable if similar characteristic lesions are present elsewhere on the body.
- Biopsy is required for definitive diagnosis.

WARD TIP

All new vulvar lesions, whether symptomatic or asymptomatic, require biopsy.

TREATMENT

- Topical steroid ointment—goal is to decrease itching and scratching/rubbing.
- Topical vitamin D analogs (creams and ointments).

Persistent Vulvar Pain

- A common, complex gynecologic condition that may be caused by a specific disorder or may be idiopathic.
  - Vulvar pain initiated by a specific disorder may be due to infectious, inflammatory, neoplastic, neurologic, traumatic, iatrogenic, or hormonal causes.

- Vulvodynia is idiopathic vulvar pain of at least 3 months duration without a clear identifiable cause.
- Most common signs and symptoms include vulvar pain, dyspareunia, tenderness, and erythema.

DIAGNOSIS

- A thorough history of the pain is required (inquire whether it is generalized, localized, provoked, spontaneous, timing, duration, prior treatments).
- A thorough pelvic exam and musculoskeletal exam should be done, and infection or other possible sources of pain should be ruled out. Vulvodynia is a diagnosis of exclusion.
- Cotton swab test: Lightly touch the vulvar vestibule with a cotton-tipped applicator. The diagnosis is made by identifying areas of pain and classifying as mild, moderate, or severe.
- Other possible diagnostic tests include vulvar biopsy and/or fungal culture to rule out other causes of vulvar pain.

TREATMENT

- A multidisciplinary, individualized approach is necessary. The care team may include sexual counselors/clinical psychologists, physical therapists, and pain management specialists.
- Vulvar care measures to minimize vulvar irritation, such as wearing 100% cotton undergarments, avoiding vulvar irritants (dyes, perfumes, etc.), and cleaning the vulva with water only.
- Biofeedback and pelvic floor physical therapy.
- Medications:
  - Tricyclic antidepressants.
  - Anticonvulsants, i.e., gabapentin.
  - Topical treatment, i.e., lidocaine ointment (extended use or prior to intercourse), or topical estrogen cream.
  - Intralesional treatment.
  - Pudendal nerve blocks and botulinum toxin.
- Surgery: If unresponsive to nonsurgical treatment and the pain is localized to the vestibule, vestibulectomy is an option, though with risk of recurrence.

WARD TIP

The Bartholin glands (also known as vestibular glands) are located at the 5 and 7 o'clock positions of the inferolateral vestibule (area between the labia minora just below the hymenal ring).

Vulvar Cysts

BARTHOLIN'S CYST/ABSCESS

A 35-year-old G2P2 patient presents for evaluation of a tender nodule noted 3 days ago at the opening of the vagina, on the right. The patient reports some discomfort during intercourse several days ago, but didn't discover the nodule until yesterday morning, and reports that it is becoming increasingly uncomfortable to walk. What is the most likely diagnosis?
Answer: Bartholin abscess.

- The Bartholin glands are two pea-sized glands, located at the 4 o'clock and 8 o'clock positions in the vulva whose main function is to secrete mucous to provide vaginal and vulvar lubrication.
- A normal Bartholin gland is not palpable.
- A Bartholin cyst occurs when the orifice of the Bartholin duct becomes obstructed and mucous produced by the gland accumulates. It is usually sterile.

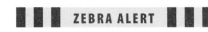

EXAM TIP

A Bartholin abscess is usually polymicrobial in origin, and the most common organisms include *Escherichia coli*, *Staphylococcus aureus*, *Enterococcus*, and Group B *Streptococcus*.

WARD TIP

Vulvar sebaceous cysts have been reported in association with female genital cutting (circumcision).

- A Bartholin abscess may occur when the Bartholin cyst becomes infected and forms an abscess.
- Both Bartholin cysts and abscesses can cause pain and require treatment.
- A Bartholin cyst may be asymptomatic.

DIAGNOSIS

- Vulvar examination with visual inspection and palpation of the Bartholin gland; cysts and abscesses are usually unilateral.
  - A Bartholin cyst usually presents as a nontender, soft, cystic mass.
  - A Bartholin abscess may be tender, warm, and fluctuant on exam with surrounding erythema and edema.
- Patients with Bartholin cysts or abscesses are usually afebrile.

TREATMENT

- If a cyst is asymptomatic, it may be monitored conservatively. However, if the patient is over age 40, or if there are findings suggestive of malignancy, an excisional biopsy should be performed to exclude malignancy.
- Abscesses require incision and drainage, with either of the following:
  - Marsupialization (suturing the edges of the incised cyst to prevent re-occlusion).
  - Word catheter (a catheter with an inflatable tip left in the gland for 10–14 days to aid healing via an epithelialized tract that allows drainage).
- The purulent material should be cultured for aerobic bacteria; although typically polymicrobial in nature, Bartholin abscesses may also be associated with community-acquired methicillin-resistant *Staphylococcus aureus* (MRSA).
- Inflammatory symptoms generally arise from infection and can be treated with antibiotics and sitz baths.
- Definitive treatment with excision of the entire Bartholin gland and duct may be done if less invasive methods have failed.

SEBACEOUS CYSTS (EPIDERMOID CYST)

- The most common vulvar cyst.
- Presents as a subcutaneous, keratin-filled cyst originating from a hair follicle, caused by occlusion of pilosebaceous ducts.
- Exam may show a palpable, nontender, smooth mass. If expressed, a yellow, thick, cheesy material is extruded.
- Usually asymptomatic and most cysts do not require treatment.
- If it becomes infected, it can be treated with incision and drainage.

HIDRADENITIS SUPPURATIVA (HS)

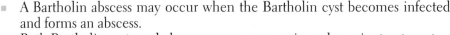

A 30-year-old G3P3 Black patient presents with painful inflammation described as "boils" of her bikini line. She is afebrile. On exam, there are draining sinuses and scarring of the skin. What is the most likely diagnosis?

Answer: Hidradenitis suppurativa (HS) is most commonly found in intertriginous areas of the body, such as the mons pubis, the genitocrural folds, buttocks, and axillae. Women are four times more likely than men to develop HS.

- This condition is a chronic inflammatory follicular occlusive disease involving the follicular portion of the folliculopilosebaceous unit.
- Most commonly presents in reproductive-age women, and in the United States, the prevalence is disproportionally high among Black women.

- The clinical presentation of HS varies from recurrent painful inflamed nodules/abscesses to draining sinus tracts and bands of severe scar/pit formation.

DIAGNOSIS

- History and physical exam; biopsy may be helpful if the diagnosis is uncertain.

TREATMENT

- Patient education and support is an important part of treatment, as HS can be psychologically distressing.
- Recommend smoking cessation and weight loss if indicated. (HS is more common in patients who smoke cigarettes and are obese.)
- Topical treatment: Topical clindamycin reduces inflammatory lesions.
- Oral antibiotics i.e., tetracyclines are indicated if topical therapy does not achieve disease control.
- Anti-androgenic agents such as oral contraceptive pills, spironolactone, or finasteride (exclude pregnancy first).
- Acute lesions that are symptomatic may be treated with intralesional injection of corticosteroids.
- Severe refractory cases can be treated by excision of the infected skin.

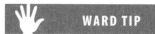

WARD TIP

Excision of refractory HS can be disfiguring and typically requires a long recovery period.

OTHER RARE CYSTS

- **Cyst of canal of Nuck:** A hydrocele (persistent processus vaginalis); contains peritoneal fluid.
- **Skene's duct cyst:**
  - Very rare and very small.
  - Ductal occlusion and cystic formation of the Skene's (paraurethral) glands occur, and patients have discomfort.
- Treatment:
  - If asymptomatic, supportive treatment.
  - If symptomatic, excision of cyst.

NOTES

Gestational Trophoblastic Disease

EXAM TIP

All genetic material in complete mole is paternal (no maternal DNA).

Gestational trophoblastic disease (GTD) is a general term that encompasses a spectrum of interrelated conditions originating from abnormal proliferation of trophoblasts of the placenta. These include complete and partial hydatidiform moles. Gestational trophoblastic neoplasia (GTN) are gestational malignant neoplasms that include invasive moles, gestational choriocarcinomas, and placental site trophoblastic tumors (PSTT).

Hydatidiform Mole

COMPLETE MOLE

A 22-year-old G1P0 patient at 12 weeks' gestation presents with vaginal bleeding and an enlarged-for-dates uterus on exam. Her blood pressure is 160/90, there are no fetal heart sounds, and an ultrasound shows a "snowstorm pattern." After dilation and curettage (D&C), what would most likely be the karyotype?
Answer: 46,XX in a complete mole.

EXAM TIP

DNA of a partial mole is both maternal and paternal triploidy.

ZEBRA ALERT

Because of the very high β-HCG levels with molar pregnancy, women may present with hyperemesis gravidarum or symptoms of thyroid storm. (See Table 30-1)

A complete mole forms when a maternal ova devoid of deoxyribonucleic acid (DNA) "empty egg" is "fertilized" by the sperm. Note—no fetus is present in a complete mole. Diagnosis is made with ultrasound (Figure 30-1). The ultrasound appearance is described as a snowstorm. Grossly, the mole looks "grapelike," as multiple connected cystic structures (Figure 30-2).

COMPLETE MOLE KARYOTYPE

- Most have karyotype 46,XX, resulting from sperm penetration and subsequent DNA replication.
- Some have 46,XY, believed to be due to two paternal sperms simultaneously penetrating the ova.
- The β-human chorionic gonadotropin (β-HCG) value may be higher as compared to a partial mole and both are WAY higher than a normal pregnancy.

RISK FACTORS

- Maternal age <15 or >35
- History of a prior molar pregnancy

EXAM TIP

The treatment for partial and complete molar pregnancy is prompt removal of intrauterine contents with D&C.

EXAM TIP

Partial mole usually contains a fetus or fetal parts.

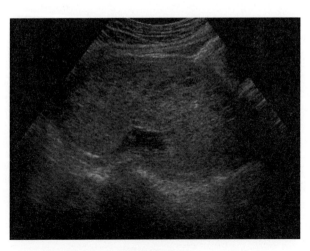

FIGURE 30-1. Complete mole on ultrasonography.

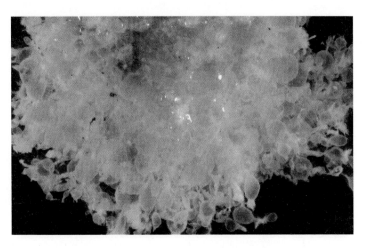

FIGURE 30-2.   **Gross pathology specimen for a complete mole.**

PARTIAL MOLE

- A mole with a fetus or fetal parts (see Figure 30-3).
- Women with partial (incomplete) molar pregnancies tend to present later than those with complete moles.

KARYOTYPE

Usually 69,XXY and contains both maternal and paternal DNA.

EPIDEMIOLOGY

One in 50,000 pregnancies in the United States.

INVASIVE MOLE

- A variant of hydatidiform mole that invades the myometrium or blood vessels.
- It is by definition a malignant GTN and can spread to extrauterine sites. Note that 20% of patients will develop malignant sequelae after a complete hydatidiform mole, and 1–5% following a partial mole.
- The treatment involves complete metastatic workup and appropriate malignant/metastatic therapy (see section on Metastatic Workup). A D&C is not recommended for treatment, because of the increased risk of uterine perforation. Chemotherapy is the usual treatment.

HISTOLOGY OF HYDATIDIFORM MOLE

- Trophoblastic proliferation
- Hydropic degeneration (swollen villi)
- Lack/scarcity of blood vessels

SIGNS AND SYMPTOMS

- The most common symptom is abnormal painless bleeding in the first trimester.
- Passage of villi (vesicles that look like grapes).
- Preeclampsia <20 weeks.
- Hyperemesis gravidarum or thyroid storm.
- Uterus large for gestational age.
- High hCG level for gestational age.

EXAM TIP

A young woman who passes grapelike vesicles from her vagina should be suspected of having a hydatidiform mole.

WARD TIP

The development of preeclampsia before 20 weeks is suspicious for the presence of a molar pregnancy.

WARD TIP

GTD secretes hCG, lactogen, and thyrotropin.

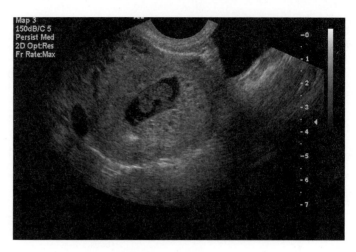

FIGURE 30-3. Partial mole on ultrasonography.

TABLE 30-1. Complications of Untreated Molar Pregnancy

COMPLICATION	PATHOLOGY
Hyperemesis gravidarum	Really high HCG
Thyroid storm/hyperthyroidism	Cross reactivity of β-subunit of TSH-R with HCG
Preeclampsia	Very rare, unknown

hCG, human chorionic gonadotropin; TSH, thyroid-stimulating hormone.

DIAGNOSIS

- Elevated hCG (usually >100,000 mIU/mL) and 15–25% theca lutein cysts visualized (secondary to the high β-HCG levels)
- Absence of fetal heartbeat
- Ultrasound: "Snowstorm" pattern
- Pathologic specimen: Grapelike vesicles
- Histologic specimen

TREATMENT OF COMPLETE OR PARTIAL MOLES

- D&C to evacuate and terminate pregnancy.
- hCG monitoring: Weekly until negative for 3 weeks, then monthly until negative for 6 months.
  - If the hCG level rises, does not fall, or falls and then rises again, the molar pregnancy is considered malignant GTN.
- Contraception should be used during the follow-up period. A rising hCG should prompt evaluation for a new pregnancy versus GTN.
- Administer RhoGAM for RH negative patients.

METASTATIC WORKUP

Perform if concerned for malignant GTN
- GTN is clinically staged.
- CXR, computed tomography (CT) of brain, lung, liver, and kidneys.
- Labs: CBC, comprehensive metabolic panel, clotting studies, and blood type, Rh, and antibody screen.

INVASIVE MOLE

Develops after 15–20% of complete moles and 1–5% of partial moles

TREATMENT OF INVASIVE MOLE

- Chemotherapy with methotrexate or actinomycin D (as many cycles as needed until hCG levels return to negative).
- Treatment based on stage and score (Tables 30-2 and 30-3, and section below on treatment of choriocarcinoma—it is the same).
- These tumors are very sensitive to chemotherapy, and the prognosis is generally excellent.
- If childbearing complete, may treat with hysterectomy ± chemotherapy (fewer cycles needed).

RECURRENCE RISK

1–2% percent in subsequent pregnancy.

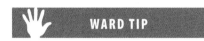

WARD TIP

Staging, risk scoring, and treatment are the same for invasive mole and choriocarcinoma.

TABLE 30-2.   FIGO Prognostic Scoring System (2009)

	SCORE			
RISK FACTOR	0	1	2	4
Age (years)	≤40	>40	–	–
Pregnancy	Hydatidiform mole	Abortion	Term	–
Interval from pregnancy event to treatment (in months)	<4	4–6	7–12	>12
hCG (pre-treatment) (IU/mL)	<1000	1000–10,000	10,000–100,000	>100,000
Largest tumor size uterus (in cm)	<3	3–4	>5	–
Site of metastases	Lung	Spleen Kidney	GI	Brain Liver
Number of metastasis	0	1–4	5–8	>8
Prior chemotherapy agent	–	–	Single	≥2 drugs

Scores are added to give the prognostic score.

GI, gastrointestinal; hCG, human chorionic gonadotropin.

TABLE 30-3.   FIGO Staging of GTN

Stage I	Disease confined to uterus
Stage II	GTN extends beyond uterus but limited to genital structures (ovary, vagina)
Stage III	GTN in lungs with or without genital tract involved
Stage IV	All other metastatic sites

GTN, Gestational trophoblastic neoplasia.

TABLE 30-4. Treatment According to Score/Prognostic Factors (World Health Organization)

Low risk (score <7)	Single-agent therapy (methotrexate)
High risk (score >7)	Multiple-agent therapy (EMACO therapy—etoposide, MAC, and vincristine)

Choriocarcinoma

May occur after a molar or non-molar and normal pregnancy. Most aggressive type of GTN.

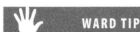
A 31-year-old G2P2 patient, 5 months after a vaginal delivery, reports to the emergency department with nausea, vomiting, and abnormal vaginal bleeding. Her pregnancy test is positive. A D&C was performed and the histology revealed sheets of trophoblastic cells and no chorionic villi. What is her diagnosis? What is the next step in management?
Answer: Choriocarcinoma. The workup includes evaluation for metastatic disease.

HISTOPATHOLOGY

Choriocarcinoma has characteristic sheets of trophoblasts with extensive hemorrhage and necrosis, and unlike the hydatidiform mole, choriocarcinoma has no villi. These tumors metastasize early. Common sites for metastasis include vagina, lung, liver, and brain.

EPIDEMIOLOGY

Incidence is about 1 in 16,000 pregnancies.

DIAGNOSIS—AFTER ANY PREGNANCY (MOLAR, MISCARRIAGE, OR NORMAL)

- Increasing or plateauing β-hCG levels.
- Absence of fetal heartbeat.
- Uterine size/date discrepancy.
- Specimen (sheets of trophoblasts, no chorionic villi).
- A full metastatic workup is required when choriocarcinoma is diagnosed.

TREATMENT AND PROGNOSIS OF CHORIOCARCINOMA

- Chemotherapy: Methotrexate or actinomycin D (as many cycles as needed until hCG levels return to negative).
- If childbearing complete, hysterectomy + chemotherapy (fewer cycles needed).
- Remission rate is near 100%.
- Treatment is determined by the patient's risk (high or low) or prognostic score. (See Table 30-4.)
- Low-risk patients (score <7) can be treated with single-agent chemotherapy.
- High-risk patients (score >7) can be treated with multiagent chemotherapy, as they have a higher chance of being resistant to single-agent chemo.
- Chemotherapy is continued until after the hCG levels are negative. hCG levels are monitored for 1 year after normalization. All patients are placed on reliable contraception during this time of monitoring.
- Serial β-hCGs every 2 weeks until negative; then every 3 months, then monthly for 1 year. Give 1–2 additional cycles after first negative β-hCG.
- Risk of recurrence: <1%.

WARD TIP

Nonmetastatic choriocarcinoma has almost a 100% remission rate following chemotherapy.

EXAM TIP

Sheets of trophoblasts = Choriocarcinoma

Placental Site Trophoblastic Tumor (PSTT)

- A rare form of GTD.
- Can develop several months to years after the antecedent pregnancy.
- Characterized by infiltration of the myometrium by intermediate trophoblasts, which stain positive for human placental lactogen. There are no chorionic villi present.
- Unlike other GTDs, hCG is only slightly elevated.

TREATMENT

- Hysterectomy plus multiagent chemotherapy.
- Prognosis is poor if there is tumor recurrence or metastasis.
- Treatment based on FIGO staging alone (Tables 30-2 and 30-4).
- World Health Organization (WHO) risk score is not helpful in PSTT.

NOTES

CHAPTER 31

Sexually Transmitted Infections and Vaginitis

Sexually transmitted infections (STIs), also known as venereal diseases or sexually transmitted diseases (STDs), are a major source of morbidity. The group includes bacteria, viruses, parasites, and protozoan infections that are transmitted by close contact. Transmission occurs via mucous membranes of the vulva, vagina, penis, rectum, mouth, throat, respiratory tract, or eyes.

WARD TIP

Rarely is a single organism responsible for PID, but always think of chlamydia and gonorrhea first (these are most common).

WARD TIP

Requirement for a clinical diagnosis of PID:
1. Lower abdominal or pelvic pain
2. Adnexal, uterine, or cervical motion tenderness on exam

WARD TIP

Remember, any reproductive-aged (approximately 15–55 years) female who presents with abdominal or pelvic pain should always get a urine pregnancy test.

WARD TIP

Positive lab tests are not necessary for diagnosis. PID is a *clinical* diagnosis.

Pelvic Inflammatory Disease (PID)

 A sexually active 21-year-old G1P1 patient presents with a 10-day history of lower abdominal pain and vaginal discharge. The patient also reports nausea and vomiting. Her temperature is 101.4°F (38.6°C). Examination demonstrates cervical motion tenderness, uterine tenderness, and bilateral adnexal tenderness. She is diagnosed with PID. What is the most appropriate treatment for this condition?

Answer: Inpatient cefoxitin/cefotetan + doxycycline. Criteria for hospital admission include vomiting and fever.

DEFINITION

Inflammation of the female upper genital tract (uterus, tubes, ovaries, ligaments) caused by ascending infection from the vagina and cervix. PID may lead to tubal scarring and an increased risk of ectopic pregnancy and/or infertility. Each year approximately 1 million patients in the United States experience an episode of symptomatic PID. PID affects 10% of female individuals in reproductive years.

COMMON CAUSATIVE ORGANISMS
- *Neisseria gonorrhoeae.*
- *Chlamydia trachomatis.*
- *Mycoplasma genitalium.*
- *Gardnerella vaginalis, Peptostreptococcus, Bacteroides, Escherichia coli,* and *Streptococcus.*
- Most PID infections are polymicrobial.

DIAGNOSIS
Physical Exam
- Lower abdominal or pelvic pain.
- Adnexal, uterine, or cervical motion tenderness on exam.
- Other findings may support the diagnosis:
  - Oral temperature >101°F (38.3°C).
  - Purulent cervical or vaginal discharge.
- It should also be noted that PID can be asymptomatic or subclinical. In these cases, PID sequelae (adhesions or hydrosalpinx) are most often identified later during evaluation for infertility or abdominal surgery for other indications.

Additional Testing That Supports Diagnosis
- Gram stain of discharge with gram-negative diplococci.
- Presence of abundant white blood cells (WBCs) on microscopy of vaginal secretions.
- Pelvic abscess (i.e., tubo-ovarian abscess or TOA).
- Elevated WBC count.
- Culture evidence of *N. gonorrhoeae* or *C. trachomatis.*
- **Laparoscopy**
  - Not often performed to diagnose PID, but may be helpful in patients who do not respond to antibiotic therapy, or in whom the diagnosis is not clear and other diagnoses need to be excluded (i.e., appendicitis).

- Reveals pus draining from the fallopian tubes, edema, adhesions, purulent drainage in the cul-de-sac.
- Ten percent of patients with acute PID will develop perihepatic inflammation, known as ***Fitz–Hugh–Curtis syndrome***. "Violin string" adhesions can be seen at the liver capsule on laparoscopy with this syndrome. Often seen months to years later during laparoscopy for other indications.

RISK FACTORS

- Age <25 years
- Multiple sexual partners
- STI in the partner
- Unprotected intercourse
- History of STI or PID

CRITERIA FOR HOSPITALIZATION

- Peritonitis or surgical emergency cannot be excluded.
- Gastrointestinal (GI) symptoms, i.e., nausea, vomiting (inability to take oral meds).
- Abscess (TOA or pelvic).
- Uncertain diagnosis.
- Outpatient treatment failure.
- Immunocompromised.
- High fever >100.9°F (38.3°C), severe pain.

TREATMENT

- Inpatient:
  - Cefoxitin/cefotetan + doxycycline.
  - Clindamycin + gentamicin.
- **Outpatient:**
  - Ceftriaxone + doxycycline ± metronidazole.
  - Cefoxitin + probenecid + doxycycline ± metronidazole.
  - Sexual partners should also be treated empirically.

Optimal treatment duration is not well studied; most experts suggest total treatment duration is 14 days.

- **Adjunctive care:**
  - Refrain from intercourse until completed antibiotic therapy.
  - Screen for other STIs.
  - Vaccinate against hepatitis B and HPV if the patient has not been vaccinated previously.

Gonorrhea

A 19-year-old G2P2 patient presents with known exposure to gonorrhea 7 days prior. The patient reports an ↑ in vaginal discharge for the past day, but denies any other symptoms. On physical exam, you notice minimal vaginal discharge. You obtain a nucleic acid amplification test (NAAT) for gonorrhea. What is the next step?

Answer: Treat the patient empirically. Since the patient notes to a recent exposure to gonorrhea, do not wait for the result to come back. In female patients, asymptomatic infection is common and symptoms may not begin until 7–21 days after exposure.

Gonorrhea can cause infection of the urethra, cervix, pharynx, or anal canal. It is caused by the gram-negative diplococcus, *N. gonorrhoeae*. It is the second

WARD TIP

Intrauterine devices (IUDs) do NOT increase the risk of PID.

WARD TIP

Criteria for hospitalization for PID:
GI symptoms
Uncertain diagnosis
Peritonitis
Abscess

WARD TIP

Gonorrhea is often asymptomatic and therefore may go untreated, causing complications of adhesions/inflammation such as ectopic pregnancy, chronic pelvic pain, and infertility.

EXAM TIP

In what media does *Neisseria* gonorrhea grow?
Thayer-Martin in CO_2-enriched environment.

most common STI and can lead to PID, chronic pelvic pain, ectopic pregnancy, and infertility. Of note, patients are frequently co-infected with *C. trachomatis*. The Centers for Disease Control and Prevention (CDC) recommends annual screening for gonorrhea in all female patients age <25 or older with risk factors.

PRESENTATION

- Asymptomatic (most common, especially in female patients)
- Dysuria
- Cervicitis
- Vaginal discharge

DIAGNOSIS

- NAAT is the preferred diagnostic test
- Culture in Thayer-Martin agar
- Nucleic acid hybridization probes

TREATMENT

- Ceftriaxone 500 mg IM (intramuscular) single dose plus azithromycin 1 g PO (by mouth) single dose.
- If severe cephalosporin allergy, treat with azithromycin 2 g PO single dose and test of cure in 1 week.
- Sexual partners should also be treated.

Chlamydia

A 16-year-old G0P0 patient presents with ↑ vaginal discharge 5 days after unprotected sexual intercourse. On physical exam, a mucopurulent cervicitis is noticed. *C. trachomatis* infection is suspected. What complications are prevented by treating this patient?
Answer: Complications of a *Chlamydia* infection include PID, Fitz–Hugh–Curtis syndrome, ectopic pregnancy, infertility, pelvic adhesions, and chronic pelvic pain.

Chlamydia is an infection of the genitourinary (GU) tract, GI tract, conjunctiva, or nasopharynx, caused by *C. trachomatis*, an obligate intracellular bacteria. It is the most common STI. Of note, the CDC recommends annual screening for chlamydia in all female patients age <25 or older female patients with risk factors. Sequelae of chlamydia include PID, Fitz-Hugh–Curtis syndrome, chronic pelvic pain, ectopic pregnancy, and infertility.

PRESENTATION

- Asymptomatic (most common, especially in female patients)
- Mucopurulent vaginal discharge
- Cervicitis
- Urethritis
- Conjunctivitis

DIAGNOSIS

- NAAT of urine or vaginal/cervical swab (preferred method)
- Antigen testing (requires swab of cervix)

TABLE 31-1. Genital Ulcers

Causative Agent	Ulcer/Lesion Qualities	Other Associated Findings
Lymphogranuloma Venereum (*Chlamydia trachomatis serotype L1-3*)	Painless papules	Palpable inguinal lymph nodes
Syphilis	Painless hard chancre	Often none at that time
Herpes simplex virus 1 or 2	Painful ulcer with erythematous base	Malaise, myalgia, vulvar burning
Chancroid (*Haemophilus ducreyi*)	Soft papule that become a painful ulcer, nonindurated base, ragged/irregular edges (usually 1–3 ulcers)	Palpable inguinal nodes
Granuloma inguinale	Ulcer is rolled, elevated and round	

TREATMENT

- Doxycycline 100 mg twice per day (BID) × 7 days or azithromycin 1 g PO single dose.
- Sexual partners should be treated.

LYMPHOGRANULOMA VENEREUM

Serotypes L1–L3 of *C. trachomatis* cause **lymphogranuloma venereum**. Most commonly found in tropical areas. This is a systemic disease that can present in several forms:

- Primary lesion: **Painless** papule on genitals. (Table 31-1 describes the differential diagnosis for genital ulcers.)
- Secondary stage: Inguinal lymphadenitis with fever, malaise, and loss of appetite.
- Tertiary stage: Rectovaginal fistulas, rectal strictures.

DIAGNOSIS

Nucleated amplification testing of the cervix [NAAT, PCR (polymerase chain reaction)].

TREATMENT

Lymphogranuloma venereum: Doxycycline 100 mg BID × 21 days.

Syphilis

A 22-year-old G1P1 patient has a positive rapid plasma reagin (RPR) with a titer of 1:4. What is the next step in the workup?

Answer: Order a specific serologic test, such as the fluorescent treponemal antibody absorption test (FTA-ABS) or microhemagglutination test for *Treponema pallidum* (MHA-TP). A false-positive RPR can be seen with certain viral infections (Epstein-Barr, hepatitis, varicella, measles), lymphoma, tuberculosis, malaria, endocarditis, connective tissue disease, and pregnancy.

 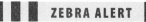 **ZEBRA ALERT**

Reiter Syndrome (due to chlamydial infection)
Classic triad of conjunctivitis, urethritis, and reactive arthritis: Can't see, can't pee, can't climb a tree.

 WARD TIP

Use azithromycin rather than doxycycline for pregnant patients with chlamydia. Doxycyline may cause discoloration of the fetal teeth if used during pregnancy (Table 31-1).

TABLE 31-2.   Stages of Syphilis

	PRIMARY	SECONDARY	LATENT	TERTIARY
Presentation	**Painless hard chancre** of the vulva, vagina, or cervix (or even anus, tongue, or fingers)	▪ **Generalized rash** (often macular or papular on the palms and soles of the feet) ▪ Condyloma lata, mucous patches with lymphadenopathy ▪ Fever, malaise	▪ Asymptomatic disease with serologic proof of infection	▪ Granulomas of the skin and bones (gummas) ▪ Cardiovascular lesions (e.g., aortic aneurysms) ▪ Neurosyphilis (e.g., tabes dorsalis, paresis, and meningovascular disease)
Timing	Appears 1 month after exposure, heals after 1–2 months	▪ Appears 1–6 months after primary chancre, regresses after 1 month	▪ **Early latent:** If syphilis was acquired <1 year prior ▪ **Late latent:** If acquired >1 year prior	▪ Presents years later

WARD TIP

Syphilis is the most likely diagnosis for a patient with painless genital lesions who later develops a rash on the palms and soles.

WARD TIP

Penicillin G is the best treatment for syphilis.

ZEBRA ALERT

A Jarisch–Herxheimer reaction is an acute self-limited febrile reaction with headache, myalgias, rah, and hypotension caused by treponemal proteins released from dying spirochetes after 1–2 hours after treatment for syphilis.

WARD TIP

Screening tests for syphilis:
▪ RPR
▪ VDRL
Confirmatory tests for syphilis:
▪ FTA-ABS
▪ MHA-TP

Syphilis is an infection caused by the spirochete *T. pallidum*. Because it can present in so many ways, syphilis is known as the great imitator (Table 31-2).

DIAGNOSIS

▪ Syphilis cannot be cultured in vitro, so must be identified by direct visualization or serology.
▪ **Screening test: Nontreponemal tests** such as RPR or Venereal Disease Research Laboratory (VDRL) test. These are inexpensive and easy to perform, but are nonspecific and can give false-positive results for many conditions.
▪ **Diagnostic test: Treponemal tests** such as FTA-ABS and MHA-TP. These tests are more expensive and complex to perform, and are used to confirm a diagnosis when the RPR/VDRL is positive.
▪ Direct visualization of spirochetes on darkfield microscopy is an additional test available.

TREATMENT

▪ **Benzathine penicillin G** for all stages, but dosing regimen differs depending on stage.
▪ Doxycycline in penicillin allergic nonpregnant patients.
▪ Treatment during pregnancy is allergic to penicillin is desensitization followed by benzathine penicillin G. It crosses the placenta to prevent **congenital syphilis**.

Genital Herpes

Genital herpes is caused most commonly by herpes simplex virus type 2 (HSV-2), though 15% of cases are due to HSV-1. HSV is a deoxyribonucleic acid (DNA) virus. Eighty percent of adults have antibodies to HSV-2, most without history of infection.

A 17-year-old G1P1 patient presents with a 5-day history of vulvar pain and discomfort with urination. On physical exam, she has a large number of bilateral ulcerated lesions on the vulva. What lab tests should be obtained?
Answer: Viral culture of ulcerated lesions to diagnose HSV.

CASE DEFINITIONS AND PRESENTATION

Patients with herpes can be asymptomatic, but may present with the following:
- **Primary infection:** Malaise, myalgias, fever, vulvar burning, or vulvar pruritus, followed by **multiple painful genital vesicles** with an erythematous base that progress to painful ulcers, usually 1–3 weeks after exposure.
- **Recurrent infection:** Recurrence from viral stores in the sacral ganglia, resulting in a *milder version* of primary infection, including vesicles.
- **Nonprimary first episode:** This is defined as **initial infection by HSV-2** in the presence of *preexisting antibodies to HSV-1* or vice versa. The preexisting antibodies to HSV-1 can make the presentation of HSV-2 milder.

COMPLICATIONS

- Aseptic meningitis.
- Urinary retention.
- Radiculitis.
- RARE: Disseminated herpes, herpes hepatitis.
- Neonatal herpes can occur if the patient has active infection (i.e., lesions) during vaginal delivery. In utero infection is very rare.

DIAGNOSIS

- Gross examination of vulva for typical lesions.
- Tzanck (cytologic) test—multinucleated giant cells (low sensitivity/specificity).
- Viral cultures of fluid from an unroofed vesicle/ulcer (first-line method, but sensitivity is only 50%).
- PCR (can also detect asymptomatic viral shedding).
- Western blot assay for antibodies against HSV.

TREATMENT

Treatment for HSV is palliative and not curative.
- **Primary outbreak:** Acyclovir 400 mg thrice per day (TID) × 7–10 days; valacyclovir 1 g BID for 7–10 days.
- **Recurrent infection:** Acyclovir 400 mg TID × 5 days; valacyclovir 1 g QD for 5 days.
- **Suppressive therapy for recurrent outbreaks:** Acyclovir 400 mg BID or valacyclovir 1g once a day (QD) (use if patient has >6 episodes a year or severe outbreaks).
- **Pregnancy:** Suppressive therapy should begin at 36 weeks of pregnancy with acyclovir 400 mg TID or valacyclovir 500 mg BID. Primary and episodic treatment same as nonpregnant.
- A vaccine is under development.
- Famciclovir is another antiviral that is dosed less frequently and can be used in pregnancy.
- Suppressive therapy decreases the frequency of outbreaks AND decreases asymptomatic shedding to prevent transmission to discordant partner.

WARD TIP

Lupus may cause false-positive RPR results.

WARD TIP

Perform a viral culture on a painful vaginal/vulvar lesion. If the result is positive for genital herpes, treat with an antiviral medication. If the lesion is crusted over, need to unroof to get good sample.

EXAM TIP

Stress, illness, and immune deficiency are some factors that predispose to herpes recurrence.

WARD TIP

Always biopsy an undiagnosed suspicious lesion in order to obtain a definitive diagnosis.

Cesarean delivery is indicated for active herpes infection or presence of prodromal symptoms.

For pregnant patients with undetectable viral load, vertical transmission is very rare. If viral load is high, cesarean delivery is protective against vertical transmission.

Human Immunodeficiency Virus (HIV) and Acquired Immune Deficiency Syndrome (AIDS)

A 30-year-old G3P3 patient presents requesting STD screening, including HIV. What test for HIV should be ordered?

Answer: Fourth-generation HIV 1/2 immunoassay. If positive, HIV-1/HIV-2 antibody differentiation immunoassay should be ordered.

HIV is an ribonucleic acid (RNA) retrovirus that causes AIDS. The virus infects CD4 lymphocytes and other cells and causes ↓ cellular immunity. Transmission occurs in a variety of ways, but the highest risk is via exposure to blood (Table 31-3).

PRESENTATION

- **Initial infection:** Mononucleosis-like illness occurring weeks to months after exposure—fatigue, weight loss, lymphadenopathy, night sweats. This is followed by a long asymptomatic period lasting months to years.
- **AIDS:** Opportunistic infections, dementia, depression, Kaposi sarcoma, wasting (Table 31-3).

DIAGNOSIS

- **Fourth-generation combined antigen/antibody immunoassay.** If positive, a second confirmatory HIV-1/HIV-2 antibody differentiation immunoassay is performed. If the second test is negative or indeterminate, then HIV viral load testing (PCR) is performed.
- **If early or acute HIV is suspected** perform fourth-generation combined antigen/antibody immunoassay PLUS HIV viral load (PCR) testing at the same time in order to pick up early HIV infection.

TREATMENT

- CD4 T-cell counts and plasma HIV-RNA viral load are measured to monitor patient's response to therapy.
- Highly active antiretroviral therapy (HAART) is used. It consists of varying combinations of nucleoside/nucleotide reverse transcriptase inhibitors (NRTIs), non-nucleoside reverse transcriptase inhibitors (NNRTIs), and protease inhibitors (PIs), and integrase strand transfer inhibitors (INSTIs).

TABLE 31-3. **Risk Factors for HIV**

BLOOD-BORNE EXPOSURES*	SEXUAL EXPOSURES*	OTHER RISKS*
Blood transfusion	Receptive anal intercourse	Concurrent STIs
Needle sharing / injection drug use	Insertive anal intercourse	(especially syphilis and HSV)
	Receptive penile-vaginal intercourse	
Percutaneous needle stick	Insertive penile-vaginal intercourse	Vertical transmission
Mucous membrane exposure (splash to eye)	Receptive or insertive penile-oral intercourse	Unprotected intercourse

*Exposures are listed in order of highest risk to lowest risk.

HSV, herpes simplex virus; STI, sexually transmitted infection.

Human Papillomavirus (HPV)

Human papillomavirus (HPV) is associated with an increasing number of malignancies, as well as with genital warts. Subtypes 6 and 11 are associated with genital warts (condylomata acuminata). Subtypes 16, 18, 31, and 33 are associated with cervical and penile cancer and some oral cancers.

A 16-year-old G0 patient reports a painless growths on her vulva. On exam, numerous irregular, colored, raised lesions are noted. What test can help to make a definitive diagnosis?

Answer: Condylomata acuminata can be diagnosed on physical exam. Biopsy can be done to confirm.

PRESENTATION

Warts of various sizes (sometimes described as cauliflower-like papules) on the external genitalia, perineum, anus, vagina, and cervix. HPV may also be asymptomatic and identified on routine pap test screening. Warts may grow during pregnancy or be worse in individuals who are immunosuppressed.

DIAGNOSIS

- Warts are diagnosed on physical exam. Biopsy can be performed for confirmation.
- Cervical dysplasia caused by HPV infection is screened via Pap test.

TREATMENT FOR WARTS

- Treatment is based on either destructive therapy, immune mediated therapy, or surgical therapy.
  - Destructive therapies: Podophyllotoxin, trichloroacetic acid, 5-fluorouracil.
  - Immune-based therapies: Imiquimod cream, interferons.
  - Surgical therapies: Cryosurgery, laser ablation, excision.
- See Chapter 24 for management/treatment of cervical dysplasia.

HPV VACCINE

HPV vaccines can help with primary prevention of HPV infection. There are multiple HPV vaccines, all of which protect against the most common subtypes that lead to malignancy (16 and 18). Other version protect against more subtypes as well. In general, the vaccine is recommended at age 11–12 but can be given as early as age 9. The vaccine consists of 2 shots given at 0 and then 6–12 months later. Ideally, the vaccine should be given before sexual debut.

Chancroid

A 21-year-old G1P1 patient presents with a painful genital ulcer on the vulva. On exam, there is an irregular, deep, well-demarcated ulcer with a gray base, along with inguinal lymphadenopathy. The culture and gram stain returns as chancroid. What is the causative organism?

Answer: *Haemophilus ducreyi.* The diagnosis is confirmed with a culture in a special medium that requires special growth conditions.

PRESENTATION

- Chancroid presents as a soft papule on external genitalia that becomes a painful ulcer (unlike syphilis, which is hard and painless) with a gray, non-indurated, base with ragged edges.
- Inguinal lymphadenopathy, or bubo, also is possible.
- Incubation period is 1 week.

ETIOLOGY

H. ducreyi, a small gram-negative rod. Uncommon in the United States.

DIAGNOSIS

- Gram stain of ulcer or inguinal node aspirate showing gram-negative rods in chains—"school of fish." The sensitivity of gram stain is low.
- Culture is a more sensitive test, but the culture media required is not widely available.
- Screen for other STIs.

TREATMENT

Ceftriaxone, ciprofloxacin, or azithromycin

EXAM TIP

A gram stain showing "school of fish" or gram-negative rods in chains is consistent with chancroid.

Pediculosis Pubis (Crabs)

A 26-year-old G1P1 patient presents after unprotected sexual intercourse with intense genital pruritus. You suspect pediculosis pubis. How do you confirm the diagnosis?

Answer: By visualizing the crab louse *Phthirus pubis*, which has a crablike appearance under microscopy.

PRESENTATION

- Pruritus in the genital area from parasitic saliva of the organism.
- Ninety percent are commonly seen in the pubic hair, but it can involve any hair-bearing area of the body, i.e., axillae.
- The incubation period is 1 month.

ETIOLOGY

Blood-sucking parasitic crab louse, *P. pubis.* The louse is typically transmitted by close sexual contact, but can less commonly be transmitted by fomites such as clothing or towels.

DIAGNOSIS

- History of pruritus
- Visualization of crabs or nits

TREATMENT

- Pyrethrin, permethrin (Nix) cream, or lindane (Kwell) shampoo.
- Proper cleaning of clothing and bedding is also necessary.
- Lindane is contraindicated in pregnancy.
- Reevaluate after 7 days.

Vaginitis and Vaginosis

A 25-year-old G2P2 patient reports a large amount of foul-smelling vaginal discharge. On physical exam, a frothy, yellow-green discharge and multiple petechiae on the cervix are noted. The wet mount of the discharge shows motile protozoa. What is the treatment of choice?

Answer: Metronidazole is the treatment of choice for trichomoniasis. In addition to the classic frothy, yellow-green malodorous discharge, petechiae are often seen on the cervix during exam (commonly called *strawberry cervix*).

A 38-year-old G0 patient reports foul-smelling vaginal discharge every month after her menses ends. On physical exam, a malodorous gray-clear discharge is noted. The wet mount of the discharge shows clue cells. What is the treatment of choice?

Answer: Metronidazole is the treatment of choice for BV.

DEFINITION

Inflammation of the vagina and cervix, often resulting in ↑ discharge and/or pruritus, and usually caused by an identifiable microbe (see Table 31-4). The

TABLE 31-4. **Vaginitis**

	PHYSIOLOGIC (NORMAL)	**BACTERIAL VAGINOSIS**	**CANDIDIASIS**	**TRICHOMONIASIS**
Clinical complaints	None	**Malodorous discharge,** especially after menses and intercourse	**Pruritus, erythema, edema,** odorless discharge, dyspareunia	**Copious, frothy discharge,** malodorous, pruritus, urethritis
Quality of discharge	**Clear** or **white**, no odor, in vaginal vault	Homogenous gray or white, thin, sticky, adherent to vaginal walls	**White, "cottage cheese–like,"** adherent to vaginal walls	**Green** to **yellow**, sticky, "bubbly" or "frothy"
pH	3.8–4.2	**>4.5**	4–4.5	**>4.5**
Microscopic findings	Epithelial cells. Normal bacteria include mostly *Lactobacillus*, with *Streptococcus epidermidis, Streptococcus* species, as well as small amounts of colonic fora	Visualize with saline. **Clue cells** (epithelial cells with bacteria attached to their surface) Bacteria include *Gardnerella (Haemophilus)* and/or *Mycoplasma*	In 10% KOH. **Budding yeast** and Pseudohyphae	In saline. **Motile, fagellated, protozoa**
"Whiff" test	Negative (no smell)	Positive (fishy smell)	Negative	Positive or negative
Treatment		Oral or topical **metronidazole;** oral or topical **clindamycin**	Oral, topical, or suppository **imidazole** (or other various antifungals)	Oral **metronidazole** (Note: Metronidazole has potential disulfram-like reaction and has a metallic taste)
Treat sexual partners?		Not necessary	Not necessary	Yes

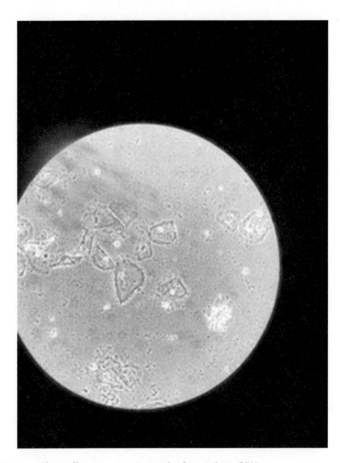

FIGURE 31-1. **Clue cells seen on wet prep in the setting of BV.**

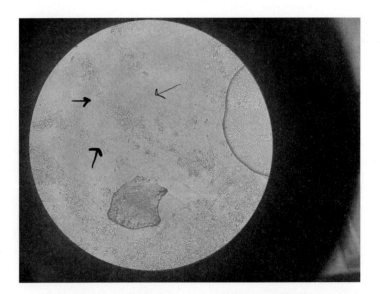

FIGURE 31-2. **Hyphae seen on wet prep in the setting of vaginal candida infection.**

EXAM TIP

If a patient has a "strawberry" appearance of the cervix or "frothy" discharge, what is the most likely diagnosis? *Trichomonas vaginitis*.

only vaginitis that is sexually transmitted is trichomoniasis. Bacterial vaginosis (BV) is due to a dysbiosis of normal vaginal flora with increased *Gardnerella* and decreased *Lactobacillus*. It is diagnosed with clue cells on a wet prep (Figure 31-1). Candidiasis is a vulvar or yeast infection, and usually presents with itching and thick white discharge, and hyphae are seen on wet prep (Figure 31-2).

ETIOLOGY

- **Antibiotics:** Destabilize the normal balance of vaginal flora.
- **Douche:** Raises the pH.
- **Intercourse:** Raises the pH.
- **Foreign body:** Serves as a focus of infection and/or inflammation.

DIAGNOSIS

- **Diagnosis** is based on microscopic findings.

WARD TIP

"Whiff" test: Combining vaginal secretions with 10% KOH. Amines associated with BV released will give a fishy odor, indicating a positive test.

WARD TIP

Clinical diagnosis depends on the examination of the vaginal secretions under the microscope

WARD TIP

The most common symptom of a patient with candidiasis (yeast infection) is itching.

WARD TIP

The most common symptom of a patient with BV is malodorous discharge.

 ZEBRA ALERT

What infection is commonly associated with a forgotten IUD? *Actinomyces:* Sulfa granules, gram positive + rod (like fungi).

NOTES

Breast Disease

Benign breast disease may be encountered after a physical exam or noted on imaging studies. Breast-related signs and symptoms are among the most common reasons patients present to obstetrics and gynecology physicians (OB/GYNs). Treatment often is focused on relief of symptoms and patient education.

Breast Anatomy

A 34-year-old G3P3 patient presents with a 3-month history of right breast pain. She reports that her mother had breast cancer at age 64, and was treated with surgery and chemotherapy. Examination reveals a 2-cm mobile, tender, cystic mass to the right of her areola. Ultrasound (US) demonstrates a simple cystic structure. What is the next step in management of this patient?

Answer: Reassure the patient that the mass is benign in nature. Continue annual clinical breast examinations (CBEs) and encourage breast self-awareness.

Breast anatomy:
- The breasts, or mammary glands, are large modified sebaceous glands located in the anterior chest wall, with a "tail" of breast tissue projecting into the axilla.
- Composed of glandular tissue (ducts and lobules), fibrous tissue, and adipose (fat) tissue. Each breast contains 15–20 lobules, which are drained by branching lactiferous ducts that converge in the subareolar region beneath the nipple. The lobules are supported by both fatty and fibrous stroma.
- Lymphatic drainage:
  - Superficial and deep lymphatic vessels.
  - Drains to regional nodes in axilla and the clavicle.
- Blood supply:
  - Primarily from internal mammary artery.
  - Lateral thoracic artery (especially upper outer quadrant).

> **EXAM TIP**
>
> In the United States, a patient's lifetime risk of developing breast cancer is 1 in 8.

Approach to Breast Concerns

- Alleviate/treat symptoms attributed to benign breast disease.
- Distinguish benign from malignant breast disease.
- Identify patients with an increased risk of breast cancer.

Approach to Breast Cancer Screening

- The goal of breast cancer screening in low-risk patients is to detect pre-clinical disease and improve survival. Traditionally, breast cancer screening methods have included self-breast examination (SBE), clinical breast examination (CBE) by a health care provider, and mammogram screening.
  - It is well established that screening tests may have both benefits (i.e., earlier detection of cancer or pre-cancer) and risks (i.e., cost, false-positive results, overdiagnosis and treatment, patient anxiety).
  - This balance of risks and benefits has led to varying opinions by many expert groups about the utility of various breast cancer screening methods.

- Most expert groups no longer recommend routine SBE. Many groups, including The American College of Obstetricians and Gynecologists (ACOG), recommend "breast self-awareness" (which may or may not include SBE). Shared decision making involves discussing pros and cons of SBE, and/or viewing SBE as a method of self-empowerment rather than screening.
- An annual CBE is no longer recommended by the American Cancer Society (ACS). However, other groups, such as ACOG and the National Comprehensive Cancer Network (NCCN), continue to recommend CBE every 1–3 years from age 25 to 39 years, and annually thereafter.
- See Chapter 33 for screening mammogram recommendations.
- **CBE:**
  - Inspect for skin changes and breast asymmetry.
  - Exam in supine and sitting position.
  - When supine, raise the ipsilateral arm above the head to flatten the breast tissue.
- Use *systematic* palpation method (concentric circle or vertical strip method).
  - Use middle three fingers to palpate the breasts.
  - Apply pressure to the breast with the pads of the fingers, progressing from superficial to deep palpation.
  - Apply gentle pressure to the nipple to look for a nipple discharge.
  - Palpate for lymph node enlargement in the axillary and supraclavicular area.

BREAST CANCER RISK ASSESSMENT

- Breast cancer is the most common cancer in U.S. females and the second leading cause of cancer deaths.
- Regular risk assessment is important to identify patients at increased risk so they may be offered appropriate screening or testing.
- Patients determined to be high risk may be candidates for modified breast imaging [with magnetic resonance imaging (MRI)], genetic testing for hereditary breast and ovarian cancer (HBOC) syndromes, or chemoprevention with medications like tamoxifen.

Common Breast Signs and Symptoms

PALPABLE BREAST MASS

Breast mass workup may include the following:
- History and physical exam of both breasts and axillae (start with the non-affected breast first).
- Assess risk factors for breast cancer to help direct the evaluation.
- Imaging (diagnostic mammogram, targeted US).
  - In general, diagnostic mammogram with US is preferred for patients over age 35, and US is preferred for patients under age 35 because the breast tissue is more dense, making mammogram less sensitive.
  - US helps to differentiate a cystic breast mass from a solid breast mass.
  - Lesions found on an imaging study require either interval follow-up with further imaging or biopsy, depending on how suspicious it appears.
- **Pathology analysis**
  - **Fine needle aspiration cytology (FNAC):** Allows analysis of cells in isolation.
  - **Core biopsy:** Histopathology evaluation allows more detail about the architecture of the tissue.

WARD TIP

Two methods to perform a breast exam:
- Concentric circle method
- Vertical strip method

EXAM TIP

Risk factors for breast cancer:
- Family history of breast cancer, ovarian cancer, or other HBOC syndrome-associated cancer (i.e., prostate cancer, pancreatic cancer)
- Known deleterious gene mutation
- Early menarche
- Late menopause
- Not breast-feeding
- Nulliparity
- Prolonged interval between menarche and first pregnancy
- Alcohol intake
- Obesity
- Increasing age
- Decreased physical activity
- Use of combined estrogen/progestin menopausal hormone therapy (MHT)

WARD TIP

- Mammogram reports are standardized using a tool called BIRADS—Breast Imaging Reporting and Data System (fifth edition).
- Findings described in a structured fashion: Density of breast tissue, presence and location of a mass or masses, calcifications, asymmetry, and any associated features.
- Findings are reported in categories 0–6, depending on the likelihood of malignancy in the obtained images:
  BIRADS 0: Insufficient or incomplete study
  BIRADS 1: Normal study
  BIRADS 2: Benign features
  BIRADS 3: Probably benign (<2% risk of malignancy)
  BIRADS 4: Suspicious features
  BIRADS 5: Probably malignant (>95% chance of malignancy)
  BIRADS 6: Malignant (proven malignant on tissue biopsy)

EXAM TIP

Physical exam findings that are suspicious for breast cancer:

- Fixed, firm, irregular mass
- Mass > 2 cm
- Asymmetry or bulging contour
- Skin changes such as dimpling or retraction
- Nipple changes such as asymmetry, new inversion/retraction

EXAM TIP

Suspicious findings (for a cancer) on mammogram:

- Spiculated focal mass (most specific)
- Clusters of calcifications
- ↑ Breast density
- Architectural distortion

WARD TIP

Simple breast cysts are the most common type of benign breast disease and are most common in patients aged 35–50 years. **Fibroadenomas** are the most common cause of breast masses in adolescent and young females.

- Both procedures are invasive and involve risks; thus, they should generally only be done when there is suspicion for malignancy. The decision to perform a biopsy is a clinical one.
- Pathologic studies may be unnecessary in young (age < 25), low-risk patients with a benign exam and reassuring imaging studies.
- The decision whether to perform FNAC or core biopsy depends on factors such as **physician** expertise, available diagnostic equipment, and site and characteristics of the lesion. See Figure 32-1.
- The **differential diagnoses** of benign breast masses:
  - **Breast cyst** is a fluid filled, round, well-circumscribed, mobile mass that may be solitary or may present with multiple masses. The size and number and associated symptoms may fluctuate. They may be painful or painless. They are most commonly found in premenopausal patients. A simple fluid-filled breast cyst is not associated with an increased risk of breast cancer, and can be followed conservatively.
  - **Fat necrosis** is usually a result of trauma to the breast with subsequent bleeding into the breast tissue. It may also occur after injection of substances into the breast such as fat or silicone, after a surgery such as breast reconstruction, or after radiation therapy. It is rare but often confused with cancer. The breast may contain a firm, tender, ill-defined mass that sometimes requires surgical excision.
  - **Fibroadenoma** is a common benign solid mass that is typically rubbery, firm, freely mobile, and well circumscribed. It is most commonly found in patients between the ages of 20–40 years.
  - **Phyllodes tumors** are rare fibroepithelial tumors that usually occur in older women (median age 40 years). They are typically larger than fibroadenomas, but have similar exam findings. They have a wide range of biologic behavior (from benign to malignant) and thus should be completely excised.
  - **Fibrocystic changes** are usually diffuse but may be prominent/organized and present with a mass. It most commonly occurs in premenopausal patients. The classic symptoms and signs include breast pain, ↑ engorgement, and excessive nodularity that is often related to the menstrual cycle. These lesions do not place the patient at ↑ risk for cancer.

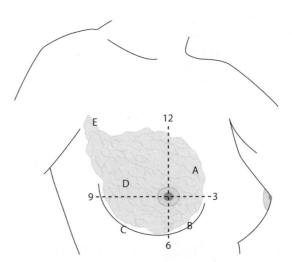

FIGURE 32-1. **Female breast quadrants. (A)** UIQ (upper inner quadrant); **(B)** LIQ (lower inner quadrant); **(C)** LOQ (lower outer quadrant; **(D)** UUQ (upper outer quadrant), majority of breast cancers are detected in this quadrant; **(E)** Tail of Spence (outer portion of breast toward the axilla).

NIPPLE DISCHARGE

- This symptom may represent either **benign** or **malignant** breast disease.
  - Benign processes are usually bilateral, only present when expressed, multiductal, and milky or green in color.
  - Discharge that is unilateral, spontaneous, and from a single duct is associated with a higher risk of malignancy and requires more thorough investigation.
- **Physiologic** nipple discharge is not pathologic and may be straw-colored, clear, green, or brown, but not bloody.
- **Galactorrhea** is bilateral milky discharge from multiple ducts outside of the pregnancy and the postpartum period. Galactorrhea may occur during pregnancy and may persist for up to 12 months postpartum or from the time of conclusion of breast-feeding. Refer to Chapter 19 for more details.
  - It is typically caused by elevated prolactin levels rather than intrinsic breast disease. Possible causes include:
    - Endocrine disorders such as hypothyroidism or prolactin-producing adenomas.
    - Medications that inhibit dopamine such as antipsychotics, antidepressants, gastrointestinal drugs, and some antihypertensives.
    - Chronic breast stimulation.
- **Intraductal papilloma** is a benign papillary tumor arising from the lining of the breast duct. The nipple discharge may be clear but is often bloody.

MASTALGIA (BREAST PAIN)

- History and physical exam, noting the cyclicity and duration of the pain. Inquire about menstrual history, hormone use, dietary habits (caffeine, tea, sodas, chocolate), and the presences of breast implants or trauma history.
- It is important to reassure patients that mastalgia is rarely a symptom of breast cancer.
- Mastalgia may be separated into three categories:
  - **Cyclical** pain is bilateral in nature and is related to normal hormonal changes related to the menstrual cycle or to contraception or other cyclically administered hormones. Pain is ↑ during the luteal phase, dissipating with menses onset.
  - **Noncyclical** pain is more likely to be unilateral, does not vary according to the menstrual cycle, and typically has a breast-related cause such as: Large breasts, mastitis, trauma, cysts, duct ectasia, inflammatory breast cancer, and some medications.
  - **Extramammary** pain is due to other sources such as costochondritis, fibromyalgia, chest wall trauma, chest wall pain due to pectoralis muscle overuse/injury, and herpes zoster.
- **Treatment** is based on the cause and may consist of reassurance, reducing intake of caffeine, treatment with nonsteroidal anti-inflammatory drugs (NSAIDs) or acetaminophen, evening primrose oil, warm compresses or ice packs, and a "support" bra. Imaging may be considered if there are suspicious physical exam findings, but is often not necessary.

EXAM TIP

Oral contraceptives may cause breast pain.

BREAST SKIN CHANGES

- On exam, the skin is inspected for edema, erythema, or retraction.
- Ulceration, eczema, and redness around the nipple can be Paget disease. Mammogram and surgery referral is warranted.

- Erythema, tenderness, and a mass lead to suspicion for **inflammatory breast cancer**. Mammogram and surgery referral is warranted.
- Warmth, tenderness, induration, and erythema may also be mastitis or a breast abscess, even in the nonlactating woman. If fluctuance is appreciated, a breast US, drainage, and antibiotics are the treatment of choice.

Female Patient Health Maintenance

Preventative services and health maintenance is an important aspect of the care of the female patient. For the purposes of this chapter, the term "female" will refer to patients with a female sex assigned at birth. Transgender and gender diverse individuals face not only harassment and discrimination in society, they are also at risk for health care inequities and barriers to accessing care. Obstetricians/gynecologists (OB/GYNs) must be aware of screening tests suggested for their patients and should strive to create an environment that is inclusive and affirming. These tools are used for the prevention and/or early detection of serious medical conditions and diseases.

Screening Tests

 A 65-year-old G2P2 postmenopausal patient presents for an annual exam. She is healthy and has no medical problems. She has never had an abnormal Pap test and her last Pap test was 3 years ago and normal with a negative test for high-risk human papilloma virus (hrHPV). She has had regular care and screening over the last 10 years. How should this patient be counseled about Pap test screening?

Answer: This patient may discontinue Pap test screening after age 65 if she meets the following criteria: (1) no history of cervical high-grade intraepithelial lesion (HSIL) for the past 25 years and (2) adequate prior screening, defined as two consecutive primary HPV tests within the past 10 years with most recent test in previous 5 years, **or** two consecutive negative co-tests (Pap and HPV) within the past 10 years with most recent test in previous 5 years **or** three consecutive negative Pap tests within the past 10 years, with most recent test in previous 3 years.

CERVICAL CANCER SCREENING GUIDELINES FOR AVERAGE-RISK PATIENTS

- Screening guidelines have changed many times over the years as more information about the natural history of cervical dysplasia and hrHPV behavior have emerged.
- Leading expert organizations including American College of Obstetricians and Gynecologists (ACOG), the American Society for Colposcopy and Cervical Pathology (ASCCP), and the U.S. Preventive Services Task Force (USPSTF) have endorsed the following recommendations as of 2021 for average-risk individuals.
  - Initiate screening at age 21.
  - Aged 21–29 years: Cytology alone every 3 years.
  - Aged 30–65 years: Any one of the following:
    - Cytology alone every 3 years.
    - FDA-approved primary hrHPV testing alone every 5 years.
    - Co-testing (cytology and hrHPV testing) every 5 years.
  - Aged >65 years: no screening after adequate negative prior screening (see above scenario).
- Hysterectomy with removal of the cervix: No screening necessary in individuals who do not have a history of high-grade cervical precancerous lesions or cervical cancer.

BREAST CANCER SCREENING GUIDELINES FOR AVERAGE-RISK PATIENTS

BREAST EXAMS

See Chapter 32 for recommendations for self-breast examination (SBE) and clinical breast exam (CBE).

MAMMOGRAPHY

- Varying opinions exist among expert organizations about mammogram screening in low-risk individuals. Leading expert organizations in this field include ACOG, USPSTF, American Cancer Society (ACS), and National Comprehensive Cancer Network (NCCN).
- Counseling and shared decision-making with patients should take into account known benefits (decreased breast cancer mortality, decreased risk of advanced cancer at time of diagnosis) and potential harms (false positive results, call-backs for additional imaging and/or biopsies, patient anxiety and distress, overdiagnosis, and overtreatment). (See Figure 33-1.)

	American College of Obstetricians and Gynecologists	U.S. Preventive Services Task Force	American Cancer Society	National Comprehensive Cancer Network
Clinical breast examination	May be offered* every 1–3 years for women aged 25–39 years and annually for women 40 years and older.	Insufficient evidence to recommend for or against.[†]	Does not recommend[‡]	Recommend every 1–3 years for women aged 25–39 years. Recommend annually for women 40 years and older.
Mammography initiation age	Offer starting at age 40 years.[§] Initiate at ages 40–49 years after counseling, if patient desires. Recommend by no later than age 50 years if patient has not already initiated.	Recommend at age 50 years.[‖] Age 40–49 years: The decision to start screening mammography in women before age 50 years should be an individual one.[¶]	Offer at ages 40–45 years.[¶] Recommend at age 45 years.[#]	Recommend at age 40 years.
Mammography screening interval	Annual or biennial[§]	Biennial[‖]	Annual for women aged 40–54 years[‡] Biennial with the option to continue annual screening for women 55 years or older[‡]	Annual
Mammography stop age	Continue until age 75 years. Beyond age 75 years, the decision to discontinue should be based on a shared decision-making process that includes a discussion of the woman's health status and longevity.	The current evidence is insufficient to assess the balance of benefits and harms of screening mammography in women 75 years and older.[†]	When life expectancy is less than 10 years[‡]	When severe comorbidities limit life expectancy to 10 years or less

*Offer in the context of a shared, informed decision-making approach that recognizes the uncertainty of additional benefits and harms of clinical breast examination beyond screening mammography.

[†]Category I recommendation

[‡]Qualified recommendation

[§]Decision between options to be made through shared decision making after appropriate counseling

[‖]Category B recommendation

[¶]Category C recommendation. The Task Force notes that "Women who place a higher value on the potential benefit than the potential harms may choose to begin screening between the ages of 40 and 49 years."

[#]Strong recommendation

Data from National Comprehensive Cancer Network. Breast cancer screening and diagnosis. Version 1.2016; Oeffinger KC, Fontham ET, Etzioni R, Herzig A, Michaelson JS, Shih YC, et al. Breast cancer screening for women at average risk: 2015 guideline update from the American Cancer Society [published erratum appears in JAMA 2016;315:1406]. JAMA 2015;314:1599–614; and Siu AL. Screening for breast cancer: U.S. Preventive Services Task Force recommendation statement. U.S. Preventive Services Task Force [published erratum appears in Ann Intern Med 2016;164:448]. Ann Intern Med 2016;164:279–96. OBSTETRICS & GYNECOLOGY

FIGURE 33-1. **Recommendations for Breast Cancer Screening in Average-Risk Patients.** (Reproduced, with permission, from Committee on Practice Bulletins—Gynecology in collaboration with Pearlman M, Jeudy M, Chelmow D. Practice Bulletin Number 179: Breast Cancer Risk Assessment and Screening in Average-Risk Women. *Obstet Gynecol.* 2017;130(1):e1-e16, Table 1.).

- Individuals under age 40 are at low risk for breast cancer.
- ACOG and NCCN currently recommend **initiating** mammogram screening beginning at age 40.
- Mammography screening may be recommended either annually or every 2 years.
- Most organizations suggest mammography screening which may be discontinued at age 75 years, or when the life expectancy is less than 10 years.

OSTEOPOROSIS (BONE DENSITY) SCREENING

- The goal is to identify individuals who are at an increased risk of pathologic (low-trauma) fracture who would benefit from interventions to mitigate that risk. A combination of bone mineral density (BMD) measurements and fracture risk assessment is used.
- Screen with Dual Energy X-Ray Absorptiometry (DEXA) BMD testing starting at age 65.
- Selective patients under age 65 should be screened if they are postmenopausal and have one or more risk factors for fracture:
  - Personal history of pathologic fracture or parental history of hip fracture.
  - Body weight <127 lb.
  - Excessive alcohol intake.
  - Current cigarette smoking.
  - Rheumatoid arthritis.
  - Glucocorticoid therapy.

COLORECTAL CANCER (CRC) SCREENING

- Colorectal cancer (CRC) is the third most common cancer in females.
- Screening of low-risk individuals is directed toward removal of adenomatous polyps and sessile serrated lesions and detection of early stage CRC.
- **High-risk patients** should begin screening earlier and more frequently.
- **Low-risk patients** must meet the following criteria:
  - **No** personal history or family history of CRC or certain types of colon polyps.
  - **No** personal history of inflammatory bowel disease (i.e., ulcerative colitis or Crohn's disease).
  - **No** confirmed or suspected hereditary CRC cancer syndrome [i.e., familial adenomatous polyposis (FAP) or Lynch syndrome (hereditary non-polyposis colon cancer or HPNCC)].
  - **No** personal history of radiation to the abdomen or pelvis to treat a prior cancer of any type.
- The American College of Surgeons recommends the following CRC screening guidelines for **low-risk** individuals:
  - Initiate screening starting at age 45 years.
  - Continue screening through age 75 years.
  - Between the ages of 75 and 85 years, the decision to continue screening should be individualized based on patient preferences, life expectancy, overall health, and prior screening history.
  - Individuals over age 85 may discontinue screening.
- **Options for CRC screening:**
  - **Stool-based tests**
    1. Highly sensitive fecal immunochemical test (FIT) every year.
    2. Highly sensitive guaiac-based fecal occult blood test (gFOBT) every year.
    3. Multi-targeted stool DNA test (mt-sDNA) every 3 years.

- **Visual (structural) exams of the colon and rectum:**
  1. Colonoscopy every 10 years.
  2. Flexible sigmoidoscopy every 5 years.
  3. Computed tomographic colonography (virtual colonoscopy) every 5 years.

SEXUALLY TRANSMITTED INFECTION (STI) SCREENING

- STIs are a major public health problem that are frequently asymptomatic but may lead to several long-term complications (i.e., pelvic pain, infertility).
- STI screening is aimed at identifying and treating individuals before they develop complications, and to identify and treat partners to prevent further transmission and reinfection.
- The Centers for Disease Control (CDC) recommends that lesbian, bisexual, transgender, and gender non-conforming individuals be assessed for risks related to STI and human immunodeficiency virus (HIV) based on current anatomy and sexual behaviors. Because of the diversity of transgender persons regarding sexual affirming procedures, hormonal use, and patters of sexual behavior, health care providers must remain aware of symptoms of common STIs and screen for asymptomatic STIs on the basis of behavior and sexual practices.
- According to the CDC in 2019, reported STIs in the United States reached an all-time high for the sixth consecutive year. Over 2.5 million cases of gonorrhea, chlamydia, and syphilis were reported in 2019.
- STI screening may be targeted at individuals from groups with a high prevalence of STIs, or may be done based on assessment of an individual's personal risk based on behaviors, including the following:
  - History of multiple sexual partners.
  - History of sex with a partner who has multiple sexual contacts.
  - Persons whose partner has an STI.
  - Personal history of STI.
  - Annual screening for all sexually active females under age 25.
  - Females with developmental disabilities.
  - Females who exchange sex for drugs or money.
  - Females who use IV drugs.
  - Females who are in a detention facility.
- HIV testing is recommended for all females aged >25 years at least once, with repeat testing based on risk factors.

WARD TIP

Routine annual screening for chlamydia and gonorrhea is recommended for all sexually active females <25 years of age. These tests are done simultaneously as the presence of one of these infections is a high risk for the presence of the other.

Health Education

Good diet and exercise are crucial for leading a healthy life. The nutritional status of a female is critical to the health of future generations and reducing the burden of chronic disease. There are many factors that determine each individual's diet and exercise requirements, which all must be considered by the OB/GYN.

NUTRITION AND EXERCISE

Recommendations are based on the U.S. Department of Agriculture and the U.S. Department of Health and Human Services' 2020–2025 *Dietary Guidelines for Americans*.

- The issues of nutrition and body weight should be emphasized during the three major transitional periods in a patient's life:

1. Puberty.
2. Pregnancy.
3. Menopause.
- An individual's body weight is determined by three major factors:
  1. Genetics and heredity, which control:
     - Resting metabolic rate.
     - Appetite.
     - Satiety.
     - Body fat distribution.
     - Predisposition to physical activity.
  2. Nutrition.
  3. Physical activity and exercise.

GOALS

- The 2020–2025 *Dietary Guidelines for Americans* provides evidence-based recommendations for eating patterns and regular physical activity. The following are recommended:
  - Follow a healthy eating pattern across the lifespan. This helps to support a healthy body weight and reduces the risk of chronic disease.
  - Focus on variety, nutrient density, and amount. Choose a variety of nutrient-dense foods from each food group in recommended amounts, including grains, vegetables, fruits, dairy, protein, and oils.
  - Limit intake of added sugars, saturated fats, alcohol, and sodium.
  - Shift to healthier food and beverage choices.
  - Avoid "pre-packaged" foods and focus on "whole foods."
- Adjust caloric intake for age and physical activity level:
  - As one ages, there is a ↓ in resting metabolic rate and loss of lean tissue and muscle mass.
- Physical activity is important for all adults. Adults should do at least 150 min/week of moderate-intensity aerobic physical activity and should also include muscle strengthening activities at least 2 days per week.

Substance Use Disorders

 A 53-year-old G1P1 patient presents for an annual exam. When asked about alcohol use, she reports that she drinks several glasses of wine every evening. How should this patient be screened for substance abuse disorder?
Answer: Using the CAGE questionnaire has been shown to be very effective in screening for problem drinking.

- Substance use disorders are a major, often underdiagnosed, health problem that can affect every aspect of a patient's life.
- Substances that are commonly used or abused include alcohol, cannabinoids, opioids, prescription medications, stimulants, and tobacco.
- The role of an OB/GYN physician is to provide universal screening for substance use disorders, regardless of age, sex, race, ethnicity, or socioeconomic status. This can be accomplished by direct questioning or via validated questionnaire.
- An example of screening would be the CAGE questionnaire. Two "yes" answers have a sensitivity of 93% and a specificity of 76% for substance use disorder (alcohol).
- Fetal alcohol spectrum disorder (FASD):

 EXAM TIP

High-fat diets have adverse effects on lipid metabolism, insulin sensitivity, and body composition.

 EXAM TIP

Exercise will ↑ the body's metabolic rate and prevent the storage of fat.

- Prenatal exposure to alcohol is the leading preventable cause of developmental disabilities and birth defects. Alcohol causes irreversible central nervous system (CNS) effects. Teratogenic effects are dose related, as "safe" threshold of alcohol consumption has not been defined.
- Teratogenic effects may vary depending on the quantity and pattern of alcohol consumption. Clinical features include fetal growth restriction, facial anomalies (short palpebral fissures, thin vermillion border, smooth philtrum), and CNS abnormalities (neurobehavioral impairment).

TOBACCO, SMOKING, AND E-CIGARETTES

- Cigarette smoking is the most preventable cause of premature death and avoidable illness in the United States and worldwide.
- Electronic cigarettes (e-cigarettes or vaping devices), which entered the U.S. market in 2006, are battery-operated devices that heat a liquid (usually containing nicotine), producing an aerosol that the user inhales.
- Screening tools for tobacco use include the **5As:**
  - Ask about tobacco.
  - Advise to quit.
  - Assess willingness to quit.
  - Assist in quit attempt.
  - Arrange for follow-up.
- Linked to lung cancer, coronary artery disease (CAD), chronic obstructive pulmonary disease (COPD), and respiratory diseases.
- **Endocrine effects:** Individuals who smoke reach menopause earlier and have ↑ risk of osteoporosis.
- **Obstetric effects:** Reduced fertility, ↑ rates of spontaneous abortion, premature delivery, low-birth-weight infants, fetal growth restriction, and placental abruption.
- Children who grow up exposed to secondhand smoke have higher rates of respiratory and middle-ear illness.

WARD TIP

CAGE Questionnaire for Alcohol substance use disorder

C—Have you ever felt like you should **CUT BACK** on your drinking?

A—Have you ever been **ANNOYED** when people criticize your drinking?

G—Have you ever felt **GUILTY** about your drinking?

E—Have you ever needed a drink first thing in the morning to steady your nerves or "cure" a hangover **(EYE OPENER)?**

EXAM TIP

Heart disease is the leading cause of death among females.

EXAM TIP

Accidents (unintentional injuries) are the leading cause of death among adolescent females.

Safer Sex Practices

Improved and successful prevention of pregnancy and STIs by more adolescents requires counseling that includes:
- Education about *both* abstinence *and also* contraception and condoms.
- Creating an accepting and safe environment for patients to discuss safer sex practices regardless of sexual preference or gender identity.
- Providing information about contraceptive options, including emergency contraception and side effects of various contraceptive methods.
- Education on safer sex practices, especially condom use, and STIs.

Physical Abuse/Violence

INTIMATE PARTNER VIOLENCE (IPV)

- IPV refers to a relationship in which an individual is victimized by actual or threatened physical, psychological, or sexual harm by a current or past intimate partner.

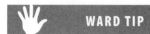

- IPV may occur among individuals with any sexual orientation or gender identity.
- Risk factors for IPV include female gender, younger age, lower socioeconomic status, and family or personal history of violence.
- Every female should be screened for IPV because it can be found among individuals from any background and with any type of partner.

RECOGNITION OF IPV

- Injuries to the head, eyes, neck, torso, breasts, abdomen, and/or genitals.
- Bilateral or multiple injuries.
- A delay between the time of injury and the time at which treatment is sought.
- Missed appointments.
- Inconsistencies between the patient's explanation of the injuries and the physician's clinical findings.
- A history of repeated trauma.
- The perpetrator may exhibit signs of control over the health care team, refusal to leave the patient's side to allow private conversation, and control of victim. The perpetrator may be overly attentive or verbally abusive.
- Frequent urgent visits or visits to the emergency department, often for general somatic symptoms.
- **Pregnant patients** are at an increased risk to experience IPV during the pregnancy.

DIAGNOSIS (SEE TABLE 33-1)

There are many screening questionnaires that can be used to assess IPV.

MEDICAL OBLIGATION TO VICTIMS

- Listen in a nonjudgmental manner, and assure the patient that it is not her fault, nor does she deserve the abuse.
- Assess the safety of the patient and her children (if applicable).
- If the patient is ready to leave the abusive relationship, connect her with resources such as shelters, police, public agencies, and counselors.
- If the patient is not ready to leave, discuss a safety or exit plan and provide the patient with IPV information.
- Carefully document all subjective and objective findings. The records can be used in a legal case to establish abuse.

SEXUAL ASSAULT

A 27-year-old G0P0 patient presents reporting that she was raped the night before by an acquaintance. How should this patient be counseled about options for emergency contraception following sexual assault involving unprotected intercourse (UPI)?

Answer: (1) Ulipristal acetate 30 mg up to 5 days after UPI (requires prescription). (2) Oral levonorgestrel 1.5 mg up to 72 hours after UPI [available over-the-counter (OTC)]. (3) Insertion of copper or levonorgestrel IUD within 5 days of UPI.

TABLE 33-1. Abuse Assessment Screen

1. Have you ever been emotionally or physically abused by your partner or someone important to you?
2. Within the past year, have you been hit, slapped, kicked, or otherwise physically hurt by someone?
3. Since you've been pregnant, have you been hit, slapped, kicked, or otherwise physically hurt by someone?
4. Within the past year, has anyone forced you to have sexual activities? Has anyone in the past forced you to have sexual activities?
5. Are you afraid of your partner or anyone you listed above?

Data from McFarlane J, Parker B, Soeken K, Bullock L. Assessing for Abuse During Pregnancy: Severity and Frequency of Injuries and Associated Entry Into Prenatal Care. *JAMA*. 1992;267(23):3176–3178.

- **Sexual assault** or sexual violence occurs when *any sexual contact* is performed by one person on another without that person's consent. This may range from inappropriate unwanted forced touching or kissing to verbally or physically coerced oral, vaginal, or anal penetration.
- **Rape** is defined as nonconsensual *vaginal, anal, or oral penetration (by penis, finger, or other object)* without the consent of one party, whether from physical or psychologic force, threat of force, or incapacity to consent due to age, intoxication, or mental condition. The legal definition of rape varies by state.
- The CDC has reported that lesbian, gay, bisexual, and transgender people experience sexual violence at similar or higher rates than straight people. As a community, LGBTQ people face higher rates of poverty, stigma, marginalization, and hate-motivated violence, which puts them at greater risk for sexual assault.

WARD TIP

It is estimated that the prevalence of rape, physical violence, and/or stalking by an intimate partner is 44% in lesbian and 61% in bisexual individuals, compared to 35% in heterosexual females.

RAPE TRAUMA SYNDROME

Sexual assault is the most common type of trauma experienced by females with a diagnosis of post-traumatic stress disorder (PTSD). It may result in Rape Trauma Syndrome resulting from the psychological and emotional stress of being raped.

SIGNS AND SYMPTOMS

According to the Rape, Abuse & Incest National Network (RAINN), there are three phases to Rape Trauma Syndrome. This descriptive model assumes that victims will take steps forward and backward in their healing process, healing is not a linear progression, and the experience will be different for each individual.

1. **Acute Phase**
   This phase occurs immediately after the assault and usually lasts a few days to several weeks. In this phase individuals can have many reactions but they typically fall into three categories of reactions:
   1. Expressed: This is when the survivor is openly emotional. He or she may appear agitated or hysterical; he or she may suffer from crying spells or anxiety attacks.
   2. Controlled: This is when the survivor appears to be without emotion and acts as if "nothing happened" and "everything is fine." This appearance of calm may be shock.
   3. Shocked disbelief: This is when the survivor reacts with a strong sense of disorientation. He or she may have difficulty concentrating, making decisions, or doing everyday tasks. He or she may also have poor recall of the assault.

2. **Outward Adjustment Phase**
   This phase is when the victim resumes what appears to be "normal" life but inside is suffering from considerable turmoil. There are five primary coping techniques during this phase:
   1. Minimization: Pretends that "everything is fine."
   2. Dramatization: Talking and thinking about the assault dominates their life and identity.
   3. Suppression: Refuses to discuss, acts as if the assault did not happen.
   4. Explanation: Analyzes what the perpetrator did, what the rapist was thinking or feeling.
   5. Flight: Tries to escape the pain by moving, changing jobs, changing appearance, changing relationships, etc.

3. **The Resolution Phase**
   During this phase the assault is no longer the central focus of the victim's life. The pain and negative outcomes decrease over time, and although the individual will never forget the assault, they begin to accept the rape as part of their life and choose to move on.

WARD TIP

Symptoms of Rape Trauma Syndrome may include the following:

- Anxiety and/or hypervigilance
- Mood swings and/or rage
- Phobias
- Depression
- Sleep disturbances
- Withdrawal from friends, family, and activities
- Changes in eating pattern (nausea, anorexia, compulsive eating)
- Gynecologic symptoms such as vaginal itching, pain, discharge

MANAGEMENT

Physician's Medical Responsibilities

- Requirements for forensic evaluations will vary by state. Many institutions have established programs with trained providers to provide this acute assessment and care.
- Obtain complete medical and gynecologic history.
- Assess and treat physical injuries in the presence of a female chaperone (even if the health care provider is female).
- Obtain nucleic acid amplification testing (NAAT) for gonorrhea, chlamydia, and trichomonas and serum testing for STIs (HIV, syphilis, hepatitis B/C).
- Counsel patient and provide empiric STI antibiotic prophylaxis.
- Provide preventive therapy for unwanted pregnancy (emergency contraception).
- Assess psychological and emotional status.
- Provide crisis intervention.
- Arrange for follow-up medical care and psychological counseling.

Physician's Legal Responsibilities

- Obtain informed consent for treatment, collection of evidence, taking of photographs, and reporting of the incident to the authorities.
- Accurately record events.
- Accurately describe injuries.
- Collect appropriate samples and clothing.
- Maintain the chain of command.
- Label photographs, clothing, and specimens with the patient's name; seal and store safely.

TREATMENT

- **Infection prophylaxis:** Gonorrhea, chlamydia, and trichomonas infections:
  - Ceftriaxone 500 mg IM (intramuscular) + azithromycin 1 g PO (by mouth) in a single dose to treat both gonorrhea and chlamydia.
  - Metronidazole 2 g PO single dose to treat trichomonas.
- Offer the hepatitis B vaccine and HPV vaccine (depends on immunization status).
- Offer prophylactic treatment with antiretroviral drugs for HIV prophylaxis.
- Administer Td toxoid when indicated.
- **Emergency contraception (EC):**
  - **Oral Levonorgestrel:** 0.75 mg taken 12 hours apart × 2 doses, or 1.5 mg as a single dose (available OTC) approved for use up to 72 hours after UPI.
  - **Combined estrogen-progestin pills "Yuzpe method":** 100 mg of ethinyl estradiol and 0.5 mg of levonorgestrel (or equivalent) given immediately and repeated in 12 hours.
  - **Ulipristal acetate:** Antiprogestin used in single dose of 30 mg PO up to 5 days after UPI.
  - **Copper or levonorgestrel IUD:** Insert within 5 days of UPI.

EXAM TIP

The greatest danger for IPV to occur is after a threat or an attempt to leave the relationship.

EXAM TIP

The annual incidence of sexual assault is 73 per 100,000 females.

WARD TIP

The Yuzpe method is flexible and can be employed using several types of commonly used combination oral contraceptive pills. It may be one way to make EC more available to patients who have limited access, finances, or concerns about privacy.

CHAPTER 34

Female Sexuality

Female Sexuality

Evaluation of sexuality and function should be a basic part of an annual exam. For the purposes of this review, female will refer to persons assigned a female gender at birth. In order to provide individuals with the highest quality health care, it is important for physicians and other health care providers to become familiar with terms used by lesbian, gay, bisexual, transgender, queer, intersex, asexual, and other sexual and gender minorities (LGBTQIA+). One way to provide inclusive, respectful, and affirming care is to ask patients their pronoun and their chosen name.

The Fenway Institute has provided a glossary of terms for health care teams relevant to the health care and identities of LGBTQIA+ people. Terms and definitions may change frequently and vary across communities, but a selection of terms is included below.

- **Agender:** A person who identifies as having no gender, or who does not experience gender as a primary identity component.
- **Ally:** A person who actively supports the rights of a marginalized community even though that person is not a member of that community.
- **Assigned female at birth (AFAB)/Assigned male at birth (AMAB):** (Also known as **sex assigned at birth.**) Refers to the sex that is assigned to an infant, most often based on the infants anatomical and other biological characteristics.
- **Bigender:** Describes a person whose gender identity combines two genders.
- **Bisexual:** A sexual orientation that that describes a person who is emotionally and physically attracted to women/females and men/males.
- **Cisgender:** A person whose gender identity is consistent in a traditional sense with their sex assigned at birth.
- **Gender-affirming hormone therapy:** Feminizing and masculinizing hormone treatment to align secondary sex characteristics with gender identity.
- **Gay:** A sexual orientation describing people who are primarily emotionally and physically attracted to people of the same sex and/or gender as themselves.
- **Gender affirmation:** The process of making social, legal, and/or medical changes to recognize, accept, and express one's gender identity. Social changes may include changing one's pronouns, name, clothing, and hairstyle. Legal changes may include changing one's name, sex designation, and gender markers on legal documents. Medical changes can include receiving gender-affirming hormones and/or surgeries.
- **Gender-affirming surgery (GAS):** Surgeries to modify a person's body to be more aligned with that person's gender identity. This may include **gender-affirming chest surgery** (also known as "**top surgery**") to remove and/or reconstruct a person's chest to be more aligned with that person's gender identity. Examples include feminizing surgery such as breast augmentation and masculinizing surgery such as mastectomy. **Gender-affirming Genital surgery** (also known as "**bottom surgery**") helps align a person's genitals and/or internal reproductive organs with that person's gender identity. Examples include clitoroplasty, labiaplasty, hysterectomy +/− oophorectomy, phalloplasty, and scrotoplasty.
- **Genderqueer:** An umbrella term that describes a person whose gender identity falls outside the traditional gender binary of male and female.
- **Heterosexual:** (Also known as "**straight**.") A sexual orientation that describes women who are primarily emotionally and physically attracted to men and men who are primarily attracted to women.
- **Intersectionality:** The idea that comprehensive identities are influenced and shaped by the interconnection of race, class, ethnicity, sexuality/sexual

orientation, gender/gender identity, physical disability, national origin, religion, age, and other social or physical attributes.

- **Intersex:** Describes a group of congenital conditions in which the reproductive organs, genitals, and/or other sexual anatomies do not develop according to traditional expectations for males or females.
- **Lesbian:** A sexual orientation that describes a woman who is primarily emotionally and physically attracted to other women.
- **Non-binary:** Describes a person whose gender identity falls outside of traditional gender binary structure of girl/woman and boy/man.
- **Pronouns:** Pronouns are the words people should use when they are referring to you, but not using your name. Examples include she/her/hers, he/him/his, and they/them/theirs.
- **Queer:** An umbrella term describing people who think of their sexual orientation or gender identity as outside societal norms.
- **Questioning:** Describes a person who is unsure about or exploring their sexual orientation and/or gender identity.
- **Sexual orientation:** How a person characterizes their emotional and sexual attraction to others.
- **Transgender:** Describes a person whose gender identity and sex assigned at birth do not correspond based on traditional expectations. For example, a person assigned a female sex at birth who identifies as a man.
- **Trans man/transgender man:** A transgender person whose gender identity is boy/man/male.
- **Tran woman/transgender woman:** A transgender person whose gender identity is girl/woman/female.
- **Transsexual:** A term used sometimes in the medical literature or by some transgender people to describe people who have gone through the process of medical gender affirmation treatments.

FEMALE SEXUAL RESPONSE CYCLE

The landmark studies regarding the sexual response cycle tended to favor linear models of desire, arousal, orgasm, and resolution. There is increasing recognition that this framework cannot be consistently applied to a female's sexual response, and that achieving all of these phases may not be required to achieve a satisfactory sexual experience. Sexual activity is also informed and motivated by other factors such as desire for emotional closeness and strengthening a relationship with a partner. Hormone such as estrogens and androgens also play a role in sexual physiology, aspects of which continue to be poorly understood.

SEXUAL DYSFUNCTION

The *Diagnostic and Statistical Manual of Mental Disorders*, Fifth Edition, defines four specific types of female sexual dysfunction. It is important to first clarify whether the dysfunction reported is:

- Lifelong or acquired
- Global (all partners) or situational

EVALUATION STRATEGIES

- Look for possible etiologies:
  - Medical illnesses
  - Menopausal status
  - Medication use (antihypertensives, cardiovascular meds, antidepressants, etc.)

- Rule out other psychiatric/psychological causes:
  - Life discontent (stress, fatigue, relationship issues, traumatic sexual history, guilt)
  - Major depression
  - Drug abuse
  - Anxiety
  - Obsessive-compulsive disorder

MANAGEMENT STRATEGIES

- Medical illnesses need evaluation and specific treatment.
- Screen for and treat depression with psychotherapy and/or medication.
- Reduce dosages or change medications that may alter sexual interest (i.e., switch to antidepressant formulations that have less of an impact on sexual function).
- Address menopause and hormonal deficiencies.

Types of Sexual Dysfunction

- **Female sexual interest and arousal disorder:** Lack of or decreased interest in at least three of the following, which has been persistent for a minimum of 6 months and causes clinically significant distress to the individual:
  - Interest in sexual activity
  - Sexual or erotic thoughts/fantasies
  - Initiation of sexual activity and responsiveness to a partner's initiation
  - Interest or arousal in response to internal or external sexual or erotic cues
  - Genital or nongenital sensations during sexual activity
- **Female orgasmic disorder:** Marked delay in, marked infrequency of, or absence of orgasm, or markedly reduced intensity of orgasm, which has persisted for a minimum of 6 months and causes clinically significant distress to the individual.
- **Genitopelvic pain/penetration disorder:** Persistent or recurrent presence of one or more of the following symptoms which has been present for a minimum of 6 months and causes clinically significant distress to the individual:
  - Difficulty having intercourse
  - Marked vulvovaginal or pelvic pain during intercourse or penetration attempts
  - Marked fear or anxiety about vulvovaginal or pelvic pain anticipating, during, or resulting from vaginal penetration
  - Marked tensing or tightening of the pelvic floor muscles during attempted vaginal penetration
- **Substance or medication-induced sexual dysfunction:** A disturbance in sexual function that has a temporary relationship with substance/medication initiation, dose increase, or discontinuation, and causes clinically significant distress in the individual

TREATMENT FOR SEXUAL DYSFUNCTION

Treatment varies depending on the sexual function issue(s), and there are often issues in more than one sexual domain. In general, treatment should involve both partners and may include aspects of the following:

- Couples counseling/sex therapy.
- Treatment of any underlying psychiatric disorder with medication and/or psychotherapy.
- Lifestyle changes to reduce fatigue and stress.
- Improvement of body image with exercise and/or weight loss.
- Relationship interventions i.e., "date night", use of sexual aids, masturbation education.

WARD TIP

Certain medications, especially selective serotonin reuptake inhibitors (SSRIs) may be associated with impaired sexual arousal.

WARD TIP

A diagnosis of a sexual dysfunction disorder can only be made once other causes have been ruled out such other nonsexual mental health or medical conditions, severe relationship distress or other significant stressors, and is not due to side effects of a substance or medication.

EXAM TIP

Low libido is the most common sexual problem for women.

- Treatment of ↓ lubrication with the use of topical lubricants.
- Pelvic physical therapy can be helpful for patients with dyspareunia or pelvic pain.

Sexual Arousal Disorders

- Transdermal androgen therapy may be helpful in postmenopausal patients.
- Menopausal symptoms may respond to oral or topical estrogen.
- Bupropion may be used off-label to treat sexual arousal disorders.
- Flibanserin is the first FDA-approved drug to treat female sexual arousal disorders in premenopausal patients. It is a centrally acting serotonin receptor agonist/antagonist.

Female Orgasmic Disorders

- Treatment is primarily focused on education, relationship/psychosocial interventions, masturbation education, and the use of aids such as vibrators or videos.

Genitopelvic Pain/Penetration Disorders

- Treatment depends on the suspected primary cause. Coital position changes may be helpful for all causes.
- **Genitourinary syndrome of menopause:** Primarily caused by low estrogen due to menopause, but can also be caused by anti-estrogen medications. Treatment may include:
    - Vaginal moisturizers and/or lubricants.
    - Vaginal estrogen therapy.
    - Vaginal dehydroepiandrosterone therapy.
    - Oral ospemifene (estrogen agonist/antagonist) treatment.
- **Provoked pelvic floor hypertonus (Vaginismus):** Recurrent involuntary spasm of the outer third of the vagina (perineal and levator ani muscles), interfering with or preventing coitus.
    - Pelvic physical therapy, which may include techniques such as pelvic floor exercises, muscle relaxation, massage/myofascial release, and gradual vaginal dilatation with or without biofeedback. The patient controls the pace and duration.
- **Vulvar pain syndromes:** A common cause of dyspareunia with many possible contributing factors. See Chapter 29 for more details about evaluation and treatment.

 WARD TIP

Exogenous administration of estrogen improves vaginal lubrication, atrophic conditions, hot flashes, headaches, and insomnia.

 WARD TIP

Menopause and Sexual Dysfunction
Menopause → vaginal epithelial thinning and lack of adequate lubrication → painful intercourse → ↓ sexual desire.

 EXAM TIP

Many antidepressants worsen the sexual response by increasing the availability of serotonin and decreasing dopamine.

NOTES

Ethics

Physicians in all fields of medicine encounter difficult ethical decisions. Understanding the various aspects of forensic medicine may not make these decisions easier but will likely cause the physician to more closely consider the outcomes of the decision being made.

It is the physician's responsibility to:
- Determine the patient's preferences.
- Honor the patient's wishes when the patient can no longer speak for herself.

End-of-Life Decisions

 A 35-year-old G2P2 patient is scheduled for major surgery. She would like to delineate preferences for her care, in the event that she is unable to speak for herself. What options does she have?

Answer: She can either write a living will (dictates her preferences) or appoint someone as her durable power of attorney to make decisions on her behalf.

- **Advance directives (living will and durable power of attorney for health care)** allow patients to voice their preferences regarding treatment if faced with a potentially terminal illness.
- In a **living will**, a competent adult patient may, in advance, formulate and provide a valid consent to the withholding/withdrawal of life-support systems in the event that injury or illness renders that individual incompetent to make such a decision.
- In a **durable power of attorney for health care**, a patient appoints someone to act as a surrogate decision maker when the patient cannot participate in the consent process.
- The patient's legal spouse is the *de facto* durable power of attorney for health care if no other is appointed; the spouse cannot defy the conditions of a living will or make decisions if another person has been appointed durable power of attorney.

WARD TIP

If a married person has a living will or has appointed another person to be a durable power of attorney, the spouse cannot defy the conditions.

Life-Sustaining Treatment

Any treatment that serves to prolong life without reversing the underlying medical condition.

Reproductive Issues

The ethical responsibility of the physician is:
- To identify his or her own opinions on the issue at hand.
- To be honest and fair to their patients when they seek advice or services in this area.
- To explain his or her personal views to the patient and how those views may influence the service or advice being provided.

Informed Consent

A legal document that requires a physician to obtain consent for treatment rendered, an operation performed, or many diagnostic procedures.

Informed consent requires the following conditions be met:
1. Must be **voluntary**.
2. **Information:**
   - **Risks and benefits** of the procedure are discussed.
   - **Indications** for the procedure are reviewed.
   - **Alternatives** to procedure are discussed.
   - **Consequences** of not undergoing the procedure are discussed.
   - Physician must be willing to **discuss the procedure** and answer any questions the patient has.
3. The patient must be **competent**.

Exceptions

The following are certain cases in which informed consent need not be obtained:
1. Lifesaving medical emergency.
2. Suicide prevention.
3. Normally, minors must have consent obtained from their parents. However, minors may give their own consent for certain treatments, such as alcohol detox and treatment for sexually transmitted infections.

Patient Confidentiality

The information disclosed to a physician during his or her relationship with the patient is confidential. The physician should not reveal information or communications without the express consent of the patient, unless required to do so by law.

EXCEPTIONS

- A patient threatens to inflict serious bodily harm to herself or another person
- Communicable diseases [i.e., human immunodeficiency virus (HIV)]
- Gunshot wounds
- Knife wounds

Minors

- When minors request confidential services, physicians should encourage minors to involve their parents.
- Where the law does not require otherwise, the physician should permit a competent minor to consent to medical care and should **not** notify the parents without the patient's consent.
- If the physician feels that without parental involvement and guidance the minor will face a serious health threat, and there is reason to believe that the parents will be helpful, disclosing the problem to the parents is equally justified.
- Documentation of the rationale for these types of decisions is key.

NOTES

Menopause

Menopause signifies the depletion of oocytes and manifests as the absence of menses. The changes in female hormones can have significant morbidity as well as bothersome symptoms.

Definitions

- **Menopause** is the permanent cessation of menstruation diagnosed retrospectively after 12 months of amenorrhea without any other physiologic cause.
- Menopause signifies ovarian follicular depletion, which results in ↓ estrogen production and ↑ of follicle-stimulating hormone (FSH).
- Menopause is preceded by the **menopause transition** or **perimenopause**, which begins on average four years before the **final menstrual period (FMP)**.
- Most individuals become menopausal between the ages of 45 and 55, with an average age of 51–52 years.
- The **postmenopausal period** is the time after the FMP (Figure 36-1).

Factors Affecting Age of Onset

- Genetics
- Smoking (↓ age by 2 years)—may include exposure to passive smoking
- Chemo/radiation therapy
- Hysterectomy (with ovarian conservation, possibly due to altered blood supply)

Physiology of the Menopause Transition and Menopause

OVARIAN FOLLICULAR DEPLETION

- Decline in oocyte number due to progressive atresia (via apoptosis) of the original complement of oocytes, which become **resistant to FSH**, the pituitary hormone that causes their maturation.

Stages:	−5	−4	−3	−2	−1	0	+1	+2
Terminology	Reproductive			Menopausal Transition			Postmenopause	
	Early	Peak	Late	Early	Late*		Early*	Late
				Perimenopause				
Duration of Stage:	variable			variable		(a) 1 yr	(b) 4 yrs	until demise
Menstrual Cycles:	variable to regular	regular		variable cycle length (>7 days different from normal)	≥2 skipped cycles and an interval of amenorrhea (≥60 days)	Amen x 12 mos	none	
Endocrine:	normal FSH		↑ FSH	↑ FSH			↑ FSH	

Final Menstrual Period (FMP)

*Stages most likely to be characterized by vasomotor symptoms   ↑ = elevated

FIGURE 36-1. The STRAW staging system. (Reproduced, with permission, from Soules MR, Sherman S, Parrott E, et al. Executive Summary: Stages of Reproductive Aging Workshop [STRAW]. *Fertil Steril.* 2001;76(5):874–878.)

- Menopause is characterized by an **elevated FSH** due to:
  1. ↓ inhibin (inhibin inhibits FSH secretion; it is produced in smaller amounts by the fewer oocytes).
  2. Resistant oocytes require more FSH to successfully mature, triggering greater FSH release.
  3. **↓ in estradiol levels and absence of negative feedback**.
- Androstenedione is aromatized peripherally to estrone (less potent than estradiol), which is the major estrogen in postmenopausal individuals.
- Androstenedione and testosterone levels fall. These two hormones are produced by the ovary.
- The most **important physiologic change** that occurs with menopause is the **decline of estradiol-17β** levels that occurs with the cessation of follicular maturation. Table 36-1 lists the organ systems affected by the decreased estradiol levels.

EXAM TIP

The length of the luteal phase does not change (14 days). In contrast, the follicular phase length varies between patients and at the ends of the reproductive spectrum.

OVULATION BECOMES LESS FREQUENT

Patients **ovulate less frequently** and thus experience menstrual cycle variability. This is due to a **shortened follicular phase**. The length of the luteal phase does not change. When a patient starts skipping 2 menstrual periods in a row, there is a 95% chance her FMP will be within the next 4 years.

EXAM TIP

Oligo/anovulation leads to abnormal uterine bleeding during the menopause transition.

TABLE 36-1. **Physiologic Effects of Menopause**

ORGAN SYSTEM	EFFECT OF DECREASED ESTRADIOL	AVAILABLE TREATMENT
Cardiovascular	LDL and ↓ HDL. After two decades of menopause, the risk of myocardial infarction and coronary artery disease is equal to that in men	
Bone	Osteoporosis: Estrogen receptors found on many cells mediating trabecular bone maintenance (i.e., ↓ osteoblast activity, ↑ osteoclast activity) due to ↓ estrogen levels	▪ Bisphosphonate first-line therapy ▪ Raloxifene ▪ MHT is not first-line therapy but has been shown to help ▪ Calcitonin ▪ Exercise ▪ Calcium and Vitamin D supplementation ▪ Smoking cessation
Genitourinary	Genitourinary syndrome of menopause with associated symptoms	▪ Vaginal moisturizers and lubricants ▪ Vaginal EHT ▪ Vaginal DHEA
Psychiatric	Emotional lability and depression	▪ SSRI, SNRI ▪ Psychotherapy ▪ MHT is not first-line therapy but has been shown to help

EHT, estrogen hormone therapy; DHEA, dehydroepiandrosterone; HDL, high density lipoprotein; LDL, low density lipoprotein; MHT, menopausal hormone therapy; SNRI, serotonin-norepinephrine reuptake inhibitors; SSRI, Selective serotonin reuptake inhibitors.

ESTROGEN LEVELS FALL

 A 51-year-old G4P4 patient presents with new-onset pain with intercourse and occasional vaginal itching that started 6 months ago. Workup for sexually transmitted infections (STIs) is negative, and on examination she is noted to have pale vaginal mucosa with reduced rugae. What is the major hormonal change implicated in these symptoms and findings?

Answer: There is a decline in estrogen that causes genitourinary syndrome of menopause.

COMMON SYMPTOMS OF MENOPAUSE

- **Vasomotor** (i.e., hot flushes, night sweats) and **vaginal symptoms** are the most common symptoms of menopause and are the most commonly reported bothersome symptoms.
- **These symptoms occur largely due to a decline in estrogen (estradiol-17β) levels**.
- There is a major reduction in ovarian estrogen production at 6 months before menopause.
- There is a wide variety in symptom duration, with reports of bothersome symptoms lasting anywhere from 6 months to 10 years. Most patients will stop having vasomotor symptoms within 4–5 years of onset, but a small percentage will report persistent symptoms even after age 70.
- **Hot flushes** are characterized by a sudden sensation of extreme heat, usually on the face, neck, and upper chest. These episodes usually last a few minutes and are characterized by sweating, flushing, chills, clamminess, anxiety, and/ or heart palpitations. Patients often report sleep disruption.
- **Vaginal symptoms** are caused by vaginal atrophy due to hypoestrogenism, which results in anatomic and physiologic changes in the genitourinary tract. Loss of superficial epithelial cells results in thinning of tissue, and loss of vaginal rugae and elasticity results in narrowing of the vagina. Vaginal pH becomes more alkaline, predisposing patients to infection by altering flora. Vaginal secretions decrease, predisposing patients to dyspareunia.

EXAM TIP

Primary ovarian insufficiency occurs when the ovaries stop functioning before the age of 40.

WARD TIP

The cause of vasomotor symptoms is likely multifactorial, including decreased estrogen levels, elevated FSH levels, changes in thermoregulatory mechanisms in the brain, genetic factors, and other physiologic factors including the serotonergic, noradrenergic, opioid, adrenal, and autonomic systems.

Long-Term Consequences of Menopause

BONE LOSS

- Begins during menopause transition, with highest rates of bone loss in the year leading up to the FMP and the first 2 years after.

CARDIOVASCULAR DISEASE

- Estrogen depletion increases the risk of cardiovascular disease.
- Lipid profiles worsen, contributing to cardiovascular risk factors.

BODY COMPOSITION

- Loss of muscle mass and increase in fat mass.
- Redistribution of body weight with increased risk of central obesity and metabolic syndrome.

- There is evidence that the brain and the activity of serotonin are influenced by estrogen.
- There is limited epidemiologic evidence linking decreased circulating levels of estradiol with cognitive impairment, and clinical trials on early use of hormone replacement therapy have not shown improvement in cognition.
- There is a significant increase in new-onset depression in patients during the menopausal transition, likely due to decreased circulating levels of serotonin.
- These symptoms may be exacerbated by sleep disruption during this time period.

Management of Menopausal Symptoms

 A 50-year-old G1P1 patient presents with a 3-month history of hot flushes during the day and night sweats so bad she has to change her bedding at night. On further questioning, she reports that she feels very irritable during the day because her sleep is so disrupted. Her last menstrual period (LMP) was six months ago. She is healthy and has no medical problems. What is this patient's most likely diagnosis, and what treatment is most likely to alleviate her symptoms?

Answer: This patient is experiencing the menopause transition. If her symptoms are distressing, she could be offered menopausal hormone therapy (MHT) to alleviate some of her symptoms.

Management of Vasomotor Symptoms

- Most individuals who seek therapy for vasomotor symptoms are in their late 40s or 50s and can be reassured that the absolute risk of serious complications is very low.
- **Systemic MHT** with estrogen alone, or in combination with progestin, is the most effective treatment of menopausal vasomotor symptoms.
- MHT may be considered a safe option for healthy, symptomatic patients who are younger than age 60 and who do not have contraindications to the use of MHT. After age 60, the risk of vascular complications is increased.
- The primary goal of MHT is to relieve bothersome vasomotor symptoms, but other symptoms such as sleep disturbances and mood lability often respond to estrogen as well.
  - **Estrogen Therapy (ET)** is appropriate for individuals who have undergone hysterectomy.
  - **Combination estrogen-progestin therapy** is necessary for patients with an intact uterus to prevent estrogen-associated endometrial hyperplasia or malignancy.
  - Both ET and estrogen-progestin therapy may be administered in oral or transdermal forms.
- Non-hormonal options to treat vasomotor symptoms include selective serotonin reuptake inhibitors (SSRIs), selective serotonin-norepinephrine reuptake inhibitors (SNRIs), clonidine, and gabapentin (both used off label).
- The initial results of the **Women's Health Initiative (WHI)** study published in 2002 prompted great changes in the understanding and

recommendations for MHT. It specifically demonstrated adverse effects in individuals over age 60 or greater than 10 years since menopause. The risk-benefit profile is more favorable in individuals aged 50–59, which is the age range in which patients typically present seeking treatment for menopausal symptoms.

- The WHI included patients aged 50–77, with an average age of 61 years. Thus, it is difficult to generalize these findings to younger patients who are recently menopausal.
- For patients who took combination EPT for an average of 5 years, it demonstrated a slightly increased risk of breast cancer, coronary artery disease, stroke, and venous thromboembolism (VTE) and a decreased risk of fractures and colon cancer.
- For patients who took ET only, the WHI demonstrated an increased risk of VTE, but not an increased risk of cardiovascular events or breast cancer.
- Short-term therapy (<5 years) is acceptable for menopausal symptom relief in young, postmenopausal patients. Prescribe the lowest dose that relieves the symptoms. Order a mammogram before initiating therapy and yearly thereafter.
- MHT should not be used to prevent cardiovascular disease.

MANAGEMENT OF VAGINAL SYMPTOMS

The term **Genitourinary Syndrome of Menopause (GSM)** is an umbrella term that encompasses the atrophic symptoms patients may experience in the vulvovaginal and bladder-urethral areas due to menopausal loss of estrogen.

- Symptoms and problems associated with GSM may include sexual dysfunction, dyspareunia, postcoital bleeding, and recurrent urinary tract infections.
- Initial treatment includes vaginal lubricants and moisturizers. Lubricants can be water-based or oil-based and may be used during sexual activity to treat dyspareunia and dryness. Moisturizers are typically bioadhesive products and are intended to be used routinely.
- Vaginal estrogen therapy is available in a pill, cream, or vagina ring form and may be used to treat dryness, discomfort, tissue fragility, and dyspareunia. This topical treatment does not pose the same cardiovascular and other risks as systemic treatment.
- Vaginal dehydroepiandrosterone (DHEA), also known as prasterone, is a treatment option for dyspareunia due to GSM.

OSTEOPOROSIS MANAGEMENT

- Osteoporosis is a skeletal disorder characterized by loss of bone mass, deterioration in bone microarchitecture, and a decline in bone quality, all of which lead to an increased risk of pathologic fracture. Treatment includes lifestyle modification and medical therapy.
  - **Smoking cessation** is essential for bone health, as smoking has been shown to accelerate bone loss.
  - **Weight-bearing exercise** at least 30 minutes three times per week is recommended to prevent osteoporosis and has shown a significant positive effect on bone mineral density (BMD).
  - Postmenopausal patients should get at least 1200 mg of **calcium** daily, from a combination of dietary and supplemental sources. They should also ingest a total of 800 international units of **vitamin D** daily.
  - While **MHT** has been shown to reduce osteoporosis, it is not considered to be an appropriate first-line therapy in most situations due to

the potential adverse events and the availability of other therapies with fewer potential cardiovascular risks.

- **Bisphosphonates** are a category of antiresorptive agents that are the leading treatment for osteoporosis. They work by inhibiting osteoclast resorption of bone.
- **Raloxifene** is another antiresorptive agent that is a selective estrogen receptor modulator (SERM). It has also been shown to reduce the risk of postmenopausal breast cancer in patients at high risk. It is not used as often as bisphosphonates due to possible adverse effects of VTE.
- **Calcitonin** is an antiresorptive agent available as a nasal spray or subcutaneous injection. Its benefits are not as robust in early postmenopausal patients, and it should not be used until individuals are at least 5 years postmenopausal.

MANAGEMENT OF MOOD SYMPTOMS

- While MHT has been shown to improve mood symptoms in perimenopausal and menopausal patients, it is not considered first-line treatment due to potential cardiovascular risks.
- First-line treatment is typically SSRIs and SNRIs +/− psychotherapy.

WARD TIP

Menopause wreaks HAVOC:
Hot flashes
Atrophy of the
Vagina
Osteoporosis
Coronary artery disease

EXAM TIP

Estrogen creates a hypercoagulable state due to ↑ production of hepatic coagulation factors.

NOTES

Pelvic Relaxation

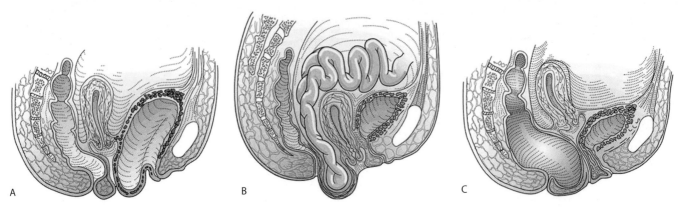

FIGURE 37-1.   **Types of prolapse: (A) cystocele, (B) enterocele, and (C) rectocele.** (Figure 37-1A: Reproduced, with permission, from Hoffman BL, Schorge JO, Halvorson LM, et al. *Williams Gynecology.* 4th ed. New York: McGraw Hill; 2020. Figure 37-1B and C: Reproduced, with permission, from DeCherney AH, Pernoll ML. *Current Obstetrics & Gynecology Diagnosis & Treatment*, 8th ed. Originally published by Appleton & Lange. Copyright © 1994 by The McGraw-Hill Companies, Inc.)

Pelvic organ prolapse (POP) is a very common benign condition which may cause symptoms that interfere with quality of life. It occurs when there is descent of one or more aspects of the vaginal walls or uterus, allowing nearby organs to herniate into the vagina. This may be classified according to the location of the herniated pelvic organ(s). POP may be described as occurring in the anterior vaginal wall (cystocele), posterior vaginal wall (rectocele), uterus/cervix, or the vaginal vault/vaginal cuff in patients who have undergone a hysterectomy (enterocele). **Uterine procidentia** occurs when there is herniation of all three compartments, including uterus, through the vaginal introitus. See Figure 37-1.

POP is most likely to present in postmenopausal patients, with a peak incidence in individuals aged 70–79 years. POP may cause a variety of distressing symptoms, including a sensation of ↑ pressure and vaginal bulge, defecatory dysfunction, voiding dysfunction, and sexual dysfunction. Diagnosis must be made by examining the patient when supine and standing. Mild descent of the pelvic organs is very common and is generally not considered to be pathologic. Asymptomatic POP generally does not require treatment. When prolapse symptoms become bothersome, treatment is warranted.

Anatomy of Pelvic Floor Support

Several crucial structures make up the support of the female pelvic floor and pelvic organs, requiring an elegant interaction between pelvic floor muscles and connective tissue attachments to the bony pelvis. The levator ani muscle complex (comprised of pubococcygeus, puborectalis, and iliococcygeus muscles) provides a firm elastic base for the organs to rest upon. Disturbance of any of the following can result in prolapse:

- Bony structure
- Endopelvic fascia (i.e., uterosacral and cardinal ligaments)
- Pelvic diaphragm
- Urogenital diaphragm
- Perineum

The function of the pelvic floor muscles includes the following:

- **Support of the abdominopelvic viscera** (i.e., bladder, intestines, uterus) through their tonic contraction

- **Resistance to increases in intra-abdominal pressure** during activities such as heavy lifting, coughing, or sneezing
- **Urinary and fecal continence** through their sphincter action around the rectum and urethra

Pelvic Organ Prolapse (POP)

 A 57-year-old G3P3 patient presents with a sensation of pressure and a bulge in her vagina that is worse at the end of the day. She is healthy and has no medical problems. Her history is significant for three vaginal deliveries proven to 8 lb, and menopause since age 52. What is the next step in the evaluation of this patient?

Answer: Take a detailed history of symptoms and perform a complete pelvic exam to assess for POP. Examine the patient in both the supine and standing positions to help determine the severity of the prolapse.

There are two main systems used for staging the degree of POP. Both systems measure the most distal portion of the prolapse during straining (Valsalva maneuver).

The **Baden–Walker System** is a reasonable clinical method to evaluate and document the exam of the pelvic compartments.

The **Pelvic Organ Prolapse-Quantification (POP-Q)** system is an international system that involves taking several measurements, is more complex but highly reliable, and is used in both clinical assessment and research. See Table 37-1.

WARD TIP

The distinction between symptomatic and asymptomatic POP is clinically relevant, since treatment is generally indicated only for women with symptoms.

TABLE 37-1. **The Pelvic Organ Prolapse-Quantification (POP-Q) Staging System of Pelvic Organ Support**

Stage 0	No prolapse is demonstrated. Points Aa, Ap, Ba, and Bp are all at −3 cm and either point C or D is between −TVL and −(TVL−2) cm [i.e., the quantitation value for point C or D is ≤−(TVL−2) cm]. Figure 37-2 represents stage 0.
Stage I	The criteria for stage 0 are not met, but the most distal portion of the prolapse is >1 cm above the level of the hymen (i.e., its quantitation value is <−1 cm)
Stage II	The most distal portion of the prolapse is ≤1 cm proximal to or distal to the plane of the hymen (i.e., its quantitation value is ≥−1 cm but ≤+1 cm)
Stage III	The most distal portion of the prolapse is >1 cm below the plane of the hymen but protrudes no further than 2 cm less than the TVL in centimeters [i.e., its quantitation value is >+1 cm but <+(TVL−2) cm]. Figure 24–4A represents stage III Ba and Figure 24–4B represents stage III Bp prolapse
Stage IV	Essentially, complete eversion of the total length of the lower genital tract is demonstrated. The distal portion of the prolapse protrudes to at least (TVL−2) cm [i.e., its quantitation value is ≥+(TVL−2) cm]. In most instances, the leading edge of stage IV prolapse will be the cervix or vaginal cuff scar. Figure 24–3C represents stage IVC prolapse.

Used, with permission, from Bump RC, Mattiasson A, Bø K, et al. The standardization of terminology of female pelvic organ prolapse and pelvic floor dysfunction. *Am J Obstet Gynecol.* 1996;175(1):10–17.

TVL, total vaginal length.

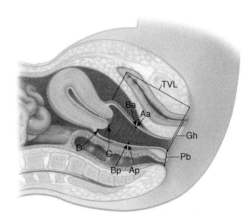

FIGURE 37-2. **Anatomic landmarks used during pelvic organ prolapse quantification (POP-Q).** Reproduced, with permission, from DeCherney AH, Pernoll ML. *Current Obstetrics & Gynecology Diagnosis & Treatment*, 8th ed. Originally published by Appleton & Lange. Copyright © 1994 by The McGraw-Hill Companies, Inc.

GRADING (BADEN-WALKER CLASSIFICATION)

Organ displacement:

To the level of the ischial spines:	Grade I
Between ischial spines and introitus:	Grade II
Up to introitus:	Grade III
Past introitus:	Grade IV

RISK FACTORS

Many conditions can cause prolapse: Disturbing the anatomical support, disrupting the innervation, or chronically increasing abdominal pressure. Modifiable risk factors such as obesity and constipation should be addressed with patients in order to reduce the risk of developing POP. Examples of conditions predisposing to POP include:

- ↑ abdominal pressure: Obesity, chronic cough (e.g., chronic obstructive pulmonary disease), heavy lifting, chronic constipation.
- Loss of levator ani function: Increasing parity, vaginal delivery
- Transection of supporting tissue: Postsurgical, i.e., hysterectomy
- Loss of innervation: Amyotrophic lateral sclerosis (ALS), paralysis, multiple sclerosis
- Loss of connective tissue: Spina bifida, myelomeningocele
- Atrophy of supporting tissues: Aging, especially after menopause

SIGNS AND SYMPTOMS

- Feeling of "pressure" or "bulge"
- Organ protrusion, especially upon exertion
- Urinary incontinence
- Groin pain
- Dyspareunia
- Spotting
- Splinting to defecate

Symptom alleviation/exacerbation is often related to gravity (i.e., better when prone, better in the morning, worse with standing, worse in evening).

DIAGNOSIS

- Diagnosis is made by direct visualization of prolapsed organ during complete pelvic examination.
- Patient should be **examined in both the supine and standing positions.**

EXAM TIP

Risk factors for developing POP:
- Advancing age
- Chronic obstruction
- Constipation
- Genetic predisposition
- Menopause
- Higher parity
- Prior surgery
- Pulmonary disease
- Tumor/mass

WARD TIP

Remember to examine the patient in **both** the supine and standing positions.

TREATMENT

Nonsurgical

- **Asymptomatic prolapse:**
  - Usually requires **follow-up**, but no immediate intervention needed.
  - **Education** and **reassurance** are appropriate.
  - Pelvic-strengthening exercises (i.e., **Kegel** maneuvers, pelvic physical therapy) and/or menopausal hormone therapy may be beneficial.
- **Symptomatic prolapse:** Lifestyle modification can help in some situations (i.e., management of underlying predisposing condition such as constipation). Can be treated with a pessary or surgically.
  - A vaginal **pessary** is a silicone device placed in the upper vagina designed to help maintain support of the pelvic organs. Over 90% of patients can successfully be fitted with a pessary. They are available in several shapes and sizes.

Surgical

- Indications for surgery: Childbearing is completed, symptoms are bothersome, and the patient has failed or declined nonsurgical treatment.
- There are several types of surgical repairs for each type of prolapse. New, minimally invasive techniques are being developed.
  - **Cystocele: Anterior colporrhaphy (anterior repair)**—bladder buttress base sutures proximal to the bladder neck.
  - **Rectocele: Posterior colporrhaphy (posterior repair)**—posterior vaginal wall reinforcement with levator ani muscles via vaginal approach.
  - **Apical prolapse:** Vaginal approach—sacrospinous ligament fixation (SSLF), uterosacral ligament suspension (USLS); and abdominal approach—sacrocolpopexy.
  - **Uterine prolapse: Hysterectomy**—a uterine prolapse often occurs in conjunction with another prolapse, so combined repairs are usually performed.
  - **LeFort procedure/colpoclesis:** Surgical obliteration of the vaginal canal in a patient who is NOT sexually active. This procedure can be performed with any type of prolapse.

WARD TIP

Pessaries are especially useful when surgery is contraindicated.

WARD TIP

Complications of POP:
- Urinary retention
- Constipation
- Urinary tract infections
- Ulcerations
- Vaginal bleeding

NOTES

Urinary Incontinence

Urinary incontinence is an involuntary loss of urine that can be due to a variety of conditions. It can cause social embarrassment, sexual dysfunction, hygiene issues, and at times significant lifestyle restrictions. It is important to differentiate between the different types of urinary incontinence with a careful history, because the management of each type is different.

Definition

Urinary incontinence is a very common condition in women, occurring in up to half of postmenopausal patients; however, the true prevalence is likely underestimated as many individuals are hesitant to seek care or discuss their symptoms with their physician.

Causes

There are four main types of urinary incontinence in women:
- Stress urinary incontinence (SUI)
- Urgency urinary incontinence
- Mixed urinary incontinence
- Overflow urinary incontinence

It can also be helpful to think of incontinence causes as being categorized as reversible and irreversible.

REVERSIBLE CAUSES

- Delirium, urinary tract infection, genitourinary syndrome of menopause (GSM), drug side effects, psychiatric illness, excessive urine production, restricted patient mobility, and stool impaction are *reversible* causes of urinary incontinence.
- It is necessary to first evaluate for these correctable causes before moving on to the more expensive and invasive workup for the irreversible causes.

IRREVERSIBLE CAUSES

Stress Incontinence

- Loss of urine (usually **small amount**) with ↑ **intra-abdominal pressure** (i.e., with coughing, laughing, exercise, other effort or physical exertion).
- Often caused by **urethral hypermotility** and/or **intrinsic sphincter deficiency**.
  - Urethral hypermobility may occur when there is insufficient support of the urethra and bladder neck by the pelvic floor musculature and vaginal connective tissue, resulting in the loss of ability of these organs to close completely against the anterior vaginal wall. Increases in intra-abdominal pressure results in the urethra failing to close properly, leading to stress incontinence.
  - Intrinsic sphincter deficiency occurs when there is a loss of the normal intrinsic urethral mucosal and muscular tone that usually keeps the urethra closed.

WARD TIP

Reversible causes of urinary incontinence—

DIAPPERS
Delirium
Infection
Atrophic vaginitis (better known as GSM)
Pharmacologic causes
Psychiatric causes
Excessive urine production
Restricted mobility
Stool impaction

WARD TIP

Stress incontinence is the most common type of incontinence in younger individuals.

Urge Incontinence

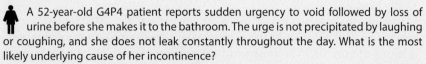

A 52-year-old G4P4 patient reports sudden urgency to void followed by loss of urine before she makes it to the bathroom. The urge is not precipitated by laughing or coughing, and she does not leak constantly throughout the day. What is the most likely underlying cause of her incontinence?

Answer: This patient is most likely to have urge incontinence that is caused by unopposed detrusor muscle contraction.

- Sudden feeling of **urgency** followed by involuntary leakage of urine (can be small or large volume loss).
- Caused by unopposed detrusor contraction. Also called "overactive bladder."
- Often accompanied with urinary frequency and nocturia.

Mixed Incontinence

Describes patients with a combination of stress and urge incontinence

Overflow Incontinence

- Constant dribbling +/− continuous leakage with inability to completely empty the bladder
- Caused by detrusor underactivity (due to a neuropathy) or urethral/bladder outlet obstruction

Evaluation

HISTORY

Ask about aforementioned symptoms, medications, medical history (diabetes mellitus, neuropathies), and impact on quality of life. It is also helpful to have the patient keep a **voiding diary** (i.e., volume, frequency, fluid intake).

PHYSICAL

- Pelvic exam: Check for pelvic organ prolapse (POP), masses, atrophic changes, and Q-tip test.
- Rectal exam: Check for impaction and rectocele; assess sphincter tone.
- Neurological exam: Assess for neuropathy.
- Cough stress test: In clinic, place patient in standing (or supine) position with full bladder. Visualize urethra and ask patient to cough to see if direct visualization of leaking from urethra is possible.
- Postvoid residual (PVR) (normal is <50–100 mL).

LABS

Urinalysis and culture to rule out urinary tract infection

Q-TIP TEST

- A cotton swab is placed in the urethra. The change in angle between the Q-tip and the woman's body is measured upon straining.
- Normal upward change is <30 degrees, and a **positive test** is one with >30-degree change.
- A **positive test indicates urethral hypermobility**.

ZEBRA ALERT

Incontinence that presents as continuous urinary leakage may be due to a fistula. This can occur as a result of:
- Prior pelvic surgery
- Obstetric trauma
- Radiation

WARD TIP

Functional incontinence: A person can recognize the need to urinate, but cannot make it to the bathroom in time because of immobility.

WARD TIP

Q-tip test: ↑ upward motion of the Q-tip is caused by loss of support from the urethrovesicular junction, indicating urethral hypermobility.

CYSTOMETRY

- Cystometry provides measurements of the relationship of pressure and volume in the bladder.
- Catheters that measure pressures are placed in the bladder and rectum, while a second catheter in the bladder supplies water to cause bladder filling.
- Measurements include post **residual volume, volumes at which an urge to void occurs, bladder compliance, flow rates**, and **capacity**.
- **Diagnoses:** Stress, urge, and overflow incontinence.

URODYNAMIC STUDIES

- A set of studies that evaluate lower urinary tract function.
- Studies may include **cystometry** (see above), **bladder filling tests, cystoscopy, uroflowmetry, and leak-point pressure tests**.
- Can help diagnose and differentiate between types of incontinence.

EXAM TIP

Stress incontinence is treated with α-adrenergic agonists and surgical repair.

Treatment

Lifestyle modification is recommended for all patients with incontinence of any type. This may include weight loss, dietary changes (i.e., reduction of caffeine, alcohol), correction of constipation, and smoking cessation. Patients may select more or less invasive treatment options (or no treatment at all) based on their severity of symptoms.

STRESS INCONTINENCE

- **Kegel exercises** strengthen pelvic floor muscles. Referral to a **physical therapist** who specializes in pelvic floor health can be beneficial.
- **Topical vaginal estrogen therapy**.
- Incontinence **pessary**.
- Surgical repair.
  - Midurethral slings are considered first-line surgical treatment due to ease of placement and excellent outcomes. May be done with a retropubic or transobturator approach.
  - Burch retropubic colposuspension is the gold standard in the literature, but is not often performed as primary treatment anymore due to similar outcomes with less invasive procedures such as midurethral slings.

EXAM TIP

Midurethral sling is the treatment of choice for stress incontinence.

URGE INCONTINENCE

- **Medications:**
  - Antimuscarinic agents (↑ bladder capacity, ↓ urge by blocking release of acetylcholine during bladder filling). Most common side effects are dry mouth and constipation.
  - Mirabegron (beta-3-adrenoreceptor agonist).
- **Timed voiding:** Patient is advised to urinate in prescribed hourly intervals before the bladder fills.
- Surgery is rarely used to treat urge incontinence.
- Avoid stimulants and diuretics (i.e., alcohol, coffee, carbonated beverages).

EXAM TIP

Urge incontinence is treated with medications, timed voiding, and lifestyle changes.

OVERFLOW INCONTINENCE

- **Due to obstruction:** Relieve obstruction.
- **Due to detrusor underactivity:** Treat possible neurological causes—diabetes mellitus and B_{12} deficiency.

Index